New Insights into Arthritis Research

New Insights into Arthritis Research

Editor: Sharlton Pierce

AMERICAN
MEDICAL PUBLISHERS
www.americanmedicalpublishers.com

AMERICAN
MEDICAL PUBLISHERS
www.americanmedicalpublishers.com

Cataloging-in-Publication Data

New insights into arthritis research / edited by Sharlton Pierce.
p. cm.
Includes bibliographical references and index.
ISBN 979-8-88740-328-1
1. Arthritis. 2. Arthritis--Research. 3. Joints--Diseases. 4. Inflammation. I. Pierce, Sharlton.
RC933 .N49 2023
616.722--dc23

American Medical Publishers,
41 Flatbush Avenue,
1st Floor, New York,
NY 11217, USA

ISBN 979-8-88740-328-1 (Hardback)

Contents

Preface

Arthritis refers to a condition characterized by the inflammation of the joints. Osteoarthritis and rheumatoid arthritis are the two major forms of arthritis. Some other types of arthritis include psoriatic arthritis, gout, fibromyalgia and septic arthritis. Pain in the joints, stiffness, redness, swelling and decreased range of motion are the most common symptoms of arthritis. Multiple factors such as age, genetic history, muscle weakness and autoimmune disorders can lead to the development of arthritis. There are several diagnostic tests for this medical condition that include physical examination, blood tests, X-ray, MRI, and CT scans. The objective of treatment is to provide effective relief from symptoms and control further joint damage. Some common treatments are medications, physical therapy, nutrient rich diet, occupational therapy, regular exercise, and hot and cold compresses. The aim of this book is to present new insights into arthritis research. It is a vital tool for all researching or studying this medical condition.

This book is a comprehensive compilation of works of different researchers from varied parts of the world. It includes valuable experiences of the researchers with the sole objective of providing the readers (learners) with a proper knowledge of the concerned field. This book will be beneficial in evoking inspiration and enhancing the knowledge of the interested readers.

In the end, I would like to extend my heartiest thanks to the authors who worked with great determination on their chapters. I also appreciate the publisher's support in the course of the book. I would also like to deeply acknowledge my family who stood by me as a source of inspiration during the project.

Editor

1

The quality of online consumer health information at the intersection of complementary and alternative medicine and arthritis

Jeremy Y. Ng*, Alexandra Vacca and Tanya Jain

Abstract

Background: Complementary and alternative medicine (CAM) use is prevalent among patients living with arthritis. Such patients often seek information online, for the purpose of gaining a second opinion to their healthcare provider or even self-medication. Little is known about the quality of web-based consumer health information at the intersection of CAM and arthritis; thus, investigating the quality of websites containing this information was the purpose of this study.

Methods: Four unique search terms were searched on Google across four English-speaking countries. We assessed the first 20 results of each search, including them if they contained CAM consumer health information for the treatment and/or management of arthritis. Eligible websites were assessed in duplicate using the DISCERN instrument, which consists of 16-items designed to assess quality.

Results: Of total of 320 webpages, 239 were duplicates, and a total of 38 unique websites were deemed eligible and assessed using the DISCERN instrument. The mean summed DISCERN scores across all websites was 55.53 (SD = 9.37). The mean score of the overall quality of each website was 3.71 (SD = 0.63), thus the majority of websites are ranked as slightly above 'fair' quality.

Conclusion: Eligible websites generally received scores better than 'moderate' in terms of overall quality. Several shortcomings included a lack of transparency surrounding references used and underreporting of risks associated with treatment options. These results suggest that health providers should be vigilant of the variable quality of information their patients may be accessing online and educate them on how to identify high quality resources.

Keywords: Arthritis, Complementary and alternative medicine, Quality of information, Consumer health information, Information assessment, DISCERN

Background

Arthritis is one of the leading causes of disability among North Americans [1], describing over 100 conditions that affect joints, tissues around the joint, and other connective tissues [2]. The two main categories of arthritis include degenerative (osteoarthritis), resulting from progressive cartilage breakdown, and autoimmune/inflammatory (rheumatoid arthritis), characterized by an immune system that attacks the synovial membrane [2]. Arthritis may also arise from infections or metabolic disorders (most commonly seen as gout) [1]. Symptoms include joint pain, swelling, stiffness, tenderness, and limited range of motion commonly found in the hands, wrists, knees, hips, ankles, and spine [2]. The condition is diagnosed with a physical exam, assessing blood or

* Correspondence: ngjy2@mcmaster.ca
Department of Health Research Methods, Evidence, and Impact, Faculty of Health Sciences, McMaster University, Michael G. DeGroote Centre for Learning and Discovery, Room 2112, 1280 Main Street West, Hamilton, ON L8S 4K1, Canada

synovial fluid tests, and by using imaging techniques such as x-rays [3]. Arthritis is most common among women. Approximately 20 million people worldwide were living with rheumatoid arthritis in 2017 with over a million new cases being diagnosed each year [4]. Although arthritis affects all ages, the risk increases as individuals grow older. If left untreated, it can negatively impact physical functioning and quality of life [2].

Many arthritis patients seek out various treatment options to help them manage and cope with their condition, one of which includes complementary and alternative medicine (CAM), which has gained popularity. CAM refers to a wide range of therapies and health care practices that are not considered mainstream or standard medical practice. "Complementary" medicine can be defined as an unconventional practice that is used in combination with conventional medicine [5], while "alternative" medicine is primarily used in place of conventional health care [5]. Furthermore, the term "integrative practice" takes place when conventional and complementary approaches are used collaboratively [5, 6]. CAM treatments are popular among patients with arthritis for a variety of reasons. A Malaysian study found that people with arthritis typically use CAM because they believe there are fewer side effects associated with such therapies in comparison to conventional medicine [7]. Studies from South Korea, India, Turkey, and Nigeria have found that the majority of patients turn to CAM therapies because they believe it helps to alleviate pain, helps control morning stiffness, and is less expensive [8–11]. One report from the United Kingdom found that approximately 60% of arthritis patients have used CAM therapies at least once [12]. One Canadian study found that 33.9% of patients with juvenile idiopathic arthritis used CAM therapies [13]. Several studies from the United States have estimated that 30–41% of adults with arthritis use CAM [14–17], while CAM use among youth with juvenile idiopathic arthritis has been found to be 72% [18]. Another study found that 40% of Australians who suffer from osteoarthritis use CAM [19]. Some of the most commonly-used CAM therapies for arthritis include dietary supplements (including glucosamine sulphate and chondroitin), chiropractic and manual therapies, massage therapy, herbal medicine, acupuncture, and meditative therapies (including yoga and tai chi). These are purportedly used to improve damaged cartilage, manage pain/stress, and increase mobility [20, 21].

One study that reviewed the quality of online content found that information relating to osteoarthritis is generally 'fair' in quality [22]. Another research study investigating the quality of complementary and integrative health information on the internet typically found that most websites did well in terms of information quality relating to ownership, currency, interactivity and navigability, while results varied for authorship, balanced information and the use of sources [23]. Another study on the quality of herbal product information on the internet found serious shortcomings in terms of providing specific safety information [24]. To our knowledge, no study has specifically focused on the quality of online information at the intersection of CAM and arthritis. The objective of this study is to analyse the quality of consumer health information on CAM therapies that a "typical" patient with arthritis may encounter online. This study is of value to both healthcare providers and researchers, as it provides them with a greater understanding and insight into what types of information patients with arthritis may be accessing on their own.

Methods

Search strategy

A cross-sectional survey of the quality of websites containing CAM consumer health information for the treatment and/or management of arthritis was undertaken. JYN developed the search strategies which were executed by AV on Google on May 5th, 2020 as follows: 'alternative medicine for arthritis', 'complementary and alternative medicine for arthritis', 'complementary medicine for arthritis', and 'integrative medicine for arthritis'. All searches were conducted on Google Chrome in incognito mode to ensure that the search results retrieved were unaffected by prior browsing history and run across four English-speaking countries: Australia (Google.com.au), Canada (Google.ca), the United Kingdom (Google.co.uk), and the United States (Google.com). This was done to obtain a more internationally representative selection of commonly-visited websites. The four search strategies were based on the most common terms used to refer to CAM [6] and were designed to be simple, so as to replicate how a "typical" patient with limited knowledge of medical or research topics may seek health-related information online. We elected to search only Google as it comprises over 90% of the search engine market share used worldwide as of August 2020 [25], thereby retrieving websites that are much more likely to be accessed and read by patients. It is worth noting that the four next most popular search engines (Bing, Yahoo!, Baidu, and Yandex) only hold between 0.44 and 2.78% of the search engine market share each [25]. Additionally, we only assessed the first 20 webpage results of each Google search, given that it is known that internet users typically only view the first page of results that are generated and may occasionally look through the second search engine results page [26]. With four search terms being generated across four countries (for a total of 16 searches and 20 websites for each), we sought to assess a total of 320 websites.

Eligibility criteria

AV and TJ reviewed the 320 websites yielded across all searches and removed all duplicates. Once all of the URLs were collected, the authors assessed the inclusion criteria for each website. Websites were screened for eligibility and included if they contained at least one webpage that contained CAM consumer health information for the treatment and/or management of arthritis. For the purpose of this study, we identified and included CAM therapies based on the operational definition provided by Cochrane, as follows: https://cam.cochrane.org/operational-definition-complementary-medicine. In addition, websites had to have been published in the English-language and be publicly available. Ineligible websites that were excluded were as follows: Wikipedia pages, videos without text content (i.e. YouTube links), Google images, broken URLs, websites published in non-English languages, eBooks, peer-reviewed journals and articles, forums, and news articles that did not contain any consumer health information. A finalized list was developed to undergo further evaluation of content.

Data extraction and website quality assessment

AV and TJ data extracted the following items: website URL, website type, types of arthritis discussed, types of CAM therapies, types of non-CAM therapies (if present), whether the website appeared in more than one search (different search terms and/or regions), whether the website was certified by Health on the Net Foundation Code of Conduct (HONcode), as well as the scores for the 16 DISCERN questions. Different webpages from the same website captured by searches were considered a single item for the DISCERN instrument quality assessment; we therefore conducted a quality assessment of websites and not individual webpages. The DISCERN instrument is divided into a series of 16 key questions including an overall rating on the quality of the information being assessed. It is designed to examine what information is being provided rather than simply looking at how it is presented. It is organized into three sections: Section 1 (Questions 1–8), which address the reliability of the source, Section 2 (Questions 9–15), which analyses the specific details regarding treatment options, and Section 3 (Question 16), which is the overall quality rating of the publication [27]. To receive a 'good' quality rating, the majority of the questions must be rated highly on a five-point rating scale ranging from 'No' to 'Yes' [27]. A rating of five indicates that the answer to the question is a definite 'Yes', while a rating of one indicates a definite 'No'. The ratings in between signify that the criterion for the question was only partially fulfilled. Questions that encompass DISCERN criteria include analysing the aims of the publication, determining if the information is relevant, identifying if sources and their dates were made explicit, judging if the information is balanced and unbiased, enabling readers to pursue further sources of information and clarifying that more than one treatment option is available, identifying areas of uncertainty, providing background information on how a treatment works, describing the benefits and risks of the treatment/lack of treatment, highlighting effects on the overall quality of life, and determining if the publication (website) supports collaborative decision-making [27]. The assessor is then asked to rate the publication's overall quality (Question 16) by taking all of these areas into account and summarizing the results based on how the majority of the questions were answered. This final question is an intuitive summary of the previous 15 items of the DISCERN instrument [27].

We developed a standardized procedure to data extract and assess each website for quality using the DISCERN assessment by first conducting a pilot test on three separate websites independently, followed by a meeting to discuss and resolve any discrepancies (JYN, AV, TJ). Following this, AV and TJ completed the data extraction and assessed the quality of consumer health information using the DISCERN instrument, for each eligible website. The individual scores were reviewed by JYN and any remaining discrepancies were resolved between AV and TJ without unduly altering original assessor ratings. Averages were calculated across the two authors' scores for every DISCERN question and for all websites assessed. In addition to the five-point scale intuitive summary score for Question 16, an overall DISCERN score sum of questions 1–15 was also calculated (ranging from a score between 15 and 75). The mean score and standard deviation were determined for each DISCERN item as well as the total mean score for all 16 items.

Results

Search results

A total of 320 webpages were reviewed, of which 239 were duplicates, and 81 were unique. Twenty-seven websites were not eligible as they were peer-reviewed academic articles ($n = 20$), Google images ($n = 3$), invalid addresses ($n = 2$), and news articles ($n = 2$). One additional website did not mention CAM treatment for arthritis from a patient/consumer health information point of view, resulting in a total of 53 eligible webpages. After collapsing webpages from the same website, a total of 38 websites were deemed eligible and assessed using the DISCERN instrument. This process is depicted in Fig. 1.

General characteristics of eligible websites

We organized eligible websites based on the following categories: commercial, government, health portal, news, non-profit, professional, and other. For a website to be categorized as commercial, it would have to either purchase or sell a product or service with the intent of

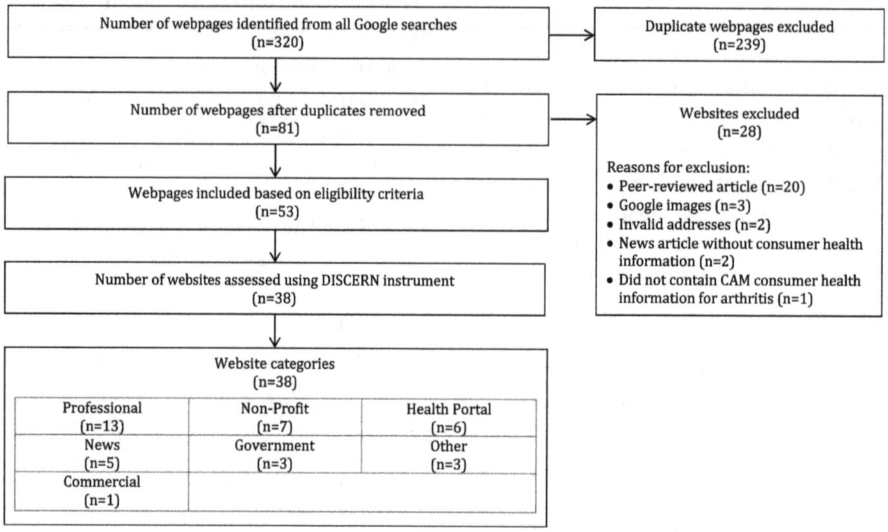

Fig. 1 Web Information Search Strategy and Assessment Flowchart

making a profit. An example of a commercial website in this study is the Praana website (https://praanaim.com/). Government websites – such as HealthLink British Columbia (https://www.healthlinkbc.ca/) – are websites that are controlled by a governmental body. A health portal is any website that primarily discusses health topics, such as WebMD (https://www.webmd.com/). The news categorization refers to websites like Medical News Today (https://www.medicalnewstoday.com/) that take information from newspapers, magazines and television and are a source of consumer health information. Non-profit websites are often linked to charities or organizations that are not aiming to make a profit, as seen with the Arthritis Foundation website (https://www.arthritis.org/). The majority of websites assessed ($n = 13$) were categorized as professional, meaning that they were either affiliated with health experts, a university/hospital, or an authorized organization, as seen in the example with the Mayo Clinic website (https://www.mayoclinic.org/). Websites that did not fit into any of the previously mentioned categories, were classified as 'other', which for example was the case for the Creaky Joints website (https://creakyjoints.org/).

Common types of CAM therapies discussed were dietary and herbal supplements, which according to the National Center for Complementary and Integrative Health, includes vitamins, minerals, herbs, botanicals, amino acids, enzymes, tissues from organs or glands, and extracts [28]. Dietary and herbal supplements were mentioned in nearly all the websites assessed aside from one ($n = 37$), proving to be the most frequent CAM therapy mentioned. Acupuncture was the next most common therapy ($n = 30$), followed by exercise ($n = 26$), when including tai chi and yoga. The overwhelming majority of websites (89.47%) also provided information about non-CAM therapies – the most common types being pharmaceutical medications and surgery. Most websites ($n = 29$) appeared in more than one search, including those that were generated from the same country but through a different search term. Table 1 depicts some of the general characteristics of the eligible websites.

DISCERN instrument ratings

The total mean score across all websites for the sum of questions 1 through 15 in the DISCERN instrument was 55.53 (SD = 9.37) out of 75. The total mean score for question 16, which assessed the overall rating of each website was 3.71 (SD = 0.63) on a five-point scale. This shows that on average, most websites achieved a moderately high overall rating. Thus, the quality of most sources was better than 'fair', but still had room for improvement in terms of obtaining the optimal standard. The Mayo Clinic and UptoDate websites scored the highest with both achieving a DISCERN score sum of 69.50. The overall quality rating was a score of 4.64 (SD = 0.05) for both of these webpages. Conversely, the Dr. Weil and Robert Schad Naturopathic Clinic websites scored the lowest, with scores of 38.00 and 32.00 respectively; the overall quality ratings were 2.53 and 2.14 respectively. A breakdown of the DISCERN instrument ratings can be viewed in Table 2, which includes the total means and standard deviations for each question.

Trends identified across resources assessed

Website aims

The DISCERN instrument considers a source to be of good quality if the aims of the publication are clearly indicated. Question 1 assesses the extent to which a

Table 1 General Characteristics of Eligible Websites

Website Name	URL	Website Category	Types of Arthritis Discussed	Types of CAM Discussed	Types of Non-CAM Therapies Discussed	Appeared in More than One Search?
Association of Accredited Naturopathic Medical Colleges	https://aanmc.org/	Professional	Osteoarthritis, inflammatory arthritis, rheumatoid arthritis, psoriatic arthritis, gout	Diet, exercise, tai chi, supplements, herbs, chiropractic, hydrotherapy, body work	Pharmaceuticals, steroid injections, surgery	Yes
American College of Rheumatology	https://www.rheumatology.org/	Non-Profit	Multiple types	Herbs, supplements, acupuncture	Pharmaceuticals	Yes
Arthritis Australia	https://arthritisaustralia.com.au/	Non-Profit	Multiple types	Acupuncture, massage, aromatherapy, vitamins, supplements, herbs	Pharmaceuticals, surgery	Yes
Arthritis Foundation	https://www.arthritis.org/	Non-Profit	Multiple types	Supplements, vitamins, acupuncture, massage, tai chi, yoga, weight loss, physical therapy, topical gels, transcutaneous electrical nerve stimulation, relaxation therapy, energy healing	Pharmaceuticals, surgery	Yes
Arthritis Health	https://www.arthritis-health.com/	Health Portal	Ankylosing spondylitis, bursitis, fibromyalgia, general arthritis, gout, juvenile arthritis, osteoarthritis, polymyalgia rheumatica, pseudogout, psoriatic arthritis, reactive arthritis, rheumatoid arthritis	Heat/cold, acupuncture, reiki healing, supplements, manual therapies, tai chi, yoga, massage, nutrition	Pharmaceuticals, surgery	Yes
Arthritis Society	https://arthritis.ca/	Non-Profit	Osteoarthritis, inflammatory arthritis, general arthritis	Heat/cold, visualization, relaxation, massage, acupuncture, meditation/mindfulness, chiropractic, herbs, supplements	Pharmaceuticals, surgery	Yes
Arthritis South Australia	https://arthritissa.org.au/	Non-Profit	Ankylosing spondylitis, fibromyalgia, gout, haemochromatotic arthritis, juvenile idiopathic arthritis, osteoarthritis, polymyalgia rheumatica, psoriatic arthritis, reactive arthritis, rheumatoid arthritis, epidemic polyarthritis, scleroderma, sjögren's syndrome, spondyloarthritis,	Acupuncture, massage, aromatherapy, vitamins, herbs, minerals	Pharmaceuticals, surgery	Yes
BMI Healthcare	https://www.bmihealthcare.co.uk/	Professional	Osteoarthritis, rheumatoid arthritis, psoriatic arthritis, general arthritis	Acupuncture, aromatherapy, massage, reflexology, yoga	Pharmaceuticals, surgery	No
Center for Holistic Medicine	http://holistic-medicine.com/	Professional	Osteoarthritis, rheumatoid arthritis	Hot/cold, diet, spinal decompression therapy, naprapathy, lasers, acupuncture	Pharmaceuticals	Yes
The Chalkboard Mag	https://thechalkboardmag.com/	News	Rheumatoid arthritis	Diet, herbs, meditation, yoga, mindfulness	Pharmaceuticals	No

Table 1 General Characteristics of Eligible Websites *(Continued)*

Website Name	URL	Website Category	Types of Arthritis Discussed	Types of CAM Discussed	Types of Non-CAM Therapies Discussed	Appeared in More than One Search?
Consumer Reports	https://www.consumerreports.org/cro/index.htm	Non-Profit	Osteoarthritis, general arthritis	Yoga, tai chi, supplements, acupuncture, massage, chiropractic, homeopathy, exercise, weight loss	No	Yes
Creaky Joints	https://creakyjoints.org	Other	Multiple types	Tai chi, acupuncture, yoga, exercise, massage, magnets, relaxation therapy, hydrotherapy, herbs, supplements, manipulation, chiropractic, weight management, physical therapy	Pharmaceuticals	Yes
Department of Family Medicine and Community Health University of Wisconsin	https://www.fammed.wisc.edu/	Professional	Osteoarthritis	Exercise, mind-body therapies, acupuncture, diet, supplements, massage	Pharmaceuticals, surgery	Yes
Dr. Weil	https://www.drweil.com/	Other	Rheumatoid arthritis, osteoarthritis, general arthritis	Exercise, relaxation techniques, hypnotherapy, diet, supplements	Pharmaceuticals	No
Everyday Health	https://www.everydayhealth.com/	News	Multiple types	Herbs, spices, supplements, acupuncture	Pharmaceuticals	Yes
Health	https://www.health.com/	News	Multiple types	Exercise, physical therapy, mind-body therapies, counselling, supplements, hot/cold, acupuncture, massage	Pharmaceuticals	No
Healthline	https://www.healthline.com/	Health Portal	Multiple types	Herbs, massage, heat/ice, exercise, tai chi, yoga, bath & soaking therapies, stress management/mind-body medicine (biofeedback & meditation), diet, vitamin supplements, acupuncture, supportive shoes, weight management, magnets	Pharmaceuticals, surgery	Yes
HealthLink British Columbia	https://www.healthlinkbc.ca/	Government	General arthritis	Supplements, vitamins, acupuncture, massage, topicals, tai chi, yoga	Pharmaceuticals, assistive devices	No
Integrative Medicine Center of Western Colorado	https://imcwc.com/	Professional	General arthritis	Herbs, vitamins, minerals, enzymes, oils	Pharmaceuticals	Yes
Integrated Medical Solutions of Knoxville	https://www.integratedmedicalsolutionsknox.com/	Professional	General arthritis	Exercise, chiropractic, diet, supplements, acupuncture	Injections	Yes
Johns Hopkins Arthritis Center	https://www.hopkinsarthritis.org/	Professional	Rheumatoid arthritis, psoriatic arthritis, ankylosing spondylitis, gout, osteoarthritis	Supplements, diet, acupuncture, magnets, hydrotherapy, homeopathy, tai chi,	Pharmaceuticals, surgery	Yes

Table 1 General Characteristics of Eligible Websites *(Continued)*

Website Name	URL	Website Category	Types of Arthritis Discussed	Types of CAM Discussed	Types of Non-CAM Therapies Discussed	Appeared in More than One Search?
				yoga, mind-body therapy, energy medicine		
Markham Integrative Medicine	https://integrative-medicine.ca/	Other	Rheumatoid arthritis	Diet, supplements, herbs, sauna therapy	No	Yes
Mayo Clinic	https://www.mayoclinic.org/	Professional	Ankylosing spondylitis, gout, juvenile idiopathic arthritis, osteoarthritis, psoriatic arthritis, reactive arthritis, rheumatoid arthritis, septic arthritis, thumb arthritis	Acupuncture, supplements, yoga, tai chi, massage, heat/cold	Pharmaceuticals, surgery, assistive devices	Yes
Medical News Today	https://www.medicalnewstoday.com/	News	General arthritis	Aquatic exercise, tai chi, yoga, hot/cold therapy, mindfulness meditation, massage, supplements, diet, herbs	Pharmaceuticals	Yes
National Center for Complementary and Integrative Health	https://www.nccih.nih.gov/	Government	Rheumatoid arthritis, osteoarthritis, gout	Mind-body practices, supplements, herbs, acupuncture, massage, tai chi, yoga, relaxation therapies, diet	No	Yes
National Health Service United Kingdom	https://www.nhs.uk/	Government	Osteoarthritis, rheumatoid arthritis, ankylosing spondylitis, cervical spondylosis, fibromyalgia, gout, psoriatic arthritis, enteropathic arthritis, reactive arthritis, secondary arthritis, polymyalgia rheumatica, juvenile idiopathic arthritis	Diet, supplements, acupuncture, massage, chiropractic, osteopathy	Pharmaceuticals, injections, surgery	Yes
Nursing Times	https://www.nursingtimes.net/	News	Rheumatoid arthritis, osteoarthritis	Acupuncture, homeopathy, herbs, osteopathy	Pharmaceuticals	Yes
Philadelphia Integrative Medicine	https://philly-im.com/	Professional	Rheumatoid arthritis	Mind-body techniques, nutrition, acupuncture, supplements, exercise, eliminating toxins	Pharmaceuticals	Yes
Praana	https://praanaim.com/	Commercial	Rheumatoid arthritis	Vitamins, exercise, diet, supplements, mind-body approach	Pharmaceuticals	Yes
Practical Pain Management	https://www.practicalpainmanagement.com/	Health Portal	Fibromyalgia, inflammatory arthritis, rheumatoid arthritis, juvenile idiopathic arthritis, osteoarthritis, polymyalgia rheumatica	Yoga, massage, dietary supplements, acupuncture, balneotherapy, mind-body therapies, chiropractic, relaxation techniques, prayer, naturopathy	Pharmaceuticals, injections, monitoring with lab tests	Yes
Robert Schad Naturopathic Clinic	https://rsnc.ca/	Professional	Rheumatoid arthritis, osteoarthritis	Nutrition, supplements, herbs, traditional Chinese medicine, homeopathic medicine, physical medicine	No	No

Table 1 General Characteristics of Eligible Websites *(Continued)*

Website Name	URL	Website Category	Types of Arthritis Discussed	Types of CAM Discussed	Types of Non-CAM Therapies Discussed	Appeared in More than One Search?
Spine Universe	https://www.spineuniverse.com/	Health Portal	Rheumatoid arthritis, ankylosing spondylitis, fibromyalgia, juvenile idiopathic arthritis, osteoarthritis	Acupuncture, herbs, massage, relaxation, mind-body therapies	Pharmaceuticals	Yes
St. Luke's Hospital	https://www.stlukes-stl.com/	Professional	Osteoarthritis, rheumatoid arthritis, gout, fibromyalgia, scleroderma,	Supplements, herbs, acupuncture, chiropractic, physical therapy, hydrotherapy, homeopathy, yoga, tai chi, exercise	Pharmaceuticals, surgery, braces, splints	No
Up To Date	https://www.uptodate.com/	Health Portal	Inflammatory and non-inflammatory arthritis	Acupuncture, mind-body techniques, exercise, diet, supplements, herbs, vitamins, homeopathy, magnets, mind-body therapies	Pharmaceuticals	Yes
University of Wisconsin-Madison Health	https://www.uwhealth.org/	Professional	General arthritis	Supplements, vitamins, acupuncture, massage, topicals, tai chi, yoga	Pharmaceuticals, assistive devices, surgery	No
Versus Arthritis	https://www.versusarthritis.org/	Non-Profit	Osteoarthritis, gout, rheumatoid arthritis, spondyloarthritis, ankylosing spondylitis, psoriatic arthritis, juvenile idiopathic arthritis	Diet, exercise, meditation, psychological exercises, acupuncture, yoga, body techniques, herbals	Pharmaceuticals, surgery	Yes
WebMD	https://www.webmd.com/	Health Portal	Osteoarthritis, rheumatoid arthritis, juvenile rheumatoid arthritis, infectious arthritis, ankylosing spondylitis, bone spurs, gout, systemic lupus	Heat/cold, magnets, acupuncture, aromatherapy, biofeedback, deep breathing, exercise, massage, meditation, progressive muscle relaxation, tai chi, herbals, topical creams, gels, patches, visualization, yoga, supplements, chiropractic	Pharmaceuticals, injections, surgery	Yes
Zanjabee	http://www.zanjabee.com/	Professional	Osteoarthritis	Diet, exercise, relaxation techniques, heat/cold, acupuncture, massage, supplements, herbs, Ayurveda	Pharmaceuticals, injections, joint replacement/ surgery	No

website fulfils this requirement. The vast majority of websites ranked above average for this question with a total mean score of 4.53 (SD = 0.56). The "About" page of a website typically included this information in the form of a mission/vision statement, or it could sometimes be found in the introduction of an article. It is here where most websites identified their target audience and what kind of information users could expect to find within the resource.

Use of references

Question 4 of the DISCERN instrument evaluates whether or not the sources used to compile the information on the website are made clear to the viewer. To achieve a good ranking for this question, the website should include both in-text citations and a reference list at the end of the article. Twenty-two out of 38 websites scored a 3 or below on this question, meaning that the majority of websites did not include both in-text citations and a formal reference list. The total mean score was 2.76 (SD = 1.51). Some websites included a reference list but failed to have in-text citations and vice versa, while others showed no evidence of referencing at all. Only 4 websites achieved a perfect ranking of 5 for this question.

Table 2 DISCERN Instrument Ratings and HONcode Search

Section		SECTION 1 Is the publication reliable?							
DISCERN Question		**1. Are the aims clear?**	**2. Does it achieve its aims?**	**3. Is it relevant?**	**4. Is it clear what sources of information were used to compile the publication (other than the author or producer)?**	**5. Is it clear when the information used or reported in the publication was produced?**	**6. Is it balanced and unbiased?**	**7. Does it provide details of additional sources of support and information?**	**8. Does it refer to areas of uncertainty?**
Mayo Clinic	https://www.mayoclinic.org/	5.00	4.50	4.50	4.00	5.00	5.00	4.50	5.00
UpToDate	https://www.uptodate.com/	5.00	5.00	5.00	5.00	5.00	5.00	5.00	5.00
Medical News Today	https://www.medicalnewstoday.com/	4.50	5.00	4.50	4.50	5.00	4.00	4.50	5.00
Johns Hopkins Arthritis Center	https://www.hopkinsarthritis.org/	5.00	5.00	4.50	5.00	5.00	5.00	5.00	5.00
National Center for Complementary and Integrative Health	https://www.nccih.nih.gov/	5.00	5.00	5.00	4.00	5.00	5.00	4.50	5.00
St. Luke's Hospital	https://www.stlukes-stl.com/	3.00	5.00	5.00	4.00	5.00	5.00	4.50	5.00
WebMD	https://www.webmd.com/	5.00	5.00	5.00	4.00	4.00	5.00	4.50	5.00
Department of Family Medicine and Community Health University of Wisconsin	https://www.fammed.wisc.edu/	4.50	5.00	5.00	4.00	4.00	4.00	3.50	5.00
Arthritis Health	https://www.arthritis-health.com/	4.50	4.50	4.50	5.00	5.00	5.00	5.00	5.00
Everyday Health	https://www.everydayhealth.com/	4.50	5.00	4.50	3.00	4.00	3.00	2.50	5.00
Healthline	https://www.healthline.com/	4.50	5.00	4.50	4.00	4.50	4.00	5.00	5.00
Practical Pain Management	https://www.practicalpainmanagement.com/	4.50	5.00	4.00	4.00	4.50	3.50	4.00	5.00
Spine Universe	https://www.spineuniverse.com/	4.50	4.00	4.50	2.50	3.50	3.50	3.00	3.00
National Health Service United Kingdom	https://www.nhs.uk/	4.50	4.00	4.00	3.50	5.00	2.00	5.00	5.00
Arthritis Society	https://arthritis.ca/	5.00	5.00	5.00	2.00	1.50	3.00	3.00	4.00
The Chalkboard Mag	https://thechalkboardmag.com/	5.00	5.00	4.50	4.50	4.00	2.50	5.00	1.50
Arthritis Foundation	https://www.arthritis.org/	5.00	5.00	4.50	3.00	2.5.00	3.00	2.50	4.00
BMI Healthcare	https://www.bmihealthcare.co.uk/	4.00	4.00	3.50	4.50	2.00	3.00	5.00	1.50
Versus Arthritis	https://www.versusarthritis.org/	4.50	5.00	5.00	1.50	2.00	4.00	3.00	4.50
Nursing Times	https://www.nursingtimes.net/	5.00	5.00	4.00	5.00	5.00	5.00	1.50	5.00
Arthritis Australia	https://arthritisaustralia.com.au/	5.00	4.00	4.00	3.00	3.00	2.50	5.00	5.00
Praana	https://praanaim.com/	4.00	4.00	4.50	4.00	3.00	2.00	5.00	4.50
Arthritis South Australia	https://arthritissa.org.au/	5.00	3.50	4.00	1.00	2.00	2.50	5.00	5.00
Health	https://www.health.com/	5.00	4.50	3.50	1.00	2.50	2.50	1.00	5.00

Table 2 DISCERN Instrument Ratings and HONcode Search *(Continued)*

Section		**SECTION 1 Is the publication reliable?**							
DISCERN Question		**1. Are the aims clear?**	**2. Does it achieve its aims?**	**3. Is it relevant?**	**4. Is it clear what sources of information were used to compile the publication (other than the author or producer)?**	**5. Is it clear when the information used or reported in the publication was produced?**	**6. Is it balanced and unbiased?**	**7. Does it provide details of additional sources of support and information?**	**8. Does it refer to areas of uncertainty?**
Markham Integrative Medicine	https://integrative-medicine.ca/	3.50	3.00	3.00	1.50	1.00	2.50	5.00	5.00
American College of Rheumatology	https://www.rheumatology.org/	4.50	3.00	3.00	1.00	2.50	3.00	5.00	5.00
HealthLink British Columbia	https://www.healthlinkbc.ca/	4.50	3.00	4.00	1.00	2.50	4.00	2.00	5.00
University of Wisconsin-Madison Health	https://www.uwhealth.org/	5.00	3.50	4.00	1.00	2.50	4.00	1.00	5.00
Creaky Joints	https://creakyjoints.org	4.50	3.00	4.00	1.00	1.00	2.00	3.00	5.00
Consumer Reports	https://www.consumerreports.org/cro/index.htm	5.00	2.50	3.00	3.00	3.00	2.00	4.00	5.00
Association of Accredited Naturopathic Medical Colleges	https://aanmc.org/	5.00	3.00	5.00	3.00	2.50	2.50	4.00	1.00
Integrative Medicine Center of Western Colorado	https://imcwc.com/	5.00	3.50	3.50	1.00	1.00	1.00	2.00	5.00
Philadelphia Integrative Medicine	https://philly-im.com/	4.50	2.00	2.50	1.50	4.00	2.50	4.00	5.00
Zanjabee	http://www.zanjabee.com/	4.00	3.50	4.00	1.00	1.00	2.00	1.50	1.50
Center for Holistic Medicine	http://holistic-medicine.com/	4.00	3.50	3.50	1.00	2.50	2.00	4.00	1.50
Integrated Medical Solutions of Knoxville	https://www.integratedmedicalsolutionsknox.com/	3.50	3.00	3.50	1.00	1.00	3.00	1.50	1.00

Table 2 DISCERN Instrument Ratings and HONcode Search *(Continued)*

Section	SECTION 2 How good is the quality of information on treatment choices?							SECTION 3 Overall Rating of the Publication			HONcode Search
DISCERN Question	**9. Does it describe how each treatment works?**	**10.Does it describe the benefits of each treatment?**	**11. Does it describe the risks of each treatment?**	**12. Does it describe what would happen if no treatment is used?**	**13. Does it describe how the treatment choices affect overall quality of life?**	**14. Is it clear that there may be more than one possible treatment choice?**	**15. Does it provide support for shared decision-making?**	**16. Based on the answers to all of the above questions, rate the overall quality of the publication as a source of information about treatment choices**	**Standard Deviation of Overall Score (Q16)**	**DISC ERN Score (Sum of Q1-Q15)**	**Is it certified by HONcode (yes/no)**
Mayo Clinic	4.00	5.00	3.00	5.00	5.00	5.00	5.00	4.64	0.05	69.50	Yes
UpToDate	4.00	4.50	4.00	2.00	5.00	5.00	5.00	4.64	0.05	69.50	Yes
Medical News Today	4.00	5.00	2.50	5.00	4.00	5.00	5.00	4.50	0.14	67.50	Yes
Johns Hopkins Arthritis Center	3.00	4.50	3.00	2.50	5.00	5.00	4.50	4.47	0.00	67.00	No
National Center for Complementary and Integrative Health	3.00	5.00	4.50	4.00	2.00	5.00	5.00	4.47	0.09	67.00	No
St. Luke's Hospital	3.00	4.50	3.50	3.50	5.00	5.00	5.00	4.43	0.14	66.00	No
WebMD	3.00	4.50	3.00	5.00	2.50	5.00	5.00	4.37	0.05	65.50	Yes
Department of Family Medicine and Community Health University of Wisconsin	3.50	5.00	4.50	5.00	2.50	5.00	5.00	4.37	0.05	65.50	No
Arthritis Health	4.00	4.50	3.00	1.00	3.50	5.00	5.00	4.30	0.14	64.50	Yes
Everyday Health	3.50	5.00	3.00	5.00	4.00	5.00	5.00	4.14	0.09	62.00	Yes
Healthline	2.50	5.00	3.50	1.50	2.50	5.00	5.00	4.10	0.04	61.50	Yes
Practical Pain Management	3.50	5.00	2.00	2.50	4.00	5.00	5.00	4.10	0.24	61.50	Yes
Spine Universe	4.00	5.00	3.50	5.00	4.50	5.00	5.00	4.03	0.14	60.50	Yes
National Health Service United Kingdom	5.00	5.00	4.00	2.00	1.00	5.00	5.00	4.10	0.14	60.00	No
Arthritis Society	5.00	5.00	3.00	5.00	3.00	5.00	5.00	3.97	0.05	59.50	No
The Chalkboard Mag	3.50	4.50	1.50	3.00	5.00	5.00	5.00	3.97	0.05	59.50	No
Arthritis Foundation	4.50	5.00	3.50	1.00	4.50	5.00	5.00	3.87	0.09	58.00	No
BMI Healthcare	3.50	5.00	1.50	5.00	5.00	5.00	5.00	3.84	0.05	57.50	No
Versus Arthritis	4.00	4.50	4.00	2.00	3.00	5.00	5.00	3.80	0.00	57.00	No
Nursing Times	1.00	3.50	3.50	2.00	1.50	4.50	5.00	3.77	0.14	56.50	No
Arthritis Australia	4.00	4.00	4.00	1.00	1.50	5.00	5.00	3.74	0.09	56.00	Yes
Praana	1.50	3.00	1.50	5.00	5.00	4.00	5.00	3.74	0.09	56.00	No

Table 2 DISCERN Instrument Ratings and HONcode Search *(Continued)*

Section	SECTION 2 How good is the quality of information on treatment choices?							SECTION 3 Overall Rating of the Publication			HONcode Search
DISCERN Question	**9. Does it describe how each treatment works?**	**10.Does it describe the benefits of each treatment?**	**11. Does it describe the risks of each treatment?**	**12. Does it describe what would happen if no treatment is used?**	**13. Does it describe how the treatment choices affect overall quality of life?**	**14. Is it clear that there may be more than one possible treatment choice?**	**15. Does it provide support for shared decision-making?**	**16. Based on the answers to all of the above questions, rate the overall quality of the publication as a source of information about treatment choices**	**Standard Deviation of Overall Score (Q16)**	**DISC ERN Score (Sum of Q1-Q15)**	**Is it certified by HONcode (yes/no)**
Arthritis South Australia	5.00	5.00	5.00	1.00	1.50	5.00	5.00	3.70	0.04	55.50	No
Health	3.00	5.00	2.00	2.00	4.50	5.00	5.00	3.44	0.05	51.50	No
Markham Integrative Medicine	3.50	4.00	3.50	3.00	4.00	4.00	5.00	3.44	0.23	51.50	No
American College of Rheumatology	2.50	3.00	4.00	1.00	3.00	5.00	5.00	3.37	0.05	50.50	No
HealthLink British Columbia	2.00	3.50	2.50	3.00	3.00	5.00	5.00	3.34	0.19	50.00	No
University of Wisconsin-Madison Health	2.00	3.50	2.50	3.00	3.00	5.00	5.00	3.34	0.19	50.00	No
Creaky Joints	3.50	4.00	3.50	2.00	2.50	5.00	5.00	3.27	0.19	49.00	No
Consumer Reports	2.50	4.00	2.50	1.00	1.00	5.00	5.00	3.30	0.04	48.50	No
Association of Accredited Naturopathic Medical Colleges	4.00	5.00	1.50	1.00	2.50	5.00	2.50	3.17	0.05	47.50	No
Integrative Medicine Center of Western Colorado	3.50	4.50	2.00	3.00	2.00	5.00	4.50	3.10	0.14	46.50	No
Philadelphia Integrative Medicine	2.00	3.00	2.00	1.00	3.00	5.00	2.50	2.97	0.05	44.50	No
Zanjabee	4.00	4.50	1.00	4.00	3.00	5.00	4.00	2.94	0.19	44.00	No
Center for Holistic Medicine	4.00	4.50	1.00	3.00	1.00	5.00	3.00	2.90	0.04	43.50	No
Integrated Medical Solutions of Knoxville	3.00	5.00	1.00	4.00	1.50	5.00	3.00	2.67	0.19	40.00	No
Dr. Weil	2.00	2.50	1.00	5.00	1.50	5.00	1.50	2.53	0.00	38.00	No
Robert Schad Naturopathic Clinic	2.00	3.50	1.00	1.00	4.00	4.00	2.00	2.14	0.09	32.00	No
TOTAL Means	3.30	4.38	2.78	2.92	3.16	4.91	4.54	3.71	0.10	55.53	
TOTAL Standard Deviations	0.97	0.72	1.13	1.54	1.33	0.28	0.98	0.63	0.07	9.37	

Risks associated with treatment

To achieve a high ranking for question 11 of the DISC ERN instrument, a website must include a description of the risks associated with each treatment that is discussed. The mean score for this question was 2.78 (SD = 1.13). None of the sources assessed received a perfect score of 5, which is of concern given that patients should be made aware of what to expect from a treatment, especially if any adverse side effects are known. Many websites did not provide enough detail about the disadvantages of a treatment, or only mentioned the risks for some of the CAM therapies discussed but failed to provide adequate details.

Variety of treatment options

The overwhelming majority of websites analysed in this study scored highly on question 14 of the DISCERN instrument. The question assesses whether or not a source demonstrates that there are various treatment options for arthritis patients. Thirty-four out of the 38 websites assessed received a perfect score of 5, and no website was graded lower than 4. This provided a mean score of 4.91 (SD = 0.28). Various forms of CAM therapies were often discussed, including dietary and herbal supplements, acupuncture, exercise, and manual therapies. Most of the websites provided additional information regarding conventional treatment options as well, such as pharmaceuticals, surgery, steroid injections and assistive devices.

Shared decision-making

Question 15 of the DISCERN instrument assesses the extent to which a website provides patients with support for shared decision-making. The majority of the websites assessed received a high ranking, with a mean score of 4.54 (SD = 0.98). Only 4 websites scored below a 3 for this question. Most websites recommended that patients do not take any dietary and herbal supplements without first consulting with their physician, stating that such products may interact with medications or potentially cause harm. Many sources also contained disclaimers about how website content should not be a substitute for professional medical advice and making healthcare decisions in collaboration with a healthcare provider.

Recommended websites for patients and consumers

The websites that scored highest in this study (an overall ranking of 4 or above for Question 16) may serve as good quality sources for practitioners to recommend to arthritis patients who seek additional CAM consumer health information about arthritis. These websites were similar in the sense that they typically scored a high rating above 4 across many of the DISCERN questions. Each of the highest scoring websites received a score of 5 for question 8 (which assesses whether the website refers to any areas of uncertainty with the treatment) and question 14. Furthermore, these websites clearly outlined areas of uncertainty in the research known about the disease, and highlighted the various treatment options that are available to arthritis patients. The majority of these websites provided clear cited sources and, in our judgement, provided information which remained unbiased. Many of these websites also referred consumers to further material on the topic discussed, and provided sufficient details surrounding the impacts a treatment option could have on a patient's overall quality of life. Additional details about these websites are provided in Table 3.

Discussion

The purpose of this study was to assess the quality of online CAM consumer health information for the treatment and/or management of arthritis. Given the high prevalence of CAM use among patients with arthritis and their increasing reliance on the internet for health information, it is important to critically evaluate the online resources that this unique patient population accesses. This is especially crucial given the fact that nearly half of all arthritis patients who utilize CAM therapies do not disclose this to their physicians [29]. Healthcare providers should, therefore, be aware of the online information that their patients may consult, either as a second opinion or in their absence, to help them navigate appropriate resources and discern between websites of high quality and those providing misinformation or unsafe recommendations.

The present study found that the majority of eligible websites assessed were of 'fair' quality. Twenty-one out of the 38 sources analysed received a moderate overall score (ranging from 2.90–3.97 out of 5). The total mean score of 3.71 (SD = 0.63) and average DISCERN score of 55.53 (SD = 9.37) suggests that most websites were slightly above adequate quality but still had some shortcomings. It should be noted that 14 out of 38 websites achieved a high overall ranking of 4 or above and can be deemed of 'good' quality. The websites that scored highest in this study may serve as useful resources to healthcare providers who seek to recommend high-quality resources for their patients. While no websites assessed received an overall score below 2 (i.e. 'poor' quality), three websites ranked below moderate (ranging from 2.14–2.67), suggesting that these websites had some serious shortcomings (including a lack of transparency in terms of the sources used, dates of the articles, areas of uncertainty, and the risks associated with each treatment while also not providing further reading).

This study also found that the majority of sources outlined the aims of the website, provided a wide variety of treatment options, and encouraged the use of shared decision-making between the patient and those who are involved in their care. In particular, adequate discussion surrounding different treatment options are beneficial for

Table 3 Recommended Websites for Patients and Consumers

Website Name	URL	DISCERN Score (Sum of our 75.00)	Overall DISCERN Score (Question 16, out of 5.00)	Website Category	Target Audience	Frequency of Updates
Mayo Clinic	https://www.mayoclinic.org/diseases-conditions/arthritis/diagnosis-treatment/drc-20350777	69.50	4.64	Professional	Healthcare providers, researchers, patients/public, prospective employees/volunteers	Website states that content is updated regularly following a schedule and whenever necessary to reflect new/revised findings. The precise frequency of updates is not clear.
UpToDate	https://www.uptodate.com/contents/complementary-and-alternative-therapies-for-rheumatoid-arthritis-beyond-the-basics	69.50	4.64	Health Portal	Healthcare providers, researchers, patients/public	The content is updated daily.
Medical News Today	https://www.medicalnewstoday.com/articles/325760 https://www.medicalnewstoday.com/articles/324446	67.50	4.50	News	Healthcare providers, researchers, patients/public	Website states that content is continually reviewed and updated. The precise frequency of updates is not available.
Johns Hopkins Arthritis Center	https://www.hopkinsarthritis.org/patient-corner/disease-management/ra-complementary-alternative-medicine/	67.00	4.47	Professional	Healthcare providers, patients/public	Information on the precise frequency of website updates is not clear.
National Center for Complementary and Integrative Health	https://www.nccih.nih.gov/health/rheumatoid-arthritis-in-depth	67.00	4.47	Government	Healthcare providers, researchers, patients/public	Website states that some parts are updated daily while other areas of the website may not be updated for weeks or months.
St. Luke's Hospital	https://www.stlukes-stl.com/health-content/medicine/33/000118.htm	66.00	4.43	Professional	Healthcare providers, patients/public	Information on the precise frequency of website updates is not clear.
WebMD	https://www.webmd.com/rheumatoid-arthritis/rheumatoid-arthritis-natural-treatments#1 https://www.webmd.com/osteoarthritis/features/alternative-arthritis-treatments#1 https://www.webmd.com/rheumatoid-arthritis/features/complementary-therapy#1	65.50	4.37	Health Portal	Healthcare providers, researchers, patients/public	Website states that corrections and updates to the material happen regularly, but information on the precise frequency of website updates is not clear.
Department of Family Medicine and Community Health University of Wisconsin	https://www.fammed.wisc.edu/integrative/resources/modules/osteoarthritis/	65.50	4.37	Professional	Healthcare providers, researchers, patients/public, prospective medical students	Information on the precise frequency of website updates is not clear.
Arthritis Health	https://www.arthritis-health.com/treatment/alternative-treatments/integrative-medicine-arthritis-pain-relief https://www.arthritis-health.com/treatment/alternative-treatments	64.50	4.30	Health Portal	Healthcare providers, patients/public	Information on the precise frequency of website updates is not clear.
Everyday Health	https://www.everydayhealth.com/	62.00	4.14	News	Healthcare providers, patients/public	Information on the precise frequency of website updates is not clear.

Table 3 Recommended Websites for Patients and Consumers *(Continued)*

Website Name	URL	DISCERN Score (Sum of our 75.00)	Overall DISCERN Score (Question 16, out of 5.00)	Website Category	Target Audience	Frequency of Updates
Healthline	https://www.healthline.com/	61.50	4.10	Health Portal	Healthcare providers, patients/ public	Website states that articles are updated when new information becomes available. Information on the precise frequency of website updates is not clear.
Practical Pain Management	https://www.practicalpainmanagement.com/	61.50	4.10	Health Portal	Healthcare providers, patients/ public	Website states that content is updated regularly. Information on the precise frequency of website updates is not clear.
Spine Universe	https://www.spineuniverse.com/	60.50	4.03	Health Portal	Healthcare providers, patients/ public	The content is updated daily.
National Health Service United Kingdom	https://www.nhs.uk/	60.00	4.10	Government	Healthcare providers, researchers, patients/public	The content is updated daily.

patients, so that they may be aware of the options that are available to them. While it is reassuring that numerous websites encourage patients to consult their healthcare providers before making any treatment decisions on their own, practitioners and researchers should be cautioned that the majority of websites did not report all of the risks that are associated with each CAM treatment and did not always provide explicit details about the references used to support their claims made about these therapies. These findings illuminate an aspect of patient behaviour outside of a clinical setting, given that many are unaware that various CAM therapies may lack efficacy and/or safety [30]; it is well-documented in the literature that, for example, many patients believe that natural remedies do not have any harmful side effects or that "natural equals safe", which is an issue that healthcare providers need to be cognizant of and should strongly advocate that their patients discuss their use of or concerns associated with CAM with them as opposed to self-medicating [30].

To our knowledge, this is the first study to assess the quality of websites containing CAM consumer health information specifically in the context of arthritis. Despite this, our findings can be compared to other studies that have assessed the quality of consumer health information on related topics. A previous study analysed the readability and quality of online information on osteoarthritis, including conventional forms of treatment. This study found that website information was considered 'fair' and that the readability was either equivalent to or more challenging than the recommended standard, as outlined by both the Journal of the American Medical Association and the DISCERN criteria [22, 31]. Prior to this, another study found that 44% of web search results related to arthritis promoted alternative medicine and that 80% of these websites had clear financial aims [32]. Another study also highlighted the importance of recommending websites that draw on evidence-based medical literature; an example of such information could include a systematic review that identified the quantity and assessed the quality of CAM recommendations for osteoarthritis and rheumatoid arthritis evidence-based clinical practice guidelines [33]. Guidelines and other evidence-based resources could be used as a starting point for the improvement of consumer health information on websites such as the ones we assessed in the present study.

Additionally, several studies have evaluated the quality of online CAM information as it relates to other conditions. A recent study assessed the quality of online consumer health information at the intersection of CAM and low back pain using the DISCERN instrument, finding that quality was quite variable across different websites. The authors found that the mean overall rating across all websites was 3.47 (SD = 0.70), while the summed DISCERN scores ranged from 25.5-68.0, with a mean of 53.25 (SD = 10.41) [34]. Another study also used the DISCERN instrument to evaluate information provided on chronic pain websites, and found that the overall quality of most were of moderate quality with several shortcomings. The overall average DISCERN score for this study was 55.90 (however, they scored this total to include question 16, out of 80) [35].

Strengths and limitations

One strength of the present study included the fact that we specifically searched Google across four different English-speaking countries (Australia, Canada, the

United Kingdom and the United States) in order to yield a more internationally-representative sample of websites. Another strength of this study included the use of the DISCERN instrument, which has been found to be both reliable and valid in assessing the quality of consumer health information [36]. Additional strengths include the fact that we also piloted conducting data extractions and applying the DISCERN instrument; during the pilot and full-assessments, both steps were conducted independently and in duplicate, before all three authors met to discuss and resolve discrepancies.

One limitation includes the fact that our search only captured a cross-sectional snapshot of website information; since the internet is a dynamic source that is subject to change, the results from this study may differ if replicated across future searches. Additionally, since the search strategy for this study only included the first 20 websites that were generated for each search term, less popular websites remain unassessed for quality. Furthermore, if different search terms were used, variable results could have been generated. Yet another limitation would include the fact that the internet searches were only conducted in English, as were the eligibility criteria, thereby excluding all websites that were written in other languages. Studies on the quality of non-English online consumer health information are also limited, thus it is unclear as to whether our findings are generalizable to non-English websites and their respective patient populations that access and read them. Multimedia platforms like videos and images were excluded, even though these may also contribute to an understanding of patient health-seeking behaviour in the context of CAM information for arthritis. Furthermore, the DISCERN instrument is primarily designed to assess the quality of health information, as opposed to determining the accuracy of the content or the safety of the information written in the publication [27].

Conclusion

The purpose of the present study was to assess the quality of online CAM consumer health information for the treatment and/or management of arthritis, that a 'typical' patient may access. While the internet gains increasing prominence as a source of information for CAM treatment choices, healthcare providers must be aware of the quality of consumer health information that their patients with arthritis may read and rely upon. Following a quality assessment using the DISCERN instrument, it was found that the majority of sources evaluated were slightly above average (3.71 out of 5), which suggests that patients should not solely base their CAM treatment decisions on the information found on these websites alone. Further discussion with a healthcare practitioner who can refer patients to reputable sources of consumer health information is warranted.

Abbreviation

CAM: Complementary and alternative medicine

Acknowledgements

JYN was funded by a Research Scholarship and an Entrance Scholarship from the Department of Health Research Methods, Evidence and Impact, Faculty of Health Sciences at McMaster University.

Authors' contributions

JYN: conceptualized and designed the study, collected the data, interpreted and analysed the data, drafted the manuscript, and gave final approval of the version to be published. AV: collected the data, interpreted and analysed the data, provided contributions and critically revised the manuscript, and gave final approval of the version to be published. TJ: collected the data, interpreted and analysed the data, provided contributions and critically revised the manuscript, and gave final approval of the version to be published.

References

1. Arthritis Foundation. What is arthritis?. 2020. Available from: https://www.arthritis.org/health-wellness/about-arthritis/understanding-arthritis/what-is-arthritis [cited 2020 Apr 26].
2. Arthritis Society. The truth about arthritis. Toronto; 2020. Available from: https://arthritis.ca/about-arthritis/what-is-arthritis/the-truth-about-arthritis [cited 2020 Apr 26].
3. Mayo Clinic. Arthritis.. 2019. Available from: https://www.mayoclinic.org/diseases-conditions/arthritis/symptoms-causes/syc-20350772 [cited 2020 Apr 26].
4. Safiri S, Kolahi AA, Hoy D, Smith E, Bettampadi D, Mansournia MA, et al. Global, regional and national burden of rheumatoid arthritis 1990–2017: a systematic analysis of the global burden of disease study 2017. Ann Rheum Dis. 2019;78(11):1463–71. https://doi.org/10.1136/annrheumdis-2019-215920 [cited 2020 May 3].
5. National Center for Complementary and Integrative Health. Complementary, alternative, or integrative health: what's in a name?. Maryland; 2018. Available from: https://www.nccih.nih.gov/health/complementary-alternative-or-integrative-health-whats-in-a-name [updated 2018 Jul; cited 2020 Apr 26].
6. Ng JY, Boon HS, Thompson AK, Whitehead CR. Making sense of "alternative", "complementary", "unconventional" and "integrative" medicine: exploring the terms and meanings through a textual analysis. BMC Complement Altern Med. 2016;16(134). https://doi.org/10.1186/s12906-016-1111-3 [cited 2020 May 3].
7. Mitha S, Nagarajan V, Babar MG, Siddiqui MJ, Jamshed SQ. Reasons of using complementary and alternative medicines (CAM) among elderly Malaysians of Kuala Lumpur and Selangor states: an exploratory study. J Young Pharm. 2013;5(2):50–3. https://doi.org/10.1016/j.jyp.2013.05.002 [cited 2020 Aug 12].
8. Lee M, Lee MS, Yang C, Lee S, Joo M, Shin B, et al. Use of complementary and alternative medicine by rheumatoid arthritis patients in Korea. Clin Rheumatol. 2008;27(1):29–33. https://doi.org/10.1007/s10067-007-0646-6 [cited 2020 May 4].
9. Jadhav P, Sharma Y, Nadkar M, Shelke P, Jadhav M. Assessment of use of complementary alternative medicine and its impact on quality of life in the patients attending rheumatology clinic, in a tertiary care centre in India. Indian J Med Sci. 2011;65(2):50–7. https://doi.org/10.4103/0019-5359.103961 [cited 2020 May 4].
10. Tokem Y, Parlar KS, Ozer S, Nakas D, Argon G. A multicenter analysis of the use of complementary and alternative medicine in turkish patients with rheumatoid arthritis: holistic practice review copy. Holist Nurs Pract. 2014;28(2): 98–105. https://doi.org/10.1097/HNP.0000000000000016 [cited 2020 May 4].
11. Obalum DC, Ogo CN. Usage of complementary and alternative medicine (CAM) among osteoarthritis patients attending an urban multi-specialist hospital in Lagos, Nigeria. Niger Postgrad Med J. 2011 Mar;18(1):44–7.
12. Arthritis research UK therapy complementary and alternative medicine for arthritis. Chesterfield; 2014. 2 p. Available from: https://www.versusarthritis.org/media/1336/complementary-and-alternative-medicines-information-booklet.pdf [cited 2020 Aug 12].
13. Feldman DE, Duffy C, De Civita M, Malleson P, Philibert L, Gibbon M, et al. Factors associated with the use of complementary and alternative medicine in juvenile idiopathic arthritis. Arthritis Rheum. 2004;51(4):527–532. https://doi.org/10.1002/art.20536 [cited 2020 Nov 23].

14. Zhang Y, Dennis JA, Bishop FL, Cramer H, Leach M, Lauche R, et al. Complementary and alternative medicine use by U.S. adults with self-reported doctor-diagnosed arthritis: results from the 2012 national health interview survey. PM&R. 2019;11(10):1059–1069. doi: https://doi.org/10.1002/pmrj.12124 [cited 2020 Nov 23].
15. Zhang Y, Leach MJ, Hall H, Sundberg T, Ward L, Sibbritt D, et al. Differences between male and female consumers of complementary and alternative medicine in a national US population: a secondary analysis of 2012 NIHS data. Evid Based Complement Alternat Med. 2015;2015:413173. doi: https://doi.org/10.1155/2015/413173 [cited 2020 Nov 23].
16. Mbizo J, Okafor A, Sutton MA, Burkhart EN, Stone LM. Complementary and alternative medicine use by normal weight, overweight, and obese patients with arthritis or other musculoskeletal diseases. J Altern Complement Med. 2016;22(3):227–236. doi: https://doi.org/10.1089/acm.2014.0390 [cited 2020 Nov 23].
17. Quandt SA, Chen H, Grzywacz JG, Bell RA, Lang W, Arcury TA. Use of complementary and alternative medicine by persons with arthritis: results of the national health interview survey. Arthritis Rheum. 2005;53(5):748–755. doi: https://doi.org/10.1002/art.21443 [cited 2020 Nov 23].
18. Seburg EM, Horvath KJ, Garwick AW, McMorris BJ, Vehe RK, Scal P. Complementary and alternative medicine use among youth with juvenile arthritis: are youth using CAM, but not talking about it? J Adolesc Health. 2012;51(2):200–202. doi: https://doi.org/10.1016/j.jadohealth.2012.01.003 [cited 2020 Nov 23].
19. Zochling J, March LM, Lapsley H, Cross M, Tribe K, Brooks P. Use of complementary medicines for osteoarthritis – a prospective study. Ann Rheum Dis. 2004;63(5):549–554. doi: https://doi.org/10.1136/ard.2003.010637 [cited 2020 Nov 23].
20. National Center for Complementary and Integrative Health. Rheumatoid arthritis: in depth Maryland. 2019. Available from: https://www.nccih.nih.gov/health/rheumatoid-arthritis-in-depth [cited 2020 Aug 20].
21. National Center for Complementary and Integrative Health. Osteoarthritis: in depth. Maryland. Available from: https://www.nccih.nih.gov/health/osteoarthritis-in-depth2016 [updated 2019 Jan; cited 2020 Aug 20].
22. Murray KE, Murray TE, O'Rourke AC, Low C, Veale DJ. Readability and quality of online information on osteoarthritis: an objective analysis with historic comparison. Interact J Med Res. 2019; 8(3):e12855. doi: https://doi.org/10.2196/12855 [cited 2020 Apr 27].
23. Chen AT, Taylor-Swanson L, Buie RW, Park A, Conway M. Characterizing websites that provide information about complementary and integrative health: systematic search and evaluation of five domains. Interact J Med Res. 2018;7(2):e14. doi: https://doi.org/10.2196/ijmr.9803 [cited 2020 May].
24. Owens C, Baergen R, Puckett D. Online sources of herbal product information. Am J Med. 2014;127(2):109–115. doi: https://doi.org/10.1016/j.amjmed.2013.09.016 [cited 2020 May].
25. Stat counter global stats [Image on internet]. 2020. Available from: https://gs.statcounter.com/search-engine-market-share/all/ [2020 Aug 12].
26. Chitika Insights. The value of google result positioning. Westborough: Chitika Inc. 2013:0–10 [cited 2020 May 3].
27. Charnock D. The DISCERN handbook: quality criteria for consumer health information; user guide and training resource. Abingdon: Radcliffe Medical Press; 1998. Available from: http://www.discern.org.uk/discern.pdf.
28. National Center for Complementary and Integrative Health. Dietary and herbal supplements. Maryland; 2020. Available from: https://www.nccih.nih.gov/health/dietary-and-herbal-supplements [updated 2020 Feb; cited 2020 Aug 12].
29. Yang L, Sibbritt D, Adams J. A critical review of complementary and alternative medicine use among people with arthritis: a focus upon prevalence, cost, user profiles, motivation, decision-making, perceived benefits and communication. Rheumatol Int. 2017;37(3):337–351. doi: https://doi.org/10.1007/s00296-016-3616-y [cited 2020 May].
30. National Center for Complementary and Integrative Health. Natural doesn't necessarily mean safer, or better [Internet]. Maryland; 2020. Available from: https://www.nccih.nih.gov/health/know-science/natural-doesnt-mean-better [cited 2020 Aug 12].
31. Willen RD, Pipitone O, Daudfar S, Jones JD. Comparing quality and readability of online English language information to patient use and perspectives for common rheumatologic conditions. Rheumatol Int. 2020; 40(12):2097–2103. doi: https://doi.org/10.1007/s00296-020-04664-8 [cited 2020 Aug 16].
32. Suarez-Almazor ME, Kendall CJ, Dorgan M. Surfing the net – information on the world wide web for persons with arthritis: Patient empowerment or patient deceit? J Rheumatol. 2001; 28(1):185–191. https://www.jrheum.org/content/28/1/185.long [cited 2020 Apr 26].
33. Ng JY, Azizudin AM. Rheumatoid arthritis and osteoarthritis clinical practice guidelines provide few complementary and alternative medicine therapy recommendations: a systematic review. Clin Rheumatol. 2020;39(10):2861–2873. doi: https://doi.org/10.1007/s10067-020-05054-y [cited 2020 Apr 27].
34. Ng JY, Gilotra K. Web-information surrounding complementary and alternative medicine for low back pain: A cross-sectional survey and quality assessment. Integr Med Res. 2020. doi: https://doi.org/10.1016/j.imr.2020.100692 [cited 2020 Nov 23].
35. Kaicker J, Debono VB, Dang W, Buckley N, Thabane L. Assessment of the quality and variability of health information on chronic pain websites using the DISCERN instrument. BMC Med. 2010;8(59). doi: https://doi.org/10.1186/1741-7015-8-59 [cited 2020 Aug 3].
36. Charnock D, Shepperd S, Needham G, Gann R. DISCERN: an instrument for judging the quality of written consumer health information on treatment choices. J Epidemiol Community Health. 1999;53(2):105–111. https://doi.org/10.1136/jech.53.2.105 [cited 2020 Nov 23].

2

Drug prices in Latin American countries: The case of rheumatoid arthritis biosimilars

Gabriela Bittencourt Gonzalez Mosegui[1*], Fernando Antõnanzas[2], Cid Manso de Mello Vianna[3] and Paula Rojas[4]

Abstract

Background: The objective of this paper is to analyze the prices of biological drugs in the treatment of Rheumatoid Arthritis (RA) in three Latin American countries (Brazil, Colombia and Mexico), as well as in Spain and the United States of America (US), from the point of market entry of biosimilars.

Methods: We analyzed products authorized for commercialization in the last 20 years, in Brazil, Colombia, and Mexico, comparing them to the United States of America (USA) and Spain. For this analysis, we sought the prices and registries of drugs marketed between 1999 and October 1, 2019, in the regulatory agencies' databases. The pricing between countries was based on purchasing power parity (PPP).

Results: The US authorized the commercialization of 13 distinct biologicals and four biosimilars in the period. Spain and Brazil marketed 14 biopharmaceuticals for RA, ten original, four biosimilars. Colombia and Mexico have authorized three biosimilars in addition to the ten biological ones. For biological drug prices, the US is the most expensive country. Spain's price behavior seems intermediate when compared to the three LA countries. Brazil has the highest LA prices, followed by Mexico and Colombia, which has the lowest prices. Spain has the lowest values in PPP, compared to LA countries, while the US has the highest prices.

Conclusion: The economic effort that LA countries make to access these medicines is much higher than the US and Spain. The use of the PPP ensured a better understanding of the actual access to these inputs in the countries analyzed.

Keywords: Biological products, Antirheumatic agents, Access to essential medicines and health technologies, Products registration, Drug Price

Introduction

Rheumatoid arthritis (RA) is a chronic inflammatory autoimmune disease that affects 0.3 to 1.0% of the world population. This prevalence seems to be lower in emerging countries, given the differences in age distribution among population groups, difficulty in accessing the health system, lack of diagnosis and lack of studies [1].

Biological agents used to treat moderate or severe active disease reduce inflammation and prevent joint damage [2]. These are innovative products made from living cells whose development is longer and more costly than that of traditional products. The economic risks involved in this process are high. There is no difference in obtaining a biosimilar drug, where companies assume the same strategic level as those who hold the patents or creators of the original biopharmaceutical [3]. Biosimilars are not generic drugs and may differ from reference products in manufacturing, composition and formulation [4].

In the US market, few biosimilars are available as a result of the high cost of approval and price competition from manufacturers of reference drugs [5]. The European Medicines Agency (EMA) has authorized the first biosimilar in over than10 years, and since then, there has been an intense debate about access, penetration with regard to originals and the prescription of these

* Correspondence: gabrielamosegui@uol.com.br
[1]Department of Health and Society, Community Health Institute, Fluminense Federal University, Rua: Marquês do Paraná, 303, 3° floor, annex building, Niterói, RJ CEP: 24033-900, Brazil

products in European Union (EU) countries. There are some factors that can influence the entry of biosimilars into the markets of different countries, ranging from the product itself, the therapeutic area to which the product is directed, the sanitary policy adopted, the price and therefore the access, and finally the prescriptive standards [6].

These supplies are among the top-selling drugs in the world market. In Brazil, in 2017, the revenues of companies that marketed biopharmaceuticals was R$ 15,409, 519,216 or US$ 491,707,322 [7]. Four of the twenty substances with the highest revenues this year in the Brazilian market were biological, with three of them (adalimumab, infliximab, and etanercept) used for RA [7]. All of these therapeutic options already have biosimilars on the market [8–10]. In 2013, biosimilars accounted for approximately 25% of the total biological sales, the patents of which having expired in the EU. In 2015, the biosimilar market amounted to US$ 490 million in the EU-5, Germany, Spain, France, Italy and the United Kingdom [6].

According to Zozoya and González [11] some studies have tried to estimate the economy magnitude produced with biosimilar introduction. In Spain, this saving was between 300 and 2800 million euros between 2007 and 2020. In Latin America, the regulation and penetration of these drugs varies considerably [12], and most of the available studies focus on the normative issue, not on prices] [4, 12–15].

The importance of biosimilars in public health is related to the costs of the original medicines and the demographic and epidemiological profiles of the population. Their adoption can lead to considerable cost savings [15]. It is crucial to the political debate to have concrete data on how the biosimilar market is evolving and how it will behave in the future, given the high degree of innovation in the sector and the speed of incorporation of new technologies demanded by society and health systems. The objective of this paper is to analyze the prices of biological drugs in the treatment of RA in three LA countries, namely, Brazil, Colombia and Mexico, as well as in Spain and the United States of America (US), from the point of market entry of biosimilars.

Methods

The records and prices of biological products of the antirheumatic class used in the treatment of RA, approved from 1998 in Brazil, Colombia and Mexico, were analyzed. An initial list of medicines for the treatment of RA released annually in the US market by the Food and Drug Administration (FDA) has been created [9]. Registration information on these drugs has been taken from Brazilian drug regulatory agencies - *Agência Nacional de Vigilância Sanitária* (Anvisa), from Colombia - *Instituto Nacional de Vigilância de Medicamentos y Alimentos* (Invima), from Spain (*Consejo General de Colegios Oficiales de Farmacéuticos*) and from Mexico - *Comisión Federal para la Protección contra Riesgos Sanitarios* (Cofepris) [16–19]. RA treatment guides from each of these countries were reviewed and consulted in pursuit of other therapeutic possibilities that had not been captured to complement the registration data [2].

From the product lists launched between 1998 and 2019, 14 authorized in Spain and Brazil, 16 in the US, and 13 in Mexico and Colombia, a sample of 10 antirheumatic biological drugs common to all these countries was defined for the treatment of RA. These were listed by authorization year, pharmaceutical form(s), and similar packaging. Biosimilars authorized in this period were also included. For these inputs, the date taken corresponded to when the first manufacturer registered the product by searching data information in Anvisa, Cofepris, Consejo General of Official Colleges of Pharmaceuticals and Invima, by year of publication and by consulting the records [16–19]. The year of marketing authorization publication guided price monitoring. The drug associations were excluded. The unit of analysis of the study was the product, considering the same concentrations and packaging.

Price research was carried out on the official bases of each of these countries, except for the US. The values identified were the retail reference values for the year 2019. In Brazil, the prices on the Anvisa website [20] were consulted. The standard set for Brazil was the maximum consumer price (MCP), which refers to 18% of the tax on the circulation of goods and services. In the US, market prices were captured from Drugs.com [21], and in Spain, from *Consejo General de Colegios Oficiales de Farmacéuticos* [19]. Colombian prices were obtained from reference price listings from 2019 for the month/ base September in the Digital Institutional Repository of the Ministry of Health [22]. In Mexico, reference prices for patented drugs were obtained from an official price list [23]. Complementary consultation was made at the Government-recommended site for 2019 only [24].

For products with different quantities of pharmaceutical units per package, for the same pharmaceutical form and concentration, the price of the package with the largest quantity or cheapest presentation was taken. Only two drug samples differed in presentation and concentration, and both were reduced to the smallest unit of presentation for comparison.

All prices were converted to US dollars using the Central Bank of Brazil exchange rates [25]; the purchasing power or purchasing power parity (PPP) was used as another price comparator. PPP conversion factor is a currency converter and spatial price deflator that controls for price level differences between countries. PPP values for 2019 were used, the latest available from the World Bank [26, 27].

This study did not require institutional review board approval or informed consent, as it was based on public data and did not involve patient records.

Results

The immunobiological drugs and biosimilar drugs analyzed, which are simultaneously registered and appear in official lists as well as in the clinical protocols of the 3 LA countries, are listed in the following table.

The registered year of publication guided the price monitoring developments in subsequent years. In the US, the FDA registered 13 distinct biologicals in the period and 4 biosimilars. Spain and Brazil recorded the 14 selected RA drugs in the period: 10 originals and 4 biosimilars. Colombia and Mexico registered 3 biosimilars in addition to 10 biologicals [9, 18, 20, 28]. Biosimilars approved for commercialization include adalimumab, etanercept, infliximab and rituximab. The FDA approved all these biosimilars, but only infliximab is marketed. Adalimumab is authorized only in Spain, while etanercept and infliximab are approved in the three LA countries and in Spain. Rituximab is not in Invima, the Colombian registration system.

There is no average difference between the release time in the US and that in other countries that deserves consideration as an indication of the greater "availability" of these inputs in one country or another. Marketing authorizations for biopharmaceuticals and biosimilars in the US are from 2002. Although Spain, Brazil and Colombia have approved biological agents for RA since the 1990s, we concentrate on those from 2014, 2009 and 2015, respectively; additionally, Mexico has approved them since 2013. For biosimilars, Spain has adopted them since 2013, Brazil since 2014, Colombia since 2006 and Mexico since 1999.

Table 1 shows the prices in US dollars and PPP of medicines per package in the analyzed markets.

The blank cells in Table 2 represent data not found in the queried databases. Regarding the prices of biological medicines used for RA, the US is the most expensive

Table 1 Prices comparison of RA biological agents registered between 1998 and 2019 in Brazil, Colombia, Spain, United States (US) and Mexico, in US dollars (US$) per presentation and PPP. Source: [19–27]

Drug	Dosage forms (DF)	US (US$/DF)	Spain (US$/DF)	PPP Spain	Brazil (US$/DF)	PPP Brazil	Colombia (US$/DF)	PPP Colombia	Mexico (US$/DF)	PPP Mexico
Abatacept	250 mg, injection powder	1167,3	447,2	636,5	450,2	812,5	324,4	823,8	431,8	902,5
Adalimumab	40 mg/0.8 mL (1 ea)	5411,3	1256,9	1788,9	2729,0	4925,6	796,4	2022,4	516,9	1080,5
Adalimumab (biosimilar)	40 mg/0.8 mL (1 ea)		1256,9	1788,9						
Baricitinib	2 mg tablets (30 tablets)	2240,4	1155,5	1644,4	920,9	1662,0			894,2	1869,0
Certolizumabe pegol	200 mg in 1 mL, injection, kit	9054,7	1164,4	1657,1	691,3	1247,7	703,5	1786,7	1059,4	2214,4
Etanercept	50 mg/mL (0.98 mL, 1 mL), Solution Prefilled Syringe, Subcutaneous	5411,2	848,7	1207,9	1255,1	2265,3	831,2	2110,8	1188,1	2483,4
Etanercept (biosimilar)	50 mg/mL (0.98 mL, 1 mL), Solution Prefilled Syringe, Subcutaneous		848,7	1207,9	899,1	1622,7	415,6	1055,4		
Golimumab	50 mg/0.5 mL (0.5 mL)	5030,1	1359,6	1934,9	1316,6	2376,2	829,4	2106,3	1298,2	2713,4
Infliximab	100 mg (1 ea)	1228,70	687,0	977,8	1365,5	2464,7	390,2	990,9	713,1	1490,4
Infliximab (biosimilar)	100 mg (1 ea)	997,4	568,8	809,5	862,8	1557,3			400,4	836,8
Rituximab	10 mg/mL (10 mL)	1998,7	633,5	901,6	673,9	1216,3	451,9	1147,6	865,9	1809,9
Rituximab (biosimilar)	10 mg/mL (10 mL)		546,5	777,8	404,9	730,7				
Tocilizumab	20 mg/4 mL (4 mL), Solution, Intravenous	476,9	215,3	306,3	165,8	299,3	97,2	246,9	192,6	402,6
Tofacitinib	5 mg tablets (60 tablets)	4687,3	1020,5	1452,4	1893,2	3417,1	810,2	2057,5	940,3	1965,3

Table 2 Innovative and biosimilar drugs used to treat rheumatoid arthritis (RA), approved from 1998 to 2019, in the countries analyzed

Drugs	Registration year	Country
Abatacept	2005	US
	2007	Brazil
	2012	Spain
	2016	Mexico
	2018	Colombia
Adalimumab	2002	US
	2003	Brazil/Colombia
	2010	Mexico
	2018	Spain
Adalimumab	2018	Spain
Biosimilar	2019	Brazil/Colombia
	2015	US
Baricitinib	2017	Spain/Mexico
	2018	US/Brazil
	2019	Colombia
Certolizumabe pegol	2009	US
	2011	Brazil
	2016	Colombia
	2017	Spain/Mexico
Etanercept	1999	Mexico
	2002	US
	2003	Brazil
	2006	Spain
	2007	Colombia
Etanercept biosimilar	2006	Colombia
	2013	Brazil/Mexico
	2016	US
	2017	Spain
Golimumab	2009	US
	2011	Brazil/Colombia
	2013	Spain
	2014	Mexico
Infliximab	1999	Spain
	2000	Colombia
	2001	US
	2007	Brazil
	2016	Mexico
Infliximab	2014	Spain/Mexico
Biosimilar	2013	US
	2015	Brazil
	2017	Colombia
Rituximab	1998	Brazil/Spain
	1999	Colombia

Table 2 Innovative and biosimilar drugs used to treat rheumatoid arthritis (RA), approved from 1998 to 2019, in the countries analyzed *(Continued)*

Drugs	Registration year	Country
	2006	US
	2017	Mexico
Rituximab	2017	Spain/Mexico
Biosimilar	2019	Brazil
Tocilizumab	2009	Brazil/Mexico
	2010	US
	2014	Spain
	2015	Colombia
Tofacitinib	2012	US
	2013	Mexico
	2014	Brazil
	2018	Colombia/Spain

country. Spain's price behavior seems intermediate when compared to the three LA countries. Brazil has the highest LA prices, followed by Mexico and Colombia, which have the lowest prices. When comparing US prices to Spanish prices in dollars, Spain has lower priced drugs.

For biosimilars, adalimumab is marketed only in Spain and has the same value as the original drug (US$ 1256.9). The biosimilar etanercept has the same price as its original in Spain (US$ 848.7) but is cheaper in Brazil and Colombia than the innovative drug (by 28.4 and 50%, respectively). This biosimilar is, in turn, more expensive in both LA countries than in Spain. Infliximab is the only biosimilar of this class marketed in the US and has a difference of minus 18.8% from the value of the original product. Spain, Brazil and Mexico also have lower prices for this biosimilar (17.2; 36.8; and 43.9%, respectively) than that of the innovative drug. Only Spain and Brazil trade the biosimilar rituximab, with prices up to approximately 40% cheaper than that of the original.

Prices were also correlated between countries, based on the PPP, when considering that the purchasing capacity changes compared to prices previously analyzed. Still under this interpretation, the US, which exhibited higher prices for biological drugs for the treatment of RA, maintains the highest PPP values, all higher than those of Spain and the LA countries, except for infliximab in Brazil and Mexico. The PPP for Spain is lower than that of the Latin American countries, except for adalimumab in Mexico, tocilizumab in Brazil and Colombia, biosimilar rituximab in Brazil and biosimilar etanercept in Colombia. The PPP values of Brazil are similar to those of Mexico, considering the absolute and relative number of medicines in each of these countries. Colombia's PPP values are lower than in Mexico and Brazil. The three LA countries have PPP values higher than those of Spain and lower than US drug prices.

Discussion

The main objective of this study was to analyze the evolution of the prices of biosimilar medicines in three LA countries, Spain and the US. Prices between countries were also compared on the basis of the PPP, which links drug values to differences in purchasing power levels. Our study points to a much lower affordability for the citizens of LA countries (as their prices, corrected by the PPP, were higher than in Spain, a wealthier country). This trend of the acquisition effort is not repeated in the United States, which has the highest PPP among the 5 countries. Putrik and collaborators [29] investigated the availability, accessibility and acceptability for synthetic and biological drugs in European countries, relating them to the socioeconomic status, well-being and health status of patients with RA. The prices of biological drugs for RA differed by up to 7.3 and 1.3 times, respectively, after adjusting for the PPP, between countries.

The findings of this paper should be carefully interpreted. For the price analysis of medicines, international comparisons should be cautious, as wholesale prices may produce misleading information [30]. Biological agents are only one drug class among many existing in the analyzed countries. We tried to compare the prices of drugs that coincided with each other in presentation, concentration, formulation, and manufacturer, but the periods in which they were available on the market are different. An ideal price analysis would control all these features. Sales data on these inputs would be important. The use of official databases, rather observing their structure, with information gaps that limit the progress of evaluations from these data, should be evaluated. There is a loss in the comparison between the PPP of the LA countries given the heterogeneity of the markets and inaccuracy in the data depicted.

In addition to the great potential of the data available for health services, there is the scarcity of studies of this type and the complexity of exploring background information with so many particularities and differences.

Recent registration approvals, nonmarketing of the product or even the absence of distributors may be behind the absence of a drug in the market. These trends, registration approval characteristics, and the marketing itself provide important information for prescribers, patients, and the industry [31]. None of the drugs analyzed appear in the Mexican government's price comparison [32]. In Mexico, biosimilar approvals were found prior to those of the original products, somewhat illustrating the lack of clarity of the database [16]. Marketing approval for unregistered but sale-authorized biological agents in the European Union, the US, Canada, and Australia can be obtained in the respective countries [28]. Differences in legislation and database updating or completion may explain the different approval dates of biologics as approved biosimilars before their originals. In Colombia, Bernal-Camargo and collaborators [13] point to problems in the classification of Invima-registered biosimilars, which, due to legal, information, availability and access barriers, make informed consumption difficult for the population.

Some biosimilar products, although approved for the US market, are not sold. These are licensing agreements with the original manufacturer that would allow the biosimilar to be launched later, up to 5 litigations, such as one of etanercept's biosimilars [33].

The high prices for medicines in the American market are not new. Mexico and Colombia may have lower prices than those in Brazil due to differences in input costs, tariff barriers, taxes, market power, industry regulation, healthcare systems or consumer preferences [34].

The economic impact of biosimilars on sanitary systems can be achieved through direct savings associated with lower prices. By competing with the original products, they eventually bring down the price of biological medicines [35]. According to Zozaya, and Gonzalez [11], the price difference between a biosimilar and its original ranges from 6 to 37% in Europe. In addition, discounts on purchases often apply. In Spain, where the price of reference biologicals should equal the lowest price of their biosimilar counterparts, average discounts are 20% [6, 35]..

Conclusions

The study compared biosimilar and biological drug prices and registration times for RA. Biosimilar market penetration of these RA drugs differs greatly from country to country, varying even within the commercialized therapeutic classes. The use of biosimilars may increase the viability of treatment of many patients in health care systems in emerging countries, where potential cost savings are highly valued.

The PPP strategy ensured a better understanding of access to biological products for RA. The economic effort of the United States and Spain is much less than that of these LA countries. Although the price of some of these drugs is lower in LA countries, the effort to obtain them is much higher and the differences noted are greater when converted into PPP units. Tracking the prices of these drugs as patents are lost can be a way to avoid monopolies. One step has already been taken regarding health regulation; other larger ones should take place regarding pricing and agreements with the pharmaceutical industry.

Acknowledgements

Carolina Foundation and Tordesillas Group for GBGM three months scholarship.

Authors' contributions

GBGM had substantial contributions to the conception and design of the work, analysis and interpretation of data, draft the paper and revised it. FA had substantial contributions to the conception and design of the work, interpretation of data and revision of the final manuscript. CMMV had contribute with the analysis and interpretation of data and revision of the final manuscript. PR had contribute with the analysis and interpretation of data and revision of the final manuscript.

We agreed both to be personally accountable for the author's own contributions and to ensure that questions related to the accuracy or integrity of any part of the work, even ones in which the author was not personally involved, are appropriately investigated, resolved, and the resolution documented in the literature.

All authors read and approved the final manuscript as they have approved the submitted version.

Author details

[1]Department of Health and Society, Community Health Institute, Fluminense Federal University, Rua: Marquês do Paraná, 303, 3° floor, annex building, Niterói, RJ CEP: 24033-900, Brazil. [2]Department of Economy and Company, Economy Faculty, University of La Rioja, Calle la Cigüeña, 60, 26006 Logroño, La Rioja, Spain. [3]Department of Health Policy, Planning and Management, Health Medicine Institute, Rio de Janeiro Estadual University, Rua São Francisco Xavier 524 – Maracanã, Bloco D, 7° floor, Rio de Janeiro, RJ 20550-013, Brazil. [4]Department of Economy and Company, Economy Faculty, University of La Rioja, Calle la Cigüeña, 60, 26006 Logroño, La Rioja, Spain.

References

1. Burgos-Vargas R, Catoggio LJ, Galarza-Maldonado C, Ostojich K, Cardiel MH. Current therapies in rheumatoid arthritis: a Latin American perspective. Reumatol Clínica English Ed. 2013;9(2):106–12. https://doi.org/10.1016/j.reumae.2013.01.007.
2. Brasil. Ministério da Saúde. Coordenação de Gestão de Protocolos Clínicos e Diretrizes Terapêuticas. Protocolo Clínico e Diretrizes Terapêuticas da Artrite Reumatoide . Brasilia; 2020 [access 2020 Nov 19]. p. 171. Available from: http://conitec.gov.br/images/Consultas/Relatorios/2020/Relatrio_Artrite_Reumatoide_CP_21_2020.pdf
3. Zozaya N, Pérez-Camarero S, Martínez-Galdeano L. La regulación y financiación de los medicamentos biosimilares en la OCDE. Madrid: Weber. Org.Es.; 2017. Report No.: 01/2017. Available from: http://weber.org.es/wp-content/uploads/2018/04/La_Regulacion_y_financiacion_de_los-biosimilares_en_la-OCDE_weber.pdf
4. Castañeda-Hernández G, Szekanecz Z, Mysler E, Azevedo VF, Guzman R, Gutierrez M, et al. Biopharmaceuticals for rheumatic diseases in Latin

America, Europe, Russia, and India: innovators, biosimilars, and intended copies. Jt Bone Spine. 2014;81(6):471–7 Available from: https://linkinghub.elsevier.com/retrieve/pii/S1297319X14000992.

5. Levenhagen K, Davies C, Perdomo M, Ryans K, Gilchrist L. United Rheumatology Clinical Practice Guideline. Vol. 97; 2019.
6. Quintiles IMS Institute. The Impact of Biosimilar Competition in Europe . 2017. p. 33. Available from: https://www.medicinesforeurope.com/wp-content/uploads/2017/05/IMS-Biosimilar-2017_V9.pdf
7. Agência Nacional de Vigilância Sanitária (Anvisa). Anuário Estatístico do Mercado Farmacêutico . 2018 [access 2019 Nov 1]. p. 28. Available from: http://portal.anvisa.gov.br/documents/374947/3413536/Anuário+Estatístico+do+Mercado+Farmacêutico+-+2017/3179a522-1af4-4b4c-8014-cc25a90fb5a7
8. México: Instituto Mexicano del Seguro Social. Diagnóstico y Tratamiento de Artritis Reumatoide del Adulto . Delegación Cuauhtémoc; 2010 [access 2019 Nov 1]. p. 97. Available from: http://www.imss.gob.mx/sites/all/statics/guiasclinicas/195GRR.pdf
9. CenterWatch. FDA Approved Drugs - Listings in Rheumatology . 2019 [access 2019 Nov 1]. p. 2. Available from: https://www.centerwatch.com/directories/1067-fda-approved-drugs/topic/110-rheumatology
10. Brasil. Ministério da Saúde. Secretaria de Atençao a Saúde. Portaria N° 996, de 30 Dde Setembro de 2015 . 2015 [access 2019 Nov 8]. Available from: http://bvsms.saude.gov.br/bvs/saudelegis/sas/2015/prt0996_30_09_2015.html
11. Zozoya N, González A. El irresistible ascenso del mercado de los biosimilares. Gestión Clínica y Sanit . 2018;(1):59–63. Available from: http://weber.org.es/wp-content/uploads/2018/10/Artículo_el-irresistible-acceso-de-los-biosimilares.pdf
12. Mysler E, Scheinberg M. Biosimilars in rheumatology: a view from Latin America. Clin Rheumatol. 2012;31(9):1279–80.
13. Bernal-Camargo DR, Gaitán-Bohórquez JC, León-Robayo ÉI. Biosimilar medicines in Colombia: an approach from the informed consumption. Rev Ciencias la Salud. 2018;16(2):311–39 Available from: https://revistas.urosario.edu.co/index.php/revsalud/article/view/6772.
14. Garcia R, Araujo DV. The regulation of biosimilars in Latin America. Curr Rheumatol Rep. 2016;18(3):1–8 Available from: https://pubmed.ncbi.nlm.nih.gov/26951254/.
15. Gomes EBP, Rosseto R, Pinheiro L, Hasenclever L, Paranhos J. Desenvolvimento de biossimilares no Brasil. Fronteiras. 2016;5(1):31–42.
16. Comisión Federal para la Protección contra Riesgos Sanitarios (Cofepris). Listados de Registros Sanitarios de Medicamentos . Governo do México. 2019 [access 2019 Nov 1]. Available from: https://www.gob.mx/cofepris/documentos/registros-sanitarios-medicamentos
17. Agência Nacional de Vigilância Sanitária (Anvisa). Consulta ao registro de medicamentos . 2019 [access 2019 Nov 1]. Available from: http://portal.anvisa.gov.br/consulta-produtos-registrados
18. Instituto Nacional de Vigilância de Medicamentos y Alimentos (Invima). Consulta Datos de Productos . Registro de Medicamentos. 2019 [access 2019 Nov 1]. Available from: https://www.invima.gov.co/consultas-registros-y-documentos-asociados
19. Consejo General de Colegios Oficiales de Farmacéuticos (España). Consulta precios medicamentos España. 2019.
20. Agência Nacional de Vigilância Sanitária (Anvisa). Consulta ao preço de medicamentos . 2019 [access 2019 Nov 1]. Available from: http://antigo.anvisa.gov.br/consulta-lista-de-preco-de-medicamento
21. Drugs.com. Buscador de preços de medicamentos . Drugs.com. 2019 [access 2019 Nov 1]. Available from: https://www.drugs.com/
22. Ministerio de Salud y Protección Social. Colombia. Base de datos de medicamentos con precio regulado o con precio de referencia . 2018. 2019 [access 2019 Aug 1]. Available from: https://actuarsalud.com/base-de-datos-de-medicamentos-con-precio-regulado-o-con-precio-de-referencia/
23. Ministerio de la Salud y Proteccion Social. Colombia. Regulación de precios de medicamentos . Ministerio de la Salud y Proteccion Social. 2019 [access 2019 Nov 1]. Available from: https://www.minsalud.gov.co/salud/MT/Paginas/medicamentos-regulacion-precios.aspx
24. San Pablo Farmacia. Buscador de preços de medicamentos . Mexico (DF). 2019 [access 2019 Nov 1]. Available from: https://www.farmaciasanpablo.com.mx/?gclid=Cj0KCQiAtf_tBRDtARIsAIbAKe1v-aDMSM4JYWV-pQx5VrkCyfphP8cN3lGOQh22WC_qn77EdrcBvDoaAm8CEALw_wcB
25. Banco Central do Brasil. Conversor de moedas e câmbio . Banco Central do Brasil. 2019 [access 2019 Nov 1]. Available from: https://www.bcb.gov.br/conversao
26. World Bank. PPP conversion factor, GDP . 2019 [access 2019 Nov 1]. Available from: https://data.worldbank.org/indicator/PA.NUS.PPP
27. Babu N. Salary Converter . 2019 [access 2019 Nov 1]. Available from: http://salaryconverter.nigelb.me/
28. Comisión Federal para la Protección contra Riesgos Sanitarios (Cofepris). Registro sanitario de producto biológico cuyo ingrediente activo no está registrado en México . Cofepris. 2019 [access 2019 Nov 1]. Available from: https://www.gob.mx/tramites/ficha/registro-sanitario-de-producto-biologico-cuyo-ingrediente-activo-no-esta-registrado-en-mexico/COFEPRIS4000
29. Putrik P, Ramiro S, Kvien TK, Sokka T, Pavlova M, Uhlig T, et al. Inequities in access to biologic and synthetic DMARDs across 46 European countries. Ann Rheum Dis. 2014;73(1):198–206.
30. Araujo DV. Preço de medicamentos na América Latina : desafios para definição de preço de referência na região . Estudo de caso : Mercosul. J Bras Econ da Saúde. 2015;55(21):86–90 Available from: http://files.bvs.br/upload/S/2175-2095/2015/v7n2/a4933.pdf.
31. MarketResearch.com. The Growing Pharmaceuticals Market: Expert Forecasts and Analysis . Rockville, MD (US). 2019 [access 1 Nov 2019]. Available from: https://blog.marketresearch.com/the-growing-pharmaceuticals-market-expert-forecasts-and-analysis
32. Mexico. Secretaria de Economia. Precios de medicamentos de patente . Ciudad de México, DF: Secretaria de Economia; 2017 [access 2019 Jun 25]. p. 9. Available from: https://datos.gob.mx/busca/dataset/precios-de-medicamentos-de-patente-de-se
33. Biosimilars Review & Report. Biosimilars, Biologics, FDA Policy and Approvals, Clinical Trials, and Specialty Pharmacy . 2019 [access 2019 Sept 20]. Available from: https://biosimilarsrr.com/biosimilars-reviews-reports/
34. Álvarez R, Alvarez R, González A. SDT 462 Análisis Comparativo de Precios de Medicamentos en América Latina Medicamentos en América Latina. 2018. Available from: http://repositorio.uchile.cl/bitstream/handle/2250/151440/Analisis-comparativo.pdf?sequence=1&isAllowed=y
35. Rodrigo J. Medicamentos biosimilares: una oportunidad para el sistema nacional de salud . Papeles de Economía Española 2019. Available from: https://www.biosim.es/wp-content/uploads/2019/06/160art20.pdf

3

An investigation about chronic prostatitis in ankylosing spondylitis

Eduardo Deves[1,2], Rodrigo Novotny[1,2], Fernando Hartmann Barazzetti[3], Mara Cristina Scheffer[3], Letícia Kramer Pacheco[3], Adriana Fontes Zimmermann[4], Ivânio Alves Pereira[4], Maria Luiza Bazzo[3] and Fabricio Souza Neves[2,5,6*]

Abstract

Background: Chronic prostatitis has been a common disease reported with high frequency in ankylosing spondylitis (AS) even from decades ago. Infectious (*Chlamydia trachomatis*) or non-infectious (uric acid) prostatitis can hypothetically trigger vertebral inflammation in AS. This study aimed to assess the features of chronic prostatitis in patients with AS compared to healthy controls.

Methods: A cross-sectional study including male patients with AS and healthy controls who agreed to undergo a prostate examination was conducted. Structured clinical interviews, prostate physical examinations, and cytological, biochemical, and microbiological tests on urinary samples collected before and after standardized prostatic massage (pre- and post-massage test) were performed.

Results: Ninety participants (45 AS patients, mean age: 52.5 ± 10.0 years, with longstanding disease, 12.4 ± 6.9 years, and 45 controls, mean age: 52.8 ± 12.1 years) were included. National Institutes of Health - Chronic Prostatitis Symptom Index (NIH-CPSI) scores were similar in the AS and control groups (4.0 [1.0–12.0] vs. 5.0 [1.0–8.5], $p =$ 0.994). The frequencies of symptoms of chronic prostatitis (NIH-CPSI Pain Domain ≥4) were also similar in both groups (23.3% vs. 22.7%, $p = 0.953$). Results of polymerase chain reaction tests for *Chlamydia trachomatis* were negative in all tested urinary samples, and uric acid concentrations and leukocyte counts were similar in all pre- and post-massage urinary samples.

Conclusions: In this study, chronic prostatitis occurred in male patients with AS, but its frequency and characteristics did not differ from those found in the healthy male population of similar age.

Keywords: Ankylosing spondylitis, Pelvic pain, Prostatitis, *Chlamydia trachomatis*, Uric acid

Background

Ankylosing spondylitis (AS) is the most common form of spondyloarthritis, mainly affecting the sacroiliac joints and spine. In severe cases, it can even cause progressive calcification and ankylosis, often in an ascending nature through its longitudinal ligaments. In addition, extra-articular manifestations may also occur, such as uveitis [1].

In 1958, Mason et al. described a strikingly high frequency (83%) of prostatitis in men with AS based on the cytological analysis of urethral fluids obtained after prostatic massage [2]. However, these results have never been reproduced since then. More recently, an Icelandic survey identified prostatitis in 27% of male patients with AS based on medical record reviews, and the authors suggested that prostatitis was the second most frequent extra-articular manifestation of AS [3].

Chronic prostatitis could not only be a consequence of AS, but also a cause of the disease. It is hypothesized that the spread of pathogen-associated molecular patterns (PAMPs) or damage-associated molecular patterns

* Correspondence: fabricio.souza.neves@ufsc.br
[2]Graduate Program in Medical Sciences (PPGCM), Health Sciences Center (CCS), Federal University of Santa Catarina (UFSC), Florianópolis, Brazil
[5]Internal Medicine Department, Health Sciences Center (CCS), Federal University of Santa Catarina (UFSC), Florianópolis, Brazil

(DAMPs) through the pelvic and vertebral lymphatic vessels from chronic prostate inflammation caused by an infectious (*Chlamydia trachomatis*) or non-infectious agent (uric acid) could induce vertebral inflammation [4].

To the best of our knowledge, the characteristics of prostatitis in AS patients have yet to be investigated and compared to a healthy control group using current standardized clinical and laboratory procedures to specifically assess these hypotheses.

The current classifications of chronic prostatitis were established in 1999 by the US National Institutes of Health (NIH) as the following: chronic bacterial prostatitis (CBP, NIH category II), inflammatory chronic prostatitis/chronic pelvic pain syndrome (CP/CPPS, NIH category IIIa), and non-inflammatory CP/CPPS (NIH category IIIb) [5]. The Meares-Stamey 4-glass test [6] or its simplified version by the Nickel's 2-glass test [7], also known as the pre- and post-massage test (PPMT), are the standard criteria for diagnosis using urinary samples collected after prostatic massage, in which NIH category II is confirmed with positive bacteriological culture results and NIH category IIIa with positive leukocyte counts. However, most men with chronic prostatitis symptoms are classified as NIH IIIb, with negative cultures and normal leukocyte counts at PPMT given the lack of biomarkers for this condition.

In this study, we first aimed to assess whether chronic prostatitis symptoms were more frequent or more severe, and whether urinary leukocyte counts at PPMT were higher in patients with AS than in healthy controls. Second, we also aimed to evaluate uric acid concentrations, bacterial growth, and presence of *Chlamydia trachomatis* in urinary samples obtained after prostatic massage in order to investigate possible causes of chronic prostatitis in this group.

Methods

We conducted a cross-sectional study including all male patients with AS attending an outpatient rheumatology public service who agreed to undergo prostate examination between 2015 and 2019. To be included in this study, these patients needed to fulfill the 1984 New York modified criteria for AS [8]. Exclusion criteria included the acute presence of urinary symptoms, use of antibiotics in the last 30 days, use of uric acid-lowering therapy, use of diuretics, and any previous diagnosis of prostatic disease. The control group comprised volunteers who attended the outpatient urology service, presenting without any current disease for prostate cancer screening.

All participants were interviewed using the validated versions of the National Institutes of Health - Chronic Prostatitis Symptom Index (NIH-CPSI) [9], International Prostate Symptom Score (IPSS) [10] and, in the AS group, the Bath Ankylosing Spondylitis Disease Activity Index (BASDAI) [11], with further calculation of Ankylosing Spondylitis Disease Activity Score (ASDAS) [12] based on serum C-reactive protein (CRP) levels (nephelometry). Erythrocyte sedimentation rate (ESR) (Westergren) and serum prostate-specific antigen (PSA) were also measured (chemiluminescence) prior to prostate palpation. Participants were defined as having prostatitis symptoms if they expressed concern of perineal pain or discomfort, and their NIH-CPSI pain domain score (ranging from 0 to 21) was ≥4 [13]. These cases were also defined as having moderate to severe prostatitis symptoms if their NIH-CPSI pain domain scores were ≥ 8 [14].

The prostate physical examination was performed in all participants by an experienced urologist (ED or CN), with a 30-s standardized prostatic massage procedure. Midstream urine samples were collected immediately before and after the prostatic massage. Leukocyte counts were performed in Neubauer chambers, cultures were performed with the seeding of urine samples in the growth medium ChromID CPS® (Biomerieux, France), and uric acid urinary concentrations were measured by uricase reaction. Polymerase chain reaction (PCR) assays for *Chlamydia trachomatis* were also performed in post-massage urinary samples of AS patients using GeneXpert CT/NG (Xpert)® (Cepheid, USA) assay. Clinical and laboratory data of participants with positive microbiological test results (cultures or PCR) were then analyzed separately from the whole group.

This study was approved by the National Committee on Ethics in Research (44,333,115.0.0000.0121), and a written informed consent was obtained from all patients. The sample size was estimated as 41 participants in each group in order to verify a difference of two points in the median NIH-CPSI score (from 4 to 6) with a 95% confidence level and 80% statistical power. Statistical analysis was performed using IBM SPSS® v20.0. Normality of data distribution was tested using the Kolmogorov-Smirnov test, and the normally distributed data are presented as mean ± standard deviation, in which differences between means were tested by Student's t-test. Non-parametric data are presented as median interquartile ranges, and the differences between medians were evaluated by Mann-Whitney *U* test. Additionally, differences between proportions were tested using the chi-square test.

Results

Ninety men were included, including 45 patients with AS and 45 controls. Regarding microbiological examination, all tested urinary samples (post-massage urine in the AS group) showed negative results for *C. trachomatis*. The cultures showed positive results with more than 10^5 colony-forming units (CFU)/mL in both pre- and post-massage samples (suggesting bacterial cystitis) in two participants - one AS patient with *Escherichia coli* and one control with *Enterococcus faecalis*. The culture result was positive in the post-massage sample and negative in the pre-massage sample (suggesting bacterial prostatitis) in one AS patient with *Enterococcus faecalis*. These patients were treated as indicated and excluded from further analysis. The clinical and blood laboratory data of the participants included in the study are presented in Table 1. All AS patients underwent regular treatment, and those who were not under treatment with anti-tumor necrosis factor (TNF) agents were using different combinations of non-steroidal anti-inflammatory drugs (NSAIDs) and non-biological disease-modifying antirheumatic drugs (DMARDs).

The urinary data comparison between the groups is presented in Table 2. All cases with symptoms of prostatitis in the AS group had leukocyte counts in post-massage samples lower than 20,000/mm^3 and were classified as non-inflammatory chronic prostatitis/chronic pelvic pain syndrome (CP/CPPS, NIH-IIIb).

Discussion

In our study, 23.3% of patients with AS had symptoms of chronic prostatitis (NIH-CPSI pain scores ≥4), which resembled the frequency of chronic prostatitis (27%) described in the 2010 epidemiological study conducted in Iceland [3]; however, chronic prostatitis symptoms were equally frequent in the control group (22.7%) of our study. The frequencies of moderate to severe prostatitis symptoms (NIH-CPSI pain scores ≥8) were also similar between the AS (14.0%) and control groups (11.4%), which resembled the overall prevalence of chronic prostatitis in the general male population, estimated to be 8.2% [15]. The median values of the NIH-CPSI and IPSS scores were also compared between the AS and control groups. In our study, post-massage urinary leukocyte counts were not elevated in chronic prostatitis cases in the AS group, which meant that all of them could be classified as non-inflammatory chronic prostatitis (NIH-IIIb classification). This was the most frequent form of chronic prostatitis and was recently conducted to the broader definition of "chronic pelvic pain syndrome" (CPPS) for this entity [16]. Thus, the characteristics of the chronic prostatitis cases in AS patients described in our study were quite similar to those expected in the general adult male population. Our results suggested that chronic prostatitis was a frequent finding in the adult male population, irrespective of the presence of AS.

Table 1 Clinical characteristics and blood laboratory tests of AS patients and controls (excluding participants with positive urinary cultures - two in the AS group and one in the control group)

	AS (*n* = 43)	Controls (*n* = 44)	p
Age (years)	52.5 ± 10.0	52.8 ± 12.1	0.882
Disease duration (years)	12.4 ± 6.9		
Anti-TNF treatment	35 (86.0%)		
BASDAI	4.9 ± 1.7		
ASDAS	2.7 ± 0.6		
NIH-CPSI	4.0 [1.0–12.0]	5.0 [1.0–8.5]	0.944
NIH-CPSI (Pain Domain) ≥ 4	10 (23.3%)	10 (22.7%)	0.953
NIH-CPSI (Pain Domain) ≥ 8	6 (14.0%)	5 (11.4%)	0.716
IPSS	6 [2.5–13.5]	2.5 [0.0–12.0]	0.105
IPSS > 8	14 (32.6%)	13 (29.5%)	0.499
PSA (ng/mL)	1.2 ± 1.1	1.8 ± 2.0	0.324
CRP (mg/L)	3.2 [2.8–3.3]	2.3 [1.0–2.6]	**0.011***
ESR (mm/h)	4 [3–5]	3 [2–5]	0.857
Uric acid (mg/dL)	5.8 ± 1.3	5.5 ± 1.2	0.624

ASDAS Ankylosing spondylitis disease activity score, *AS* Ankylosing spondylitis, *BASDAI* Bath ankylosing spondylitis disease activity index, *NIH-CPSI* National Institutes of Health - Chronic Prostatitis Symptom Index, *IPSS* International Prostate Symptom Score, *PSA* Prostate-specific antigen, *TNF* Tumor necrosis factor, *CRP* C-reactive protein, *ESR* Erythrocyte sedimentation rate. Data are presented as mean ± standard deviation (for normally distributed data), median [interquartile range] for non-parametric data

Our findings did not support the pioneering study by Mason et al., which described an impressive frequency of 83% of chronic prostatitis, defined by the presence of ≥10 polymorphonuclear leukocytes per high-power microscopy field in post-massage prostatic fluids [2]. Leukocyte counts in the post-massage samples were similar in the AS and control groups in our study. However, we may consider that current treatment of AS with anti-TNF agents may also be a therapy for chronic prostatitis, and they could have influenced our results, reducing the severity of prostatitis in the AS group (86.0% of AS patients were using anti-TNF agents) [17]. Another possible confounding factor in our study was the fact that our control group was composed of healthy men who were interested in the prostatic cancer screening. This could have led to a bias in our control group toward a higher severity of prostatitis symptoms. Before making any definitive conclusions, we believe that our findings need to be reassessed by other investigators.

Our study did not identify the etiologic factors that we tested as causative agents of prostatitis in patients with AS. All post-massage urinary samples showed negative results for *C. trachomatis* in a highly sensitive PCR assay, and uric acid concentrations did not differ between pre- and post-massage urine samples. Thus, our results did not support the hypothesis that spreading of PAMPs or DAMPs from the prostate contributes to the pathogenesis of AS [4]. However, the long duration of disease in our study group may have diminished urinary findings that could have been present in the early course of untreated disease. Prostate assessment in the early

Table 2 Comparison of pre- and post-massage urinary tests between AS patients and healthy controls (excluding participants with positive urinary cultures)

	pre-massage			post-massage		
	AS	control	p	AS	control	p
Leukocyte count (/mm^3)	2000 [1000-6000]	2000 [1000-5250]	0.603	3000 [2000-5000]	3000 [1000-11,475]	0.704
Uric acid (mg/dL)	53.3 ± 29.4	54.9 ± 24.8	0.782	55.3 ± 24.9	51.2 ± 28.9	0.480

AS Ankylosing spondylitis; Data are presented as mean ± standard deviation (for normally distributed data) or median [interquartile range] for non-parametric data

and untreated AS or undifferentiated spondyloarthtitis could be a field for further research.

Conclusions

In the present study, chronic prostatitis/chronic pelvic pain syndrome (CP/CPPS) occurred in male patients with longstanding ankylosing spondylitis (AS) under standard treatment (mainly based on anti-TNF agents); however, in this population, the frequency and characteristics of prostatic disease did not differ from those found in healthy controls of similar age.

Abbreviations

AS: Ankylosing spondylitis; ASDAS: Ankylosing Spondylitis Disease Activity Score; BASDAI: Bath Ankylosing Spondylitis Disease Activity Index; CP/CPPS: Chronic prostatitis / Chronic pelvic pain syndrome; CPSI: Chronic Prostatitis Symptom Index; DAMP: Damage-associated molecular pattern; IPSS: International Prostate Symptom Score; NIH: National Institutes of Health; PAMP: Pathogen-associated molecular pattern; PPMT: Pre- and post-massage test

Acknowledgements

Hospital Universitário Prof. Polydoro Ernani de São Thiago / Universidade Federal de Santa Catarina / Empresa Brasileira de Serviços Hospitalares (HU/UFSC/EBSERH).

Authors' contributions

ED, RN, MCS, AFZ, IAP, MLB, FSN contributed to study design. ED, RN, MLB, AFZ, IAP, FSN performed clinical procedures and contributed to data collection. FHB, MCS, LKP performed laboratorial procedures and contributed to data collection. ED and FSN analyzed data and wrote the main manuscript. All authors reviewed and contributed to the final text. The author(s) read and approved the final manuscript.

Author details

[1]Urology Service, University Hospital Prof. Polydoro Ernani de São Thiago HU/EBSERH, Federal University of Santa Catarina (UFSC), Florianópolis, Brazil. [2]Graduate Program in Medical Sciences (PPGCM), Health Sciences Center (CCS), Federal University of Santa Catarina (UFSC), Florianópolis, Brazil. [3]Laboratory of Molecular Biology, Microbiology and Serology, Health Sciences Center (CCS), Federal University of Santa Catarina (UFSC), Florianópolis, Brazil. [4]Rheumatology Unit, University Hospital Prof. Polydoro Ernani de São Thiago HU/EBSERH, Federal University of Santa Catarina (UFSC), Florianópolis, Brazil. [5]Internal Medicine Department, Health Sciences Center (CCS), Federal University of Santa Catarina (UFSC), Florianópolis, Brazil. [6]Departamento de Clínica Médica, Hospital Universitário, Universidade Federal de Santa Catarina, 3° andar, Rua Profa. Maria Flora Pausewang, Florianópolis, SC 88036-800, Brazil.

References

1. Taurog JD, Chhabra A, Colbert RA. Ankylosing Spondylitis and Axial Spondyloarthritis. N Engl J Med. 2016;374:2563–74.
2. Mason RM, Murray RS, Oates JK, Young AC. Prostatitis and ankylosing spondylitis. Br Med J. 1958;1(5073):748–51. https://doi.org/10.1136/bmj.1.5073.748.
3. Geirsson AJ, Eyjolfsdottir H, Bjornsdottir G, Kristjansson K, Gudbjornsson B. Prevalence and clinical characteristics of ankylosing spondylitis in Iceland - a nationwide study. Clin Exp Rheumatol. 2010;28(3):333–40.
4. Pöllänen R, Sillat T, Pajarinen J, Levón J, Kaivosoja E, Konttinen YT. Microbial antigens mediate HLA-B27 diseases via TLRs. J Autoimmun. 2009;32(3-4):172–7. https://doi.org/10.1016/j.jaut.2009.02.010.
5. Krieger JN, Nyberg LJ, Nickel JC. NIH consensus definition and classification of prostatitis. JAMA. 1999;282(3):236–7. https://doi.org/10.1001/jama.282.3.236.
6. Meares EM, Stamey TA. Bacteriologic localization patterns in bacterial prostatitis and urethritis. Investig Urol. 1968;5(5):492–518.
7. Nickel JC, Shoskes D, Wang Y, Alexander RB, Fowler JE, Zeitlin S, et al. How does the pre-massage and post-massage 2-glass test compare to the Meares-Stamey 4-glass test in men with chronic prostatitis/chronic pelvic pain syndrome? J Urol. 2006;176(1):119–24. https://doi.org/10.1016/S0022-5347(06)00498-8.
8. van der Linden S, Valkenburg HA, Cats A. Evaluation of diagnostic criteria for ankylosing spondylitis. A proposal for modification of the New York criteria. Arthritis Rheum. 1984;27(4):361–8. https://doi.org/10.1002/art.1780270401.
9. Novotny C, Deves E, Novotny R, Rodrigues IK, Neves FS. Cultural adaptation of the National Institutes of Health--chronic prostatitis symptom index (NIH-CPSI)--to Brazilian spoken Portuguese: NIH-CPSI (Braz). Int Braz J Urol. 2013;39(5):683–91. https://doi.org/10.1590/S1677-5538.IBJU.2013.05.11.
10. Rodrigues Netto N Jr, de Lima ML, de Andrade EF, et al. Latin American study on patient acceptance of the international prostate symptom score (IPSS) in the evaluation of symptomatic benign prostatic hyperplasia. Urology. 1997;49(1):46–9. https://doi.org/10.1016/S0090-4295(96)00372-X.
11. Shinjo SK, Gonçalves R, Gonçalves CR. Measures of clinical assessment in patients with Ankylosing spondylitis: review of literature. Rev Bras Reumatol. 2006;46(5):340–6. https://doi.org/10.1590/S0482-50042006000500007.
12. Machado P, Landewé R, Lie E, et al. Ankylosing Spondylitis Disease Activity Score (ASDAS): defining cut-off values for disease activity states and improvement scores. Ann Rheum Dis. 2011;70(1):47–53. https://doi.org/10.1136/ard.2010.138594.
13. Nickel JC, Downey J, Hunter D, Clark J. Prevalence of prostatitis-like symptoms in a population based study using the National Institutes of Health chronic prostatitis symptom index. J Urol. 2001;165(3):842–5. https://doi.org/10.1016/S0022-5347(05)66541-X.
14. Kunishima Y, Mori M, Kitamura H, Satoh H, Tsukamoto T. Prevalence of prostatitis-like symptoms in Japanese men: population-based study in a town in Hokkaido. Int J Urol. 2006;13(10):1286–9. https://doi.org/10.1111/j.1442-2042.2004.01556.x.
15. Krieger JN, Lee SWH, Jeon J, Cheah PY, Liong ML, Riley DE. Epidemiology of prostatitis. Int J Antimicrob Agents. 2008;31(Suppl 1):S85–90.
16. Magistro G, Wagenlehner FM, Grabe M, Weidner W, Stief CG, Nickel JC. Contemporary Management of Chronic Prostatitis/chronic pelvic pain syndrome. Eur Urol. 2016;69(2):286–97. https://doi.org/10.1016/j.eururo.2015.08.061.
17. Drannik GN, Gorpinchenko II, Kurchenko AI, Gusev SN. Efficacy study of new drug Mercureid (MSC-428) in anti-TNFα therapy for chronic prostatitis. Acta Sci Cancer Biol. 2019;3:9–16.

4

Ultrasonographic and resistance index evaluation of nails in psoriatic arthritis, psoriasis and control groups

Samanta Daiana De Rossi[1,2*], José Alexandre Mendonça[3], Penelope Ester Palominos[1], Charles Lubianca Kohem[1], Tania Ferreira Cestari[2] and Rafael Mendonça da Silva Chakr[1]

Abstract

Background: Nail psoriasis occurs frequently in patients with psoriatic disease, it can lead to functional impairment, pain, discomfort, decreased quality of life and can also be a predictor for the development of arthritis. Early recognition of this condition can provide early and effective treatment and prevent structural impairment. This study aims to identify nail ultrasonographic characteristics in three groups: psoriasis (PsO), psoriatic arthritis (PsA) and controls patients, to determine if the ultrasonography (US) can identify early signs of nail psoriatic impairment or local inflammation. We conducted nail US to determine nail matrix resistance index (NMRI), nail bed resistance index (NBRI), and power Doppler (PD) and grayscale (GS) parameters in these 3 groups.

Methods: Single-center, cross-sectional study. GS, PD, and spectral doppler images of bilateral 2nd and 3rd fingernails were acquired from 35 PsO, 31 PsA, and 35 controls patients. An US equipment with an 18 MHz linear transducer for GS and 8.0 MHz for PD was used. PD, NMRI, NBRI, nail plate thickness (NPT), nail bed thickness (NBT), nail matrix thickness (NMT), and morphostructural characteristics of the trilaminar structure (TS) were evaluated in saved images, blind.

Results: Mean NMRI and NBRI did not differ between groups. Linear regression analysis detected no relationships between PsO or PsA and NMRI or NBRI. Nail PD grade did not differ between groups. Type I and IV TS changes were more frequent in PsO; types II and III changes were more frequent in PsA ($p < 0.001$). NPT was greater in PsA and PsO groups than controls: PsA 0.73 ± 0.14 mm, PsO 0.72 ± 0.15 mm, Controls 0.67 ± 0.10 mm ($p = 0.001$).

Conclusion: Echographic TS characteristics of the nail plate and NPT evaluated by GS are useful and can distinguish PsO and PsA nails from controls. NMRI, NBRI, and US nail microcirculation parameters could not distinguish psoriatic nails.

Trial registration: 72762317.4.0000.5327 (Certificate of Presentation of Ethical Appreciation – CAAE - Plataforma Brasil) Avaiable in https://plataformabrasil.saude.gov.br/login.jsf.

Keywords: Doppler ultrasonography, Nails, Psoriasis, Psoriatic arthritis, Ultrasonography

* Correspondence: samantaderossi@gmail.com
[1]Division of Rheumatology, Hospital de Clínicas de Porto Alegre, Universidade Federal do Rio Grande do Sul, Porto Alegre, Brazil
[2]Divisiont of Dermatology, Hospital de Clínicas de Porto Alegre, Universidade Federal do Rio Grande do Sul, Porto Alegre, Brazil

Background

Nail involvement by psoriatic disease occurs in 40–45% of patients with skin psoriasis (PsO) and in around 80.5% of patients with psoriatic arthritis (PsA) [1, 2]. The lifetime incidence of nail involvement in psoriatic patients is estimated to be between 80 and 90% [3]. Furthermore, nail psoriasis can lead to functional impairment, pain, discomfort, decreased quality of life and can also be a predictor for the development of arthritis [4, 5]. Therefore, early recognition of this condition is essential to facilitate early and effective treatment and to prevent structural impairment.

Ultrasonography (US) is considered a highly promising method to visualize nail disease. However, there is no consensus yet about which parameters and features can provide accuracy in the evaluation of nail psoriasis [6].

Examination of the normal structure of the nail on grayscale (GS) US images can identify the nail plate (NP), the nail bed (NB), and the nail matrix (NM). The NP is a trilaminar structure (TS) comprising dorsal and ventral plates that appear as 2 hyperechoic parallel lines with a virtual hypoechoic space in between. The nail bed is a hypoechoic band between the ventral nail plate and the distal phalanx margin. The nail matrix is an isoechoic (soft gray) region at the proximal end of the nail bed in the region below the proximal nail fold. The phalanx is the deepest structure, appearing as a hyperechoic band, located immediately below the nail bed [7, 8].

US examination can detect many changes to psoriatic nails, even in the absence of clinical findings [9–13]. Wortsman et al. described and classified 4 types of US TS changes, ranging from the earliest to the most severe: focal hyperechoic involvement of the ventral plate without involvement of the dorsal plate (type I), loosening of the borders of the ventral plate (type II), appearance of wavy plates (type III), and loss of definition on both plates (type IV) (Fig. 1) [8]. The NB is usually thickened in psoriatic nails (2.0–3.0 mm) [11, 14].

Power Doppler (PD) can identify signals in psoriatic nails [14]. Gutierrez et al. have developed a scoring system to quantify PD signal activity, as follows: 0 = no signal, 1 = confluent signal in < 25% of the area evaluated, 2 = confluent signal in > 25% and < 50%, 3 = confluent signal in > 50% [15].

The Spectral Doppler (SDo) technique can differentiate between low and high peripheral resistance by assessing the movement of red blood cells in small blood vessels with low velocity flow. Peripheral resistance is expressed numerically by the Resistance Index (RI), which is assessed as the following ratio: (Qs - Qd) / Qs, where Qs represents the maximum flow velocity in systole and Qd the end diastolic flow velocity (Fig. 2). In synovitis, RI ratios range from 0 to 1, high values mean high resistance, which is normal in resting musculoskeletal tissues [16–19].

This study is designed to identify differences between PsO and PsA patients and controls in terms of NM and NB microcirculation and US nail anatomy, using GS, PD, and SDo, with a primary focus on RI measurement. If present, such differences could provide the basis for a noninvasive method for early detection of inflammation in nail apparatus of PsA and PsO patients, enabling early treatment and prevention of joint deterioration.

Methods

This was a single-center, cross-sectional, observational study, conducted in the Rheumatology and Dermatology outpatient clinics at the Hospital de Clínicas de Porto Alegre, RS, Brazil, from October 2017 to June 2018.

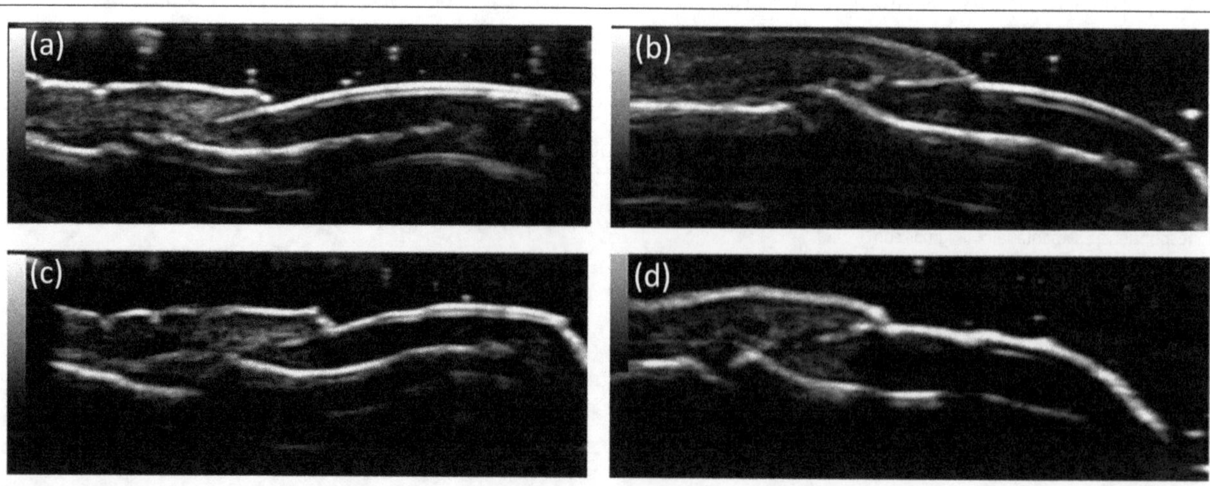

Fig. 1 Wortsman's classification of psoriatic nail changes in the trilaminar structure of nail plate. Legend: (a) hyperechoic deposits in ventral plate; (b) lost of definition of the ventral plate, (c) wavy plates, (d) loss of definition of both plates. Authors' collection

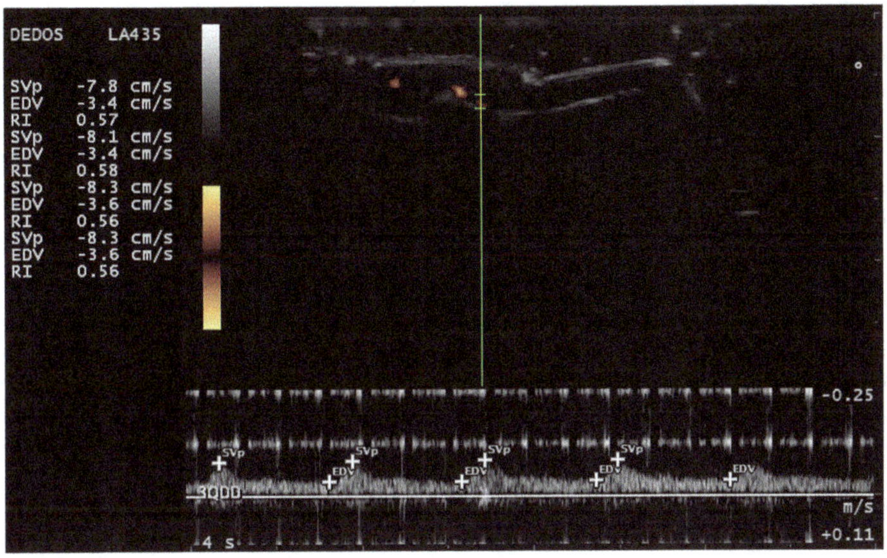

Fig. 2 RI measure by spectral doppler. Legend: SVp: maximum blood flow velocity in systole. EDV: diastolic blood flow velocity. RI: resistence index. Authors' collection

Sample size was calculated to detect an effect size of 0.36 in NMRI measures between groups, considering a Standard Deviation (SD) of 0.41 [20]. This calculation was performed using SAS Studio and considering power of 80% and $\alpha = 0.05$. Age was included as a covariate in the sample size calculation because previous studies suggest that it can influence evaluation of nail structure with Doppler [12, 21]. A low degree of correlation (0.2) was used because there is no data in the literature regarding the correlation between age and RI. The result of the sample size calculation was 81 patients, 27 in each group.

PsA patients were consecutively enrolled during their routine medical consultations. PsO patients without joint symptoms or complaints and controls were matched to the PsA group by age and gender. Participants for the control group were selected from among patients at dermatology and anesthesia outpatients clinics and hospital staff.

Participants were at least 18 years-old; to be eligible for the PsA group, they had to fulfill the CASPAR criteria [22]; for the PsO group, patients should have a diagnosis of cutaneous PsO and no signs or symptoms of present or past joint disease (arthritis, enthesitis or synovitis). Patients with fibromyalgia were excluded from the PsA group because it is difficult to differentiate between pain caused by this condition and enthesitic pain. Additional exclusion criteria for all groups included: other inflammatory joint diseases, dermatological or systemic diseases that could modify the nail structure; and severe pulmonary, vascular or hematological diseases that can interfere with circulatory evaluation [21]. Diabetes Mellitus (DM), High Blood Pressure (HBP) and smoking were not exclusion criteria for any of the groups.

The National Research Ethics Committee of Brazil approved this study under registration number 72762317.4.0000.5327, and informed consent was obtained from all participants before clinical and sonographic examinations.

Clinical evaluation

Patients answered a questionnaire about demographic and disease characteristics. On the same day, a dermatologist assessed the percentage of affected body surface area (BSA) and calculated the Psoriasis Area and Severity Index (PASI) [23] and the Nail Psoriasis Severity Index (NAPSI) [24]. Psoriatic arthritis activity was assessed by a rheumatologist during the medical consultation, using the Disease Activity in Psoriatic Arthritis (DAPSA) score [25], the Maastricht Ankylosing Spondylitis Enthesis Score (MASES) [26], the Minimal Disease Activity (MDA) criteria [27], a patient Visual Analog Scale (VAS) for pain, and a global patient VAS [28], plus blood test results for C reactive protein (CRP) and Erythrocyte Sedimentation Rate (ESR).

Ultrasonographic assessment of nails

Examinations were performed using a MyLab 50 system (Esaote Biomedica, Genova, Italy), equipped with a linear 10 to 18 MHz transducer for GS and a 6.6 to 8.0 MHz transducer for PD. The imaging parameters for Doppler ultrasound examinations were pulse repetition frequency of 700 Hz with color gain maximized for optimal sensitivity while avoiding excessive color noise.

Sonographic examinations were performed in a room with temperature between 22 °C and 26 °C, after a 10 min period at rest. The patient was seated, with forearms, hands and fingers in a neutral and relaxed position on the table and nails were scanned in the longitudinal plane. A thick gel layer was applied to provide an adequate acoustic interface and to avoid compression of the structures. The 2nd and 3rd fingernails of both hands were evaluated.

Images were saved and measures and evaluations were performed at a later date, without identification of the patient, by the same researcher who conducted the US examinations. In GS, the following structures were assessed: 1) the trilaminar appearance of the NP, graded according to Wortsman's classification of changes in psoriatic nails [8], 2) nail plate thickness (NPT), measured at the thickest point, 3) nail bed thickness (NBT), measured at the middle third of the NP, 4) nail matrix thickness (NMT), defined as the hypoechoic region below the proximal nailfold, above the cortex of the distal phalanx, determined by a perpendicular line to the bone profile [8, 12, 29] (Fig. 3).

Presence or absence of blood flow signal in the NM and the NB were evaluated in PD images and classified according to the Gutierrez score [15]. The MyLabDesktop software enables automatic calculation of RI in Spectral wave analysis of a saved image when the cursor is placed at maximum systolic velocity and end diastolic flow velocity (Fig. 2). Three measurements were taken and the arithmetic mean was considered the RI. All measurements were taken and all scores were calculated by the same researcher and agreement with an experienced sonographer was tested for 20 selected images of the nail unit. Cohen's Kappa [30] was 0.51.

Statistical analyses

Quantitative variables are expressed as mean ± SD and categorical variables as absolute frequencies and percentages. Comparisons between independent means were analyzed using ANOVA or the Kruskal-Wallis test. Associations between categorical variables were calculated using the chi-squared test or Fisher's exact test. Correlations between quantitative variables were analyzed with Spearman's correlation coefficients. Linear regression analysis was performed with each of the quantitative variables. Statistical significance was defined as a p value ≤0.05. SPSS 21.0 was used for statistical analysis.

Results

Thirty-five patients with PsO; 31 with PsA, and 35 controls were enrolled on the study. One hundred and twenty-three nails were evaluated in the PsA group (76 with clinical nail psoriasis); 139 in the PsO group (60 with clinical nail psoriasis); and 138 in the control group. Patient's demographic and disease characteristics are summarized in Table 1. No gender or age differences were found between groups.

There were no differences between the groups in terms of mean NMRI, NBRI, NBT, or NMT. There was no statistical difference between groups in nail PD grades. Mean NPT ± SD (mm) was higher in the PsA and PsO groups than in the control group: 0.73 ± 0.14 in the PsA group, 0.72 ± 0.15 in the PsO group, and 0.67 ± 0.10 in the control group ($p = 0.001$). (Table 2).

Patients undergoing systemic treatment for either PsO or PsA did not present differences in NMRI, NBRI, NPT, NBT and NMT measurements when compared to patients not undergoing systemic treatment. The same comparison was made both within and between PsO and PsA groups and no differences were found.

NPT was the only measurement to show different results when patients with clinical nail psoriasis - mean 0.75 mm (CI 0.71–0.80) - and patients without clinical nail involvement - 0.68 mm (CI 0.67–0.72) - were compared ($p = 0{,}042$). No differences were found when the same comparison was made between PsO and PsA groups.

The TS evaluation was conducted using the Wortsman classification [8]. In the control group, 137 (99.3%) nails

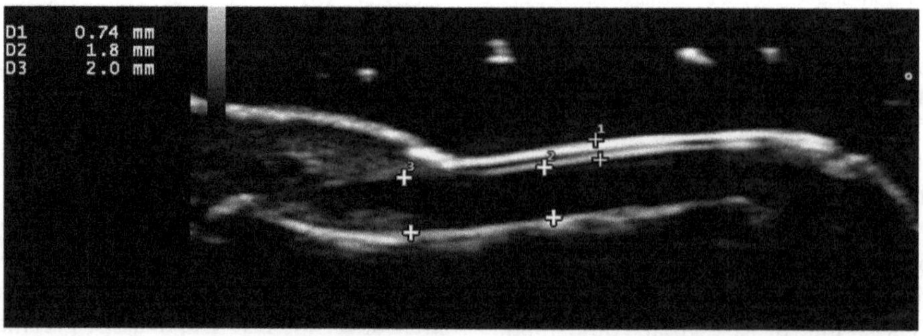

Fig. 3 Measures of nail plate, nail bed and nail matrix thickness in US gray scale. Legend: Nail plate thickness measure (1); nail bed thickness measure (2) and nail matrix thickness measure (3). Authors' collection

Table 1 Demographic and Disease characteristics in each group

	PsA (n = 31)	PsO (n = 35)	Controls (n = 35)	p value*
Gender – n(%)				
Female	16 (51.6)	18 (51.4)	21 (60.0)	0.767
Male	15 (48.4)	17 (48.6)	14 (40.0)	
Age (years) –				
mean ± SD	53.03 ± 9.64	54.46 ± 11.43	53.37 ± 10.80	0.521
Havy manual labor – n(%)	25 (80.6)	28 (80.0)	25 (71.4)	0.692
Comorbidities – n(%)				
HBP	12 (38.7)	13 (37.1)	13 (37.1)	0.99
DM	7 (22.6)	8 (22.9)	3 (8.6)	0.217
Smoking	5 (16.1)	5 (14.3)	3 (8.6)	0.627
PsO Family History– n(%)	11 (35.5)	19 (54.3)	3 (8.6)	< 0.001
Mean duration of cutaneous PsO (years) – mean ± SD	18.81 ± 10.73	16.16 ± 10.33	–	0.311
PASI – m [P25% - P75%]	(n = 13) 1.0 [0.70–4.15]	(n = 24) 3.75 [1.15–5.83]	–	0.171
With clinical nail involvment – n(%)	15 (48.4)	19 (54.3)	–	0.805
NAPSI – m [P25% - P75%]	(n = 15) 20 [4–34]	(n = 19) 11 [5–33]	–	0.891
PsO/PsA Current Treatment n(%)				
MTX	18 (58.1)	17 (48.6)	–	0.600
Phototherapy	3 (9.7)	7 (20.0)	–	0.410
Immunobiological	10 (32.3)	4 (11.4)	–	0.078
Corticosteroids	6 (19.3)	0 (0.0)	–	0.003
Any systemic treatment	27 (77.1)	21 (60.0)	–	0.029

Legend: n absolute frequency of patients, *SD* standard deviation, m median, *[P25% - P75%]* percentile 25% - percentile 75%), *PsO* psoriasis, *PsA* psoriatic arthritis, *HBP* high blood pressure, *DM* diabetes mellitus, *PASI* psoriasis area severity index, *NAPSI* nail psoriasis severity index, *MTX* methotrexate, * significance fixed on $p < 0,05$

had no TS changes. In the PsO group, 32 nails had changes in this structure, 9 type I, 5 type II, 7 type III, and 11 type IV. In the PsA group, there were also 32 nails with TS changes, 4 type I, 15 type II, 9 type III and 4 type IV.

Correlations between disease activity classifications and the variables studied were as follows: NBT with MASES ($r_s = 0.228$ $p < 0.001$); NPT with NAPSI ($r_s = 0.258$ $p < 0.001$) and with MASES ($r_s = 0.246$ $p = 0.006$). Patients in MDA (Minimal Disease Activity) had lower NPT ($r_s = -0.307$, $p = 0.002$). Patients with higher NAPSI had a higher frequency of TS changes ($r_s = 0.459$, $p < 0.001$). Trilaminar structure changes were also correlated with presence of clinical nail psoriasis ($r_s = 0.328$ $p < 0.001$) and with MASES ($r_s = 0.249$ $p = 0.006$).

Independent variables explaining the main ultrasonographic nail changes according to the linear regression model are shown in Table 3.

Discussion

Ultrasonography can be employed as a method for early detection and careful characterization of the inflammatory process in different anatomical structures and different stages of the disease in patients with PsO and PsA [11]. Since the nail apparatus can be considered a part of the musculoskeletal system and a link between joint and tegument [31], US nail evaluation has emerged as a promising tool for early identification of nail psoriasis, as a possible technique for distinguishing PsO from PsA patients and for differentiating psoriatic patients from control group patients [6].

Our study compared gray scale (NPT, NBT, NMT and TS) and power Doppler (NMRI, NBRI) nail measures among PsA, PsO, and control subjects and found that TS and NPT were different in psoriatic patients.

In previous studies, NMRI was higher in PsO patients compared to controls. The authors explained their results by the endothelial disfunction in patients with psoriasis and by capillaroscopic findings in nail folds showing greater tortuosity and decreased capillary density in psoriatic patients [18, 32, 33]. Another study found lower NMRI in PsA patients compared to control subjects, probably due to the close relationship between distal interphalangeal (DIP) enthesis and the nail matrix.

Table 2 Prevalences and means of outcomes among groups

	PsA (*n* = 123)	PsO (*n* = 139)	Controls (*n* = 138)	*p* * value
Trilaminar Structure (Wortsman's Classification) – n(%) †				
0	91 (74.0)	107 (77.0)	137 (99.3)**	**< 0.001**
I	4 (3.3)	9 (6.5)**	1 (0.7)	
II	15 (12.2)**	5 (3.6)	0 (0.0)	
III	9 (7.3)**	7 (5.0)	0 (0.0)	
IV	4 (3.3)	11 (7.9)**	0 (0.0)	
Degree of PD Nail Matrix and Bed Together– n(%)†				
0	19 (17.8)	7 (6.5)	10 (9.4)	$p = 0.133$
1	77 (72.0)	91 (85.0)	84 (79.2)	
2	7 (6.5)	8 (7.5)	8 (7.5)	
3	4 (3.7)	1 (0.9)	4 (3.8)	
NPT – mean ± SD ‡	0.73 ± 0.14[a]	0.72 ± 0.15[a]	0.67 ± 0.10[b]	**=0.001**
NBT – mean ± SD ‡	1.88 ± 0.34	1.97 ± 0.38	1.90 ± 0.31	=0.085
NMT – mean ± SD ‡	2.00 ± 0.32	2.07 ± 0.37	1.97 ± 0.36	=0.068
NMRI – mean ± SD ‡	(*n* = 84) 0.49 ± 0.06	(*n* = 95) 0.50 ± 0.07	(*n* = 91) 0.49 ± 0.06	=0.415
NBRI – mean ± SD ‡	(*n* = 46) 0.51 ± 0.07	(*n* = 83) 0.53 ± 0.07	(*n* = 79) 0.52 ± 0.06	=0.115

Legend: *n* absolute frequency of patients, *SD* standard deviation, *PsO* psoriasis, *PsA* psoriatic arthritis, *NPT* nail plate thickness, *NBT* nail bed thickness, *NMT* nail matrix thickness, *NMRI* resistance index in nail matrix, *NBRI* resistance index in nail bed. † Chi-Square Analysis of qualitative variables. ‡One-Way ANOVA $p < 0.001$,post hoc Turkey. [a], [b]: equal letters means there is no difference between means with $p > 0.05$; different letters means there is a difference between means with $p < 0.05$. * significance fixed on $p < 0{,}05$, **with statistically significant difference

According to those authors, the DIP enthesis inflammation extends into the nail matrix, resulting in vasodilatation and decreased RI [19, 20].

Our results did not confirm previous studies' findings of differences in mean NMRI between PsA, PsO, and control groups. The linear regression analysis did not show any associations between RI measures and PsO or PsA diagnoses, despite the > 80% power to detect an effect size of 0.05. This confirms the conclusion that, in our sample, there is no difference in NMRI among groups.

Analyzing mean NMRI data available in the literature, there is a considerable variation in nail RI reported by different authors, particularly for control groups [18, 20' 32, 33]. Measurement of RI is operator dependent and difficult to standardize, which makes it difficult to compare the results. More studies, with larger samples, that clarify the behavior of NMRI measurement and identify factors that can influence NMRI measures in healthy patients are important to enable study of this parameter in disease.

In larger vessels such as the renal and umbilical arteries, RI has exhibited influence from gender, age, DM, and smoking [21]. However, it still remains to be determined which factors can influence this measure in microcirculation. In the linear regression analysis, NMRI ($R^2 = 0.125$) was related to age and NBRI ($R^2 = 0.175$),

Table 3 Linear regression analysis of quantitative outcomes

Nail Matrix RI		
Variable	Standardized β	*p* value*
Multivariate model	(Adjusted R^2) = 0,125	
Age	0.002	**< 0.001**
Nail Bed RI		
Variable	Standardized β	*p* value*
Multivariate model	(Adjusted R^2) = 0,175	
Age	0.002	**< 0.001**
Gender [a]	−0.021	**0.017**
Tabagism	0.031	**0.015**
Nail Matrix Thickness		
Variable	Standardized β	*p* value*
Multivariate model	(Adjusted R^2) = 0,332	
Age	0.008	**< 0.001**
Gender [a]	0.359	**< 0.001**
Havy manual labor	0.148	**0.003**
Hand Side [b]	−0.332	**< 0.001**
Nail Bed Thickness		
Variable	Standardized β	*p* value*
Multivariate model	(Adjusted R^2) = 0,270	
Age	0.005	**< 0.001**
Havy manual labor	0.167	**< 0.001**
Hand Side [b]	−0.220	**< 0.001**
Fingernail [c]	0.142	**< 0.001**
HBP	0.140	**< 0.001**
DM	−0.113	**0.006**
Nail Plate Thickness		
Variable	Standardized β	*p* value*
Multivariate model	(Adjusted R^2) = 0,189	
PsA	0,051	**0,001**
PsO	0,041	**0,006**
Age	0.002	**< 0.001**
Havy Manual Labor	0.037	**0.012**
Hand Side [b]	0.035	**0.004**
Smoking	0.099	**< 0.001**
DM	−0.057	**0.001**

Legend: *PsO* psoriasis, *PsA* psoriatic arthritis, *RI* resistance index, *HBP* high blood pressure, *DM* diabetes mellitus.
[a]Gender: positive β: variable higher in male gender, negative β:variable higher in female gender.
[b]Hand Side: positive β: variable higher in left side, negative β: variable higher in right side.
[c]Fingernail: positive β: variable higher in 2nd fingernal, negative β: variable higher in 3rd fingernail.
* significance fixed on $p < 0{,}05$

increasing with age, and was higher in females and smokers.

Several authors have shown that NPT, NMT, and NBT were greater in psoriatic patients than controls [9, 11, 13, 14, 32, 34–38]. The present study only detected this increase in NPT. However, the mean NPT in each group was higher than those found by previous studies and it is possible that the great variation in measurements in the literature is partly related to ethnic differences [35, 36]. Larger samples could possibly reveal increases in NMT and NBT in psoriatic patients. There was no difference in NPT, NMT, or NBT between PsO and PsA patients. Our results reproduce the higher NPT measures on patients with clinical signs of nail psoriasis found in previous studies. However, our analyses did not result in higher NBT and NMT measures on these patients, as demonstrated in previous studies [32, 36, 37]..

Linear regression analysis demonstrated that NPT values were directly related (R^2 0.189) to age, presence of PsA, having PsO, right hand, heavy manual labor, and smoking habit, and inversely related to DM. A relationship between heavy manual labor and increased NPT and NBT is expected as a result of triggering of the cycle of local microdamage and repair that results in a deep Koebner phenomenon, as occurs in skin [31]. The analysis also revealed a direct relationship between NBT (adjusted for age, HBP, DM, hand side, and fingernail) and heavy manual labor ($R^2 = 0.189$).

The TS changes in the NP of psoriatic patients described by Wortsman et al. [8] were evident in the results and although the frequencies of each grade of change in each group of patients were different to those reported in previous studies [11, 36], this study was able to differentiate psoriatic patients from control patients on the basis of the presence of these changes. Presence of TS changes had direct correlations with clinical nail involvement, NAPSI, MASES, and NPT. Other authors have shown relationships between TS changes and clinical nail involvement previously [32, 38, 39].

Even though the majority of studies have reported increased PD signal in the NB and NM of psoriatic patients [11, 13, 14, 32, 36, 40], capillaroscopic evaluation of the proximal nailfold of these patients has shown decreased number and diameter of capillaries and increased vessel tortuosity [41, 42]. In our study, the grade of NMPD signal and PD assessed in the NB and NM together failed to reveal differences between groups and the NBPD signal was more frequently absent in the PsA group. Recently, Naredo et al. [34] demonstrated that neither NBPD or NMPD classified as per Gutierrez et al. [15], nor PD evaluated in the NB and NM together, could discriminate between control and psoriatic groups, or between clinically involved and clinically non-involved nails. These authors, in common with Aydin et al. [43], demonstrated that the amount of blood flow detected in control subjects is highly variable.

The discrepancies found between our results and those of previous studies may be related to the diversity in ultrasound equipment employed during the data collection phase, especially concerning frequency range, which may have affected the precision of the measurements. Some cited studies [8, 36, 33] also only focused on PsO and PsA patients with current clinical psoriatic nails, another possible cause for measurement variations.

Our study has some limitations, such as the equipment used, that had lower frequency, both for GS and PD, when compared with more recent studies, although it is high frequency. The fact that we analyzed only 4 fingernails of which patients also can be considered a limitation. Our study is the first to that compare NMRI and NBRI among these three groups (PsO, PsA, and controls).

Conclusions

In conclusion, echographic TS characteristics and NPT seem capable of distinguishing between psoriatic nails and controls nails, but not between PsO and PsA patients. Neither NMRI nor the other measures and parameters evaluated in the study could distinguish between psoriatic nails and control nails. Although US nail microcirculation parameters did not demonstrate utility for diagnostic of psoriatic nail, nail GS US is helpful and allows nails from psoriatic patients to be distinguished from those of control patients, even in the absence of clinical signs of nail psoriasis. Future studies are needed to clarify the characteristics and variations of the parameters of nail US in PsO and PsA patients, since there is no consensus to date.

Abbreviations

BSA: Body surface area; CI: Confidence interval; CRP: C reactive protein; DAPSA: Disease activity in psoriatic arthritis; DIP: Distal interphalangeal; DM: Diabetes Mellitus; ESR: Erythrocyte sedimentation rate; GS: Gray scale; HBP: High blood pressure; Hz: Hertz; MASES: Maastricht ankylosing spondylitis enthesis score; MDA: Minimal disease activity; MHz: Megahertz; NAPSI: Nail psoriasis severity index; NB: Nail bed; NBRI: Nail bed resistance index; NBT: Nail bed thickness; NM: Nail matrix; NMRI: Nail matrix resistance index; NMT: Nail matrix thickness; NP: Nail plate; NPT: Nail plate thickness; PASI: Psoriasis area and severity index; PD: Power doppler; PsA: Psoriatic Arthritis; PsO: Psoriasis; RI: Resistance Index; SD: Standard Deviation; SDo: Spectral doppler; TS: Trilaminar structure; US: Ultrasonography; VAS: Visual analog scale

Acknowledgements

Not applicable.

Authors' contributions

SDDR – Was a contributor in writing the manuscript, in collected the data and in statistical analysis. JAM – Was a contributor in writing the manuscript, in collected the data and in statistical analysis. PEP – Was a contributor in writing the manuscript and in collected the data. CLK – Was a contributor in writing the manuscript and in collected the data. TFC – Was a contributor in writing the manuscript and in collected the data. RMSC - Was a contributor in writing the manuscript, in collected the data and in statistical analysis. All authors read and approved the final manuscript.

Author details

[1]Division of Rheumatology, Hospital de Clínicas de Porto Alegre, Universidade Federal do Rio Grande do Sul, Porto Alegre, Brazil. [2]Divisiont of Dermatology, Hospital de Clínicas de Porto Alegre, Universidade Federal do Rio Grande do Sul, Porto Alegre, Brazil. [3]Department of Rheumatology, Celso Pierro Hospital, Pontifícia Universidade Católica de Campinas, São Paulo, Brazil.

References

1. Tan ES, Chong WS, Tey HL. Nail psoriasis: a review. Am J Clin Dermatol. 2012;13(6):375–88. https://doi.org/10.2165/11597000-000000000-00000.
2. Schons KR, Knob CF, Murussi N, Beber AA, Neumaier W, Monticielo OA. Nail psoriasis: a review of the literature. An Bras Dermatol. 2014;89(2):312–7. https://doi.org/10.1590/abd1806-4841.20142633.
3. Jiaravuthisan MM, Sasseville D, Vender RB, Murphy F, Muhn C. Psoriasis of the nail: anatomy, pathology, clinical presentation, and a review of the literature on therapy. J Am Acad Dermatol. 2007;57(1):1–27. https://doi.org/10.1016/j.jaad.2005.07.073.
4. Baran R. The burden of nail psoriasis: an introduction. Dermatology. 2010; 221(Suppl 1):1–5. https://doi.org/10.1159/000316169.
5. Raposo I, Torres T. Nail psoriasis as a predictor of the development of psoriatic arthritis. Actas Dermosifiliogr. 2015;106(6):452–7. https://doi.org/10.1016/j.ad.2015.02.005.
6. Mendonça JA, Aydin SZ, D'Agostino MA. The use of ultrasonography in the diagnosis of nail disease among patients with psoriasis and psoriatic arthritis: a systematic review. Adv Rheumatol. 2019;59(1):41. https://doi.org/10.1186/s42358-019-0081-9.
7. Aluja Jaramillo F, Quiasúa Mejía DC, Martínez Ordúz HM, González AC. Nail unit ultrasound: a complete guide of the nail diseases. J Ultrasound. 2017; 20(3):181–92. https://doi.org/10.1007/s40477-017-0253-6.
8. Wortsman CX, Holm EA, Jemec GB, Gniadecka M, Wulf HC. Ultrasonido de Alta Resolucion (15MHz) em el estudio de la uña psoriatica. Rev Chil Radiol. 2004;10:06–11.
9. Gisondi P, Idolazzi L, Girolomoni G. Ultrasonography reveals nail thickening in patients with chronic plaque psoriasis. Arch Dermatol Res. 2012;304(9): 727–32. https://doi.org/10.1007/s00403-012-1274-9.
10. Scarpa R, Manguso F, Oriente A, Peluso R, Atteno M, Oriente P. Is the involvement of the distal interphalangeal joint in psoriatic patients related to nail psoriasis? Clin Rheumatol. 2004;23(1):27–30. https://doi.org/10.1007/s10067-003-0817-z.
11. Sandobal C, Carbó E, Iribas J, Roverano S, Paira S. Ultrasound nail imaging on patients with psoriasis and psoriatic arthritis compared with rheumatoid arthritis and control subjects. J Clin Rheumatol. 2014;20(1):21–4. https://doi.org/10.1097/RHU.0000000000000054.
12. Arbault A, Devilliers H, Laroche D, Cayot A, Vabres P, Maillefert JF, et al. L'échographie des ongles dans le rhumatisme psoriasique : étude pilote sur la faisabilité, la reproductibilité et la validité de mesure. Rev Rhum. 2016; 83(1):37–43. https://doi.org/10.1016/j.rhum.2015.07.011.
13. Idolazzi L, Gisondi P, Fassio A, Viapiana O, Giollo A, Rossini M, et al. Ultrasonography of the nail unit reveals quantitative and qualitative alterations in patients with psoriasis and psoriatic arthritis. Med Ultrason. 2018;20(2):177–84. https://doi.org/10.11152/mu-1327.
14. Gutierrez M, Filippucci E, De Angelis R, Filosa G, Kane D, Grassi W. A sonographic spectrum of psoriatic arthritis: "the five targets". Clin Rheumatol. 2010;29(2):133–42. https://doi.org/10.1007/s10067-009-1292-y.
15. Gutierrez M, Di Geso L, Salaffi F, et al. Development of a preliminary US power Doppler composite score for monitoring treatment in PsA. Rheumatology (Oxford). 2012;51(7):1261–8. https://doi.org/10.1093/rheumatology/kes014.
16. Terslev L, Torp-Pedersen S, Qvistgaard E, Von Der Recke P, Bliddal H. Doppler ultrasound findings in healthy wrists and finger joints. Ann Rheum Dis. 2004;63(6):644–8. https://doi.org/10.1136/ard.2003.009548.
17. Terslev L, Torp-Pedersen S, Qvistgaard E, Bliddal H, Terslev L. Spectral Doppler and resistive index a promising tool in ultrasonographic evaluation of inflammation in rheumatoid arthritis. Acta Radiol. 2003;44(6):645–52. https://doi.org/10.1046/j.1600-0455.2003.00136.x.
18. Husein El-Ahmed H, Garrido-Pareja F, Ruiz-Carrascosa JC, Naranjo-Sintes R. Vessel resistance to blood flow in the nailfold in patients with psoriasis: a prospective case-control echo Doppler-based study. Br J Dermatol. 2012; 166(1):54–8. https://doi.org/10.1111/j.1365-2133.2011.10579.x.
19. Mendonça JA. As diferenças do Doppler espectral, na artrite psoriática e onicomicose. Rev Bras Reumatol. 2014;54(6):490–3. https://doi.org/10.1016/j.rbr.2014.03.029.
20. Mendonça JA, Nogueira JC, Laurido IMM, Vierhout C, Peron F, Lyrio AM. SAT0191 Can spectral doppler identify nail enthesitis in psoriatic arthritis?[Abstract]. Ann Rheum Dis. 2014;73:659.
21. Cauwenberghs N, Kuznetsova T. Determinants and prognostic significance of the renal resistive index. Pulse. 2016;3(3-4):172–8. https://doi.org/10.1159/000442445.
22. Taylor W, Gladman D, Helliwell P, Marchesoni A, Mease P, Mielants H. Classification criteria for psoriatic arthritis: development of new criteria from a large international study. Arthritis Rheum. 2006;54(8):2665–73. https://doi.org/10.1002/art.21972.
23. Frederiksson T, Pettersson U. Severe psoriasis: oral therapy with a new retinoid. Dermatologica. 1978;157(4):238–44. https://doi.org/10.1159/000250839.
24. Rich P, Scher RK. Nail psoriasis severity index: a useful tool for evaluation of nail psoriasis. J Am Acad Dermatol. 2003;49(2):206–12. https://doi.org/10.1067/S0190-9622(03)00910-1.
25. Schoels M, Aletaha D, Funovits J, Kavanaugh A, Baker D, Smolen JS. Application of the DAREA/DAPSA score for assessment of disease activity in psoriatic arthritis. Ann Rheum Dis. 2010;69(8):1441–7. https://doi.org/10.1136/ard.2009.122259.
26. Heuft-Dorenbosch L, Spoorenberg A, van Tubergen A, Landewé R, van ver Tempel H, Mielants H, et al. Assessment of enthesitis in ankylosing spondylitis. Ann Rheum Dis. 2003;62(2):127–32. https://doi.org/10.1136/ard.62.2.127.
27. Coates LC, Fransen J, Helliwell PS. Defining minimal disease activity in psoriatic arthritis: a proposed objective target for treatment. Ann Rheum Dis. 2010;69(01):48–53. https://doi.org/10.1136/ard.2008.102053.
28. Cauli A, Gladman DD, Mathieu A, et al. Patient global assessment in psoriatic arthritis: a multicenter GRAPPA and OMERACT study. J Rheumatol. 2011;38(5):898–903. https://doi.org/10.3899/jrheum.100857.
29. Cunha JS, Qureshi AA, Reginato AM. Nail Enthesis Ultrasound in Psoriasis and Psoriatic Arthritis: a Report from the 2016 GRAPPA Annual Meeting. J Rheumatol. 2017;44(5):688-90. https://doi.org/10.3899/jrheum.170146.
30. Agresti A. Modelling patterns of agreement and disagreement. Stat Methods Med Res. 1992;1(2):201–18. https://doi.org/10.1177/096228029200100205.
31. McGonagle D, Tan AL, Benjamin M. The nail as a musculoskeletal appendage - implications for an improved understanding of the link between psoriasis and arthritis. Dermatology. 2009;218(2):97–102. https://doi.org/10.1159/000182250.
32. Marina ME, Botar Jid C, Bolboaca SD, Bocsa C, Mihu CM, Tătaru AD. High-frequency sonography in the evaluation of nail psoriasis. Med Ultrason. 2016;18(3):312–7. https://doi.org/10.11152/mu.2013.2066.183.hgh.
33. Bakirci Ureyen S, Kara RO, Erturk Z, Yaldiz M. The microvascular and morphostructural changes of nails in psoriatic patients with nail disease; a link between ultrasound and videocapillaroscopy findings in the nailfold. Med Ultrason. 2018;20(2):185–91. https://doi.org/10.11152/mu-1274.
34. Naredo E, Janta I, Baniandrés-Rodríguez O, et al. To what extend is nail ultrasound discriminative between psoriasis, psoriatic arthritis and healthy subjects? Rheumatol Int. 2019;39:697–705.
35. Ally Essayed SM. al-Shatouri MA, Nasr Allah YS, Atwa MA. Ultrasonographic characterization of the nails in patients with psoriasis and onychomycosis. Egypt J Radiol Nucl Med. 2015;46(3):733–9. https://doi.org/10.1016/j.ejrnm.2015.04.009.
36. Krajewska-Włodarczyk M, Owczarczyk-Saczonek A, Placek W, Wojtkiewicz M, Wiktorowicz A, Wojtkiewicz J. Ultrasound assessment of changes in nails in psoriasis and psoriatic arthritis. Biomed Res Int. 2018;9:8251097.
37. Aydin SZ, Castillo-Gallego C, Ash ZR, et al. Ultrasonographic assessment of nail in psoriatic disease shows a link between onychopathy and distal interphalangeal joint extensor tendon enthesopathy. Dermatology. 2013; 225:231–5.
38. Acquitter M, Misery L, Saraux A, Bressollette L, Jousse-Joulin S. Detection of subclinical ultrasound enthesopathy and nail disease in patients at risk of psoriatic arthritis. Joint Bone Spine. 2017;84(6):703–7. https://doi.org/10.1016/j.jbspin.2016.10.005

39. Mondal S, Dutta S, Lahiri D, Sinha D, Sircar G, Mandal AK, et al. Assessment of nail unit structures by ultrasound in patients with psoriatic arthritis and their correlations with disease activity indices: a case–control study. Rheumatol Int. 2018;38(11):2087–93. https://doi.org/10.1007/s00296-018-4160-8.
40. Moya Alvarado P, Roé Crespo E, Muñoz-Garza FZ, López-Ferrer A, Laiz Alonso A, Vilarrassa Rull E, et al. Subclinical enthesopathy of extensor digitorum tendon is highly prevalent and associated with clinical and ultrasound alterations of the adjacent fingernails in patients with psoriatic disease. J Eur Acad Dermatol Venereol. 2018;32(10):1728–36. https://doi.org/10.1111/jdv.15035.
41. Ferrari Ribeiro C, Beatriz E, Siqueira D, Holler AP, Fabrício L, Skare TL. Periungual capillaroscopy in psoriasis Capilaroscopia periungueal em psoríase. An Bras Dermatol. 2012;87(4):550–3. https://doi.org/10.1590/S0365-05962012000400005.
42. Graceffa D, Amorosi B, Maiani E, et al. Capillaroscopy in psoriatic and rheumatoid arthritis: a useful tool for differential diagnosis. Arthritis. 2013; 2013:957480.
43. Aydin SZ, Gallego CC, Ash Z, Marzo-Ortega H, Wakefield RJ, McGonagle D. Vascularity of Nail Bed by Ultrasound to Discriminate Psoriasis, Psoriatic Arthritis and Healthy Controls.[Letter]. Clin Exp Rheumatol. 2017;35:872.

5

Brazilian recommendations for the use of nonsteroidal anti-inflammatory drugs in patients with axial spondyloarthritis

Ricardo da Cruz Lage[1*], Claudia Diniz Lopes Marques[2], Thauana Luiza Oliveira[3], Gustavo Gomes Resende[1], Charles Lubianca Kohem[4], Carla Gonçalves Saad[5], Antônio Carlos Ximenes[6], Célio Roberto Gonçalves[5], Washington Alves Bianchi[7], Eduardo de Souza Meirelles[5], Mauro Waldemar Keiserman[8], Adriano Chiereghin[9], Cristiano Barbosa Campanholo[10], André Marun Lyrio[11], Cláudia Goldenstein Schainberg[5], Lenise Brandao Pieruccetti[12], Michel Alexandre Yazbek[13], Penelope Esther Palominos[4], Rafaela Silva Guimarães Goncalves[2], Rodrigo Luppino Assad[14], Rubens Bonfiglioli[11], Sônia Maria Alvarenga Anti Loduca Lima[15], Sueli Carneiro[16], Valderílio Feijó Azevedo[17], Cleandro Pires Albuquerque[18], Wanderley Marques Bernardo[5], Percival Degrava Sampaio-Barros[5] and Marcelo de Medeiros Pinheiro[3]

Abstract

Spondyloarthritis (SpA) is a group of chronic inflammatory systemic diseases characterized by axial and/or peripheral joints inflammation, as well as extra-articular manifestations. Over some decades, nonsteroidal anti-inflammatory drugs (NSAIDs) have been the basis for the pharmacological treatment of patients with axial spondyloarthritis (axSpA). However, the emergence of the immunobiologic agents brought up the discussion about the role of NSAIDs in the management of these patients. The objective of this guideline is to provide recommendations for the use of NSAIDs for the treatment of axSpA. A panel of experts from the Brazilian Society of Rheumatology conducted a systematic review and meta-analysis of randomized clinical trials for 15 predefined questions. The Grading of Recommendations, Assessment, Development and Evaluation methodology to assess the quality of evidence and formulate recommendations were used, and at least 70% agreement of the voting panel was needed. Fourteen recommendations for the use of NSAIDs in the treatment of patients with axSpA were elaborated. The purpose of these recommendations is to support clinicians' decision making, without taking out his/her autonomy when prescribing for an individual patient.

Keywords: Spondyloarthritis, Ankylosing spondylitis, Nonsteroidal anti-inflammatory drugs, Systematic review, Meta-analysis, Guidelines

* Correspondence: ricolage@gmail.com
[1]Universidade Federal de Minas Gerais (UFMG), Alameda Álvaro Celso 175, Ambulatório Bias Fortes, 2° andar, Belo Horizonte, MG 30150-260, Brazil

Background

Spondyloarthritis (SpA) is a set of diseases that cause inflammation of the spine and peripheral joints and may have extra-articular manifestations, such as anterior uveitis, psoriasis, and inflammatory bowel disease. The main manifestation of SpA is the involvement of the entheses, attachment sites of the tendons, capsules, and ligaments to the bones, especially Achilles' tendon and plantar fascia. Frequently, axSpA patients have a genetic predisposition linked to human leukocyte antigen (HLA)-B27 and are usually seronegative for rheumatoid factor. The set of diseases consists of ankylosing spondylitis (AS), psoriatic arthritis, reactive arthritis, enteropathic arthritis and undifferentiated spondyloarthritis. Axial spondyloarthritis (axSpA) is defined as all cases involving the spine and/or sacroiliac joints, and peripheral spondyloarthritis is defined as cases involving only peripheral joints and/or peripheral entheses. When the same patient has both types of conditions, he/she should be classified by the predominant segment (predominantly axial involvement or predominantly peripheral involvement) [1–4].

AxSpA comprises the so-called radiographic form or AS, which includes patients who present sacroiliitis on simple radiography according to the modified New York criteria, and non-radiographic axial spondyloarthritis (nr-axSpA), which is diagnosed according to the presence of HLA-B27 (clinical arm) or positive sacroiliac MRI (imaging arm), according to the 2009 Assessment in Ankylosing Spondylitis (ASAS) classification criteria [1–4]. Although there is currently no consensus, the prevailing opinion is that axSpA is a single disease in which 20–30% of patients with nr-axSpA can develop radiographic changes over time (5 to 10 years) [5]. In fact, radiographic sacroiliitis artificially splits the axSpA spectrum into two groups, and it is unlikely that its presence alone is critical to the outcome [6]. Thus, the present recommendations will address axSpA as a single entity and combine all relevant data, since most of the available studies included patients with the radiographic form.

Over some decades, nonsteroidal anti-inflammatory drugs (NSAIDs) have been the basis for the pharmacological treatment of axSpA. However, with the emergence of biological agents which have brought great benefit to patients with axSpA, the discussion about the role of NSAIDs, as well as its cost/effectiveness and safety has gained attention.

Recently, the Brazilian Society of Rheumatology has published evidence based recommendations for the diagnosis and management of axSpA [7]. Our main goal in the present guideline was to specifically evaluate the role of NSAIDs for treating axSpA patients through a systematic review with meta-analysis and critical analysis of the published scientific data.

Methodology

Study design

This guideline was conducted in two phases. In the first phase, a systematic review and meta-analysis of randomized clinical trials (RCTs) were performed. In the second phase, an expert panel answered predefined questions and developed the recommendations.

Systematic review and meta-analysis

Inclusion criteria

We included RCTs, systematic reviews, and meta-analyses that have evaluated the efficacy and safety of NSAIDs, as monotherapy or in combination with TNFi or IL17i, in patients older than 18 years of age with axSpA.

Exclusion criteria

Non-randomized comparative studies, non-comparative studies, studies published only as conference abstracts, narrative reviews, animal studies, in vitro studies were excluded. Additionally, studies that evaluated the efficacy and safety of NSAIDs in populations with peripheral spondyloarthritis (psoriatic arthritis, reactive arthritis, inflammatory bowel disease) or rheumatoid arthritis were excluded.

Definition of therapeutic intervention

Studies that evaluated intervention with NSAIDs as a class (total or selective and nonselective COX-2 inhibitors), as well as studies that evaluated NSAID-specific molecules alone or in combination with TNFi or IL17i were considered.

Definition of controls

The included studies that evaluated the efficacy and safety of NSAIDs were compared to placebo or active treatment.

Efficacy outcomes

The outcomes used are shown in the Suplemmentary Material and included parameters of disease activity, functionality, and progression of axial and peripheral damage. Not all outcomes were reported in all comparisons, although most outcomes were included in each of them.

Safety outcomes

Any adverse events were considered, regardless of severity, causal relationship, and resolution, including renal, cardiovascular, gastrointestinal, neurological, dermatologic, hematologic and hepatic events.

Data sources

The search was conducted in the electronic databases MEDLINE (via PubMed), EMBASE, and the Cochrane Library. In addition, ongoing studies were searched in the Clinical Trials.gov and World Health Organization (WHO) trial registration databases. We searched for other potential studies not retrieved by the search strategies by checking the reference list of each eligible study, as well as in the electronic databases Health Technology Assessment (HTA), Database of Abstracts of Reviews of Effects (DARE), and National Institute for Health and Care Excellence (NICE), in addition to the guidelines of specialty societies.

Search strategies, eligibility assessment, data extraction and risk of bias assessment are shown in the Supplementary Material.

References eligible for meta-analyses

Through the search strategies reported above, 1915 references were retrieved (369 in Medline, 1532 in EMBASE, and 14 in the Cochrane Library) that were published from January 1, 2014 until May 31, 2018 (update date since the review by Kroon et al., 2015) [8]. After removing duplicates, 1698 references were evaluated by reading titles and abstracts, of which 1666 were excluded. Thus, 32 references were evaluated by reading their complete texts. At this stage, 29 references were excluded: 18 according to the type of study [9–26] (non-comparative studies; observational, single-arm studies; systematic reviews without meta-analysis or with overlapping studies; language other than Portuguese, English, or Spanish; and abstracts); eight according to the type of intervention [27–34] (drugs not registered in the country and anti-inflammatory agents other than NSAIDs); two according to the type of outcome [35, 36] (indirect/incomplete analyses, ineligible outcome); and one according to the type of population [37] (not AS and not spondyloarthritis). Thus, three RCTs [38–40] were considered eligible. In addition, through the search of the reference list of the studies evaluated, one RCT was manually included [41]. Therefore, four new eligible references were added to those previously analyzed by Kroon et al. (2015) [8].

Also, additional searches were performed into ClinicalTrials.gov and WHO International Clinical Trials Registry Platform databases. At ClinicalTrials.gov, 19 records were found, of which 17 reported no results. The two trials with available data, presented results before the review of Kroon et al. [8], they were not eligible. In the WHO International Clinical Trials Registry Platform, 18 reports of 15 RCT registrations were found. However, as they did not have available results, they were not included in this meta-analysis (Fig. 1).

Meta-analyses

Meta-analyses were performed for outcomes commonly reported by at least two studies. Their results are presented in the form of forest plots and are described in the text. Outcomes reported by only one study were also presented in graphical form (Supplementary Material).

Measures of association

For dichotomous variables, the measure of association used was relative risk (RR) with its respective 95% confidence interval (CI). For continuous variables, the measure of association used was the mean difference (MD) with its respective 95% CI. If the studies evaluated the same outcome, but using different scales, the measure of association used was the standardized mean difference (SMD) with its respective 95% CI.

Statistical methods

For the outcomes of dichotomous variables, the method used for the meta-analysis was the Mantel-Haenszel method. For the outcomes of continuous variables, the method used for the meta-analysis was the inverse-variance weighting.

Analytical model

The random-effects model was used when the statistical heterogeneity was significant by the Cochrane chi-squared test ($p < 0.1$). However, if the statistical heterogeneity was not significant but was moderate or high ($I^2 \geq 30\%$), the results are presented according to the random-effects model. In cases of mild statistical heterogeneity ($I^2 < 30\%$) or lack of statistical heterogeneity, the fixed-effects model was preferably used to add greater weight to the estimates from studies with larger sample sizes.

Heterogeneity

In cases of statistical heterogeneity, such heterogeneity was explored based on 2 strategies: the clinical-demographic differences of the participants among studies or study design differences and subgroup analyses. Some subgroup analyses were defined in advance because they were of clinical interest. These subgroup divisions were present or absent HLA-B27, normal or elevated C-reactive protein (CRP), normal or elevated erythrocyte sedimentation rate (ESR), present or absent syndesmophyte, and male or female sex.

The description of each included RCT, the risk of bias analyses, the evaluation of the quality of the evidence according to Grading of Recommendations Assessment, Development and Evaluation (GRADE) [42, 43] and the meta-analyses with all the forest plots are available in the Supplementary Material.

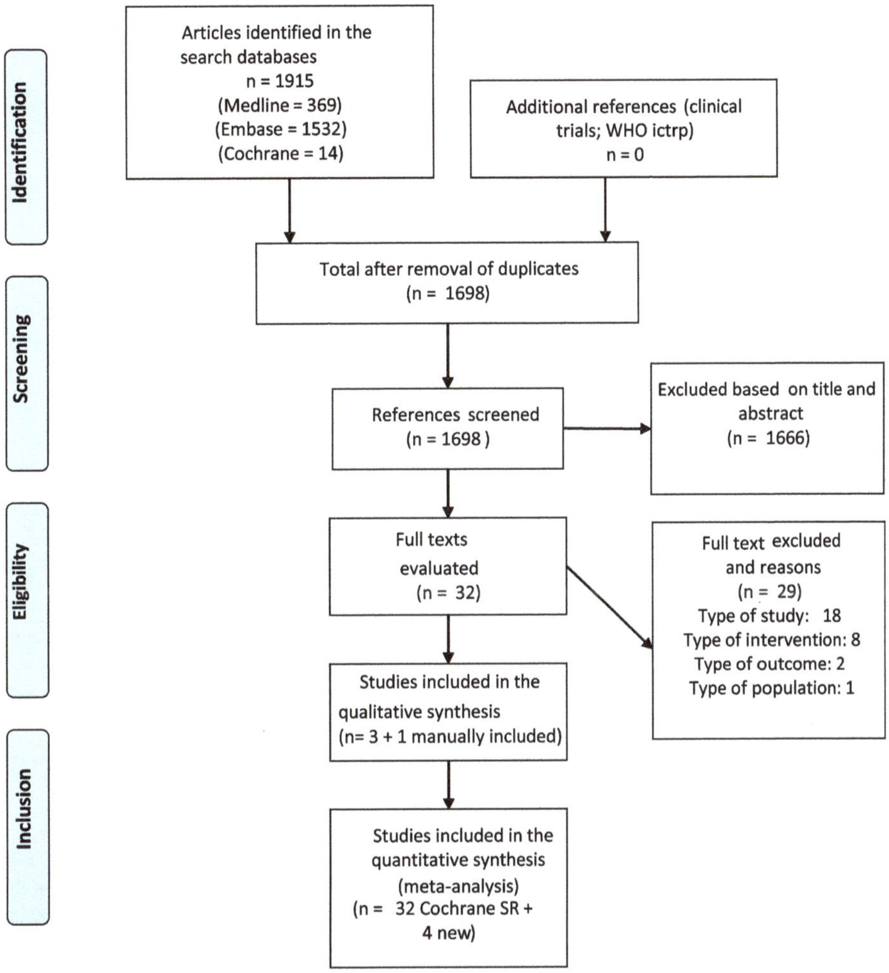

Fig. 1 PRISMA flowchart of selection and eligibility of the studies included in the systematic review (SR)

Development of recommendations

A panel of 28 rheumatologists with expertise in SpA elaborated 15 questions divided into 6 sections: efficacy and effect size, window of opportunity and treatment strategy, continuous or on demand use, radiographic progression, comparison of different NSAIDs, safety and adverse reactions. Regarding not answered questions according to the current evidence, the data from individual RCTs were reported. If necessary, a manual search for available evidences, including observational studies, was performed to support the recommendations. There was a hierarchic and standardized sequence to report available evidence: meta-analysis, individual RCTs, and finally observational studies. Observational studies were always reported as very low-quality evidence and supported conditional recommendations.

These recommendations followed the GRADE methodology. Strength of recommendation was determined by the balance between desirable and undesirable consequences of alternative management strategies, quality of evidence, variability in values and preferences, and resource use. Strong recommendations mean that most informed patients would choose the recommended management and that clinicians can structure their interactions with patients accordingly. Weak or conditional recommendations mean that patients' choices will vary according to their values and preferences, and clinicians must ensure that patients' care is in keeping with their values and preferences. The quality of evidence was assessed using GRADE for predefined key outcomes (Supplementary Material) [42, 43].

The degree of expert agreement (inter-rater reliability) was determined by the Delphi method through an online anonymous survey, and a minimum 70% agreement was needed for each recommendation.

Table 1 summarizes the Brazilian recommendations for the use of NSAIDs in patients with axSpA.

Table 1 Brazilian recommendations for the use of nonsteroidal anti-inflammatory drugs in patients with axial spondyloarthritis

Recommendations	QoE	DoA
1. EFFICACY		
Recommendation 1. In patients with active axSpA, we strongly recommend treatment with NSAIDs over no treatment, because they are effective for mitigating disease activity measures and improving functional status.	low	9.8
Recommendation 2. In patients with persistent active axSpA, we strongly recommend long-term over short-term use of NSAIDs, because they exhibit sustained symptomatic efficacy. We conditionally recommend that disease activity and adverse events should be regularly monitored, evaluating long-term risks versus benefits.	low	9.3
Recommendation 3. In patients with active axSpA, we conditionally recommend treatment with NSAIDs over no treatment for alleviate symptoms of peripheral arthritis and enthesitis, since few data have shown moderate efficacy in these clinical manifestations.	very low	8.8
2. WINDOW OF OPPORTUNITY AND TREATMENT STRATEGY		
Recommendation 4. In patients with active axSpA, we strongly recommend NSAIDs as the first-line treatment over an immunobiologic agent, considering its low cost and satisfactory efficacy. The benefit of starting an immunobiologic agent in NSAIDs-naïve patients, even in those with poor prognostic criteria, is not proven.	low	8.6
Recommendation 5. In patients with active axSpA, we strongly recommend to immediately start a NSAID after the diagnosis because early treatment may increase the response rate.	very low	8.8
Recommendation 6. In patients with active axSpA, we strongly recommend to initiate NSAIDs at full dosage over low dosage, because they exhibit a tendency for greater efficacy in achieving ASAS 20, reduction of morning stiffness, BASDAI, pain, patient global assessment of disease activity, and BASFI. We conditionally recommend that the full dosages of NSAIDs should be maintained, with adequate monitoring, until good disease control is achieved.	low	9.4
Recommendation 7. In patients with active axSpA, in the absence of a response to the first NSAID at 4 weeks, we conditionally recommend switching to a second traditional NSAID or iCOX2. If the therapeutic target is not reached with the use of NSAIDs for 12 weeks, we strongly recommend to start an immunobiologic agent.	low to high	8.6
3. CONTINUOUS OR ON-DEMAND USE		
Recommendation 8. In patients with active axSpA, we conditionally recommend to start continuous over on-demand NSAIDs until symptoms relief is achieved. After clinical improvement or the clinical target (low disease activity or remission) has been achieved, the full dosage can be reduced or switched to on-demand strategy. Before prescribing continuous NSAIDs, it is important to take into account: the patient's opinion, comorbidities and risk factors.	very low to moderate	9.4
4. RADIOGRAPHIC PROGRESSION		
Recommendation 9. Regarding radiographic progression, in patients with active axSpA, we conditionally recommend continuous over on demand use of NSAIDs. Considering controversial results among the studies, we conditionally recommend switching to on demand strategy in inactive disease. We conditionally recommend against switching NSAIDs to immunobiological therapy when there is radiographic progression without evidence of disease activity, because the risk/benefit ratio of starting an immunobiologic agent in this scenario is not clear.	Very low	8.2
5. COMPARISON AMONG NSAIDs		
Recommendation 10. In patients with active axSpA, we conditionally recommend that the choice of specific NSAI D should be based on patient's profile (age, prior toxicity, comorbidities) and on shared decision making. To date, there is no consistent evidence of efficacy and safety differences among the NSAIDs (non-selective or iCOX2) in axSpA.	low	9.6
6. SAFETY AND ADVERSE REACTIONS		
Recommendation 11. Regarding safety, in patients with active axSpA, we strongly recommend treatment with NSAIDs over no treatment, because the available evidence showed an overall good safety profile of these drugs in axSpA. We conditionally recommend that NSAIDS should be used with caution in individuals with risk factors (age > 65 years, diabetes mellitus, use of aspirin, corticosteroids and other platelet antiaggregants, renal or liver diseases). The risks and benefits of starting them should be shared and individualized according to the patient's risk profile.	low	9.0
Gastrointestinal		
Recommendation 12. In patients with active axSpA, we conditionally recommend to avoid NSAIDs (non-selective or iCOX2) and to start an immunobiologic agent in those with current or previous peptic ulcer or gastrointestinal bleeding. We conditionally recommend the use of an iCOX2 agent over a traditional NSAID in patients with gastrointestinal risk factors. We strongly recommend the use of concomitant gastroprotective drugs in symptomatic or high-risk patients.	low	8.9
Cardiovascular		
Recommendation 13. In patients with active axSpA, we conditionally recommend to avoid NSAID therapy and to start an immunobiologic agent in those with cardiovascular risk factors, mainly in those with previous acute myocardial infarction or stroke, especially if recent (past 12 months).	very low (observational studies)	8.4

Table 1 Brazilian recommendations for the use of nonsteroidal anti-inflammatory drugs in patients with axial spondyloarthritis *(Continued)*

Recommendations	QoE	DoA
Renal		
Recommendation 14. In patients with active axSpA, we conditionally recommend to avoid NSAIDs and to start an immunobiologic agent in thoses with increased risk of renal adverse events. The decision should be individualized and risk/benefits shared with the patient. We strongly recommend caution and regular monitoring of renal function, especially in high-risk individuals (elderly, hypertension, diabetes, kidney dysfunction).	very low (observa-tional studies)	9.4

NSAIDs nonsteroidal anti-inflammatory drugs, *iCOX2* selective COX-2 inhibitor, *axSpA* axial spondyloarthritis, *QoE* quality of evidence, *DoA* degree of agreement

Recommendations

Efficacy and effect size

Are NSAIDs effective for treating patients with axSpA?

Five RCTs evaluated the efficacy of conventional NSAI Ds, and three evaluated cyclooxygenase 2-selective inhibitors (iCOX2) compared to placebo. A total of 2002 patients with active AS, with a mean age between 40 and 45 years and a predominance of men (60%), were included in these studies and were followed up for 2 to 52 weeks [44–48].

There was a superiority of traditional NSAIDs over placebo for the following outcomes: pain by VAS (0–100 mm), patient global assessment (PGA) of disease activity by VAS (0–100 mm), duration of morning stiffness in minutes, C-reactive protein concentration, at least 20% improvement according to the ASAS group response criteria (ASAS 20), at least 50% improvement in pain, and the Bath Ankylosing Spondylitis Function Index (BASFI) (Table 2).

Regarding iCOX2, the meta-analyses showed superiority over placebo in the following outcomes: pain VAS, PGA, ASAS 20, and BASFI (Table 2). Individual studies showed superiority of iCOX2 over placebo in the Bath Ankylosing Spondylitis Disease Activity Index (BASDAI) [− 2.2 (− 2.74 to − 1.66)] [48], at least 50% improvement in pain [iCOX2: 47.5% vs placebo: 20%, RR: 2.41 (1.45 to 4.00)] [45], and ASAS partial remission [iCOX2: 15% vs placebo: 3%, RR: 4.65 (1.39 to 15.55)] [48]. Fig. 2 shows the subgroup analysis for pain VAS by comparing traditional NSAIDs, iCOX2, or both versus placebo.

Recommendation 1
In patients with active axSpA, we strongly recommend treatment with NSAIDs over no treatment, because they are effective for mitigating disease activity measures and improving functional status. **Quality of evidence: low; Degree of agreement: 9.8**

Do NSAIDS have sustained symptomatic efficacy in axSpA?

Most RCTs that evaluated the efficacy of NSAIDs, compared to both placebo and other NSAIDs, had a short duration (8 to 12 weeks) [13, 29, 31, 38, 40, 44, 47, 49–53]. In two long-term RCTs involving patients with AS, the sustained efficacy of NSAIDs was shown in 12 months. Van der Heijde et al. found an ASAS20 response of 52.5% with naproxen and 65% with etoricoxib compared to 20% in placebo group. The 1-year maintenance rate was 90% with etoricoxib and 79% with naproxen [48]. In another RCT, Dougados et al. evaluated the efficacy of NSAIDs in 473 patients with short- and long-term AS. At 6 weeks, 43, 50, and 47% of patients who received 20 mg of piroxicam, 15 mg of meloxicam, or 22.5 mg of meloxicam, respectively, had ≥ 50% improvement in PGA, compared to 21% for the placebo,

Table 2 Efficacy of traditional NSAIDs or iCOX2 vs. placebo in patients with axial spondyloarthritis: meta-analyses of randomized clinical trials

	TRADITIONAL NSAIDs *n*=1289	iCOX2 *n*=669
PAIN VAS (95% CI)	−16.75 (−20.28 to −13.07)	−21.68 (−35.94 to −7.42)
PGA	−17.75 (−24.39 to −11.10)	−20.82 (− 39.88 to −11.75)
ASAS20	60% vs. 23% (PbO) RR=2.49 (1.94 to 3.19)	57% vs. 20% (PbO) RR=2.51 (1.66 to 3.79)
BASFI	−9 (− 13 to −5)	−13.4 (− 17.3 to −5)
MS - SMD	−0.4 (−0.58 to −0.22)	NA
CRP mg/L	−3.37 (−6.11 to − 0.62)	NA
PAIN50%	48% vs 21% 2.25 (1.75 to 2.89)	NA

NSAIDs nonsteroidal anti-inflammatory drugs, *iCOX2* COX-2-selective inhibitors, *PAIN VAS* pain by visual analog scale 0–100 mm, *PGA* Patient Global Assessment 0–100 mm, *BASFI* Bath Ankylosing Spondylitis Function Index 0–100 mm, *MS-SMD* standardized mean difference in the duration of morning stiffness, *CRP* C-reactive protein, *PAIN50%* ≥ 50% improvement in pain, *RR* relative risk, *PbO* placebo, *N/A* meta-analysis not feasible

	Study or Subgroup	NSAIDs + iCOX2 Mean	SD	Total	Placebo Mean	SD	Total	Weight	Mean Difference IV, Random, 95% CI
	7.1.1 Nonselective NSAIDs								
1	Dougados 1994	39	25	50	57	24	95	13.8%	-18.00 [-26.44, -9.56]
2	Dougados 1999_	-32	28	120	-15	27	60	13.7%	-17.00 [-25.47, -8.53]
3	Dougados 1999	-32	27	108	-15	27	61	13.7%	-17.00 [-25.48, -8.52]
4	Dougados 2001	-21	26	90	-13	29	76	13.8%	-8.00 [-16.45, 0.45]
5	van der Heijde 2005	43.29	24.62	97	64.37	23.72	93	15.8%	-21.08 [-27.95, -14.21]
	Subtotal (95% CI)			**465**			**385**	**70.8%**	**-16.51 [-20.84, -12.17]**
	Heterogeneity: Tau² = 7.39; Chi² = 5.73, df = 4 (P = 0.22); I² = 30%								
	Test for overall effect: Z = 7.47 (P < 0.00001)								
	7.1.2 iCOX2								
6	Dougados 2001	-27	30	80	-13	29	76	12.8%	-14.00 [-23.26, -4.74]
7	van der Heijde 2005	35.8	21.86	100	64.37	23.72	93	16.4%	-28.57 [-35.02, -22.12]
	Subtotal (95% CI)			**180**			**169**	**29.2%**	**-21.68 [-35.94, -7.42]**
	Heterogeneity: Tau² = 89.57; Chi² = 6.40, df = 1 (P = 0.01); I² = 84%								
	Test for overall effect: Z = 2.98 (P = 0.003)								
	Total (95% CI)			**645**			**554**	**100.0%**	**-18.06 [-23.11, -13.00]**
	Heterogeneity: Tau² = 29.76; Chi² = 16.92, df = 6 (P = 0.010); I² = 65%								
	Test for overall effect: Z = 7.00 (P < 0.00001)								
	Test for subgroup differences: Chi² = 0.46, df = 1 (P = 0.50), I² = 0%								

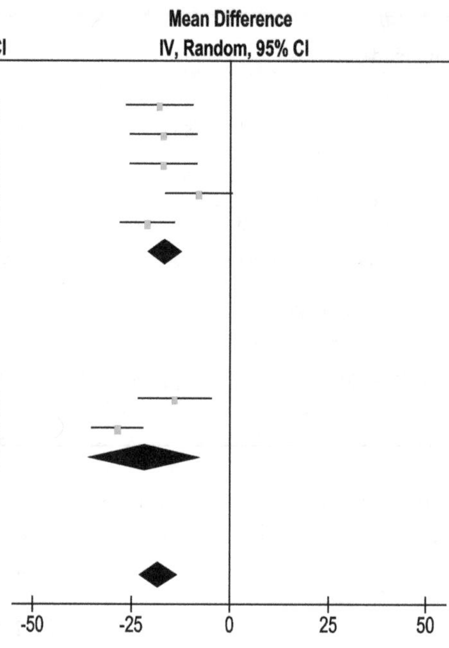

Fig. 2 Spinal pain by visual analogue scale (VAS 0–100 mm): analysis of subgroups of four randomized clinical trials of patients with ankylosing spondylitis (*n*=1199). Meta-analyses comparing traditional NSAIDs versus placebo, selective COX-2 inhibitors versus placebo, and both NSAID subtypes versus placebo. Subtitle: (1) Ximoprofen 30 mg vs placebo. (2) Meloxicam 15 mg vs placebo. (3) Piroxicam 20 mg vs placebo. (4) Ketoprofen 200 mg vs placebo. (5) Naproxen 1000 mg vs placebo. (6) Celecoxib 200 mg vs placebo. (7) Etoricoxib 90 mg vs placebo

with sustained response at 12 months. The discontinuation rate due to lack/ loss of efficacy was between 10 and 20%. Only 16% of the responders at 6 weeks had a 1-year loss of response [46].

In a German population-based cohort, almost 80% of 1080 patients with AS were on NSAIDs, of whom 71% had been taking it for more than 4 years. The NSAIDs were effective for complete or partial resolution (> 50%) of pain in 19.1 and 61.2% of patients, respectively [54]. In a Swedish cohort, 21, 108 patients with AS were analyzed for 3 years. Approximately 80% of patients used iCOX2, and 63.8% used non-selective NSAIDs for more than 50% of the follow-up time, with a good initial response rate as well as a good response rate over time [17]. In the Netherlands, Carbo et al. followed up 393 patients with AS who were anti-TNF *naïve*, of whom 254 were prescribed some TNF inhibitors (BASDAI=6.1 and ASDAS=3.8), while 139 were kept under conventional treatment (BASDAI=3.9 and ASDAS=2.4; 74% with NSAIDs). After 12 months of follow-up, both groups had similar activity scores (BASDAI=3.4 and ASDAS=2.2 vs. BASDAI=3.7 and ASDAS=2.3, respectively). Among patients who received conventional treatment, 82% maintained a sustained response with NSAIDs after 52 weeks [55]. Despite being observational studies whose primary objective was not to evaluate the response to treatment, the high rate of drug retention observed over time suggested a sustained efficacy of NSAIDs.

Recommendation 2

In patients with persistent active axSpA, we strongly recommend long-term over short-term use of NSAIDs, because they exhibit sustained symptomatic efficacy. We conditionally recommend that disease activity and adverse events should be regularly monitored, evaluating long-term risks versus benefits.

Quality of evidence: low; Degree of agreement: 9.3

Are NSAIDs effective for treating the peripheral manifestations of axSpA?

Four of the five RCTs of NSAIDs versus placebo did not evaluate the efficacy of these drugs on peripheral arthritis or enthesitis in axSpA. One RCT compared the effect of ximoprofen on peripheral arthritis at several doses with placebo as secondary outcome, and there was a significant improvement in peripheral arthritis with a moderate effect size (standardized mean difference, SMD=0.62 [95%CI: 0.26 to 0.97]) [47, 56]. From the three trials that assessed iCOX2 versus placebo, two of them excluded patients with peripheral manifestations. A *post-hoc* analysis of a study of etoricoxib and naproxen versus placebo in axSpA suggested NSAIDs were effective for treating peripheral arthritis, as assessed by question 3 of BASDAI, with an improvement on the VAS 0–100 mm of − 16.4 (− 20.3 to − 12. 6) compared to 0.9 (− 5.9 to 7.6) for placebo, as well as in enthesitis (question 4 of BASDAI), with a shift of − 21.3 (− 25.2 to −

17.5) with NSAID versus – 6.5 (– 13.3 to 0.4) with placebo in patients with concomitant peripheral arthritis, and of – 27.6 (– 30.8 to – 24.5) versus – 7.3 (– 12.9 to – 1.8) in those without concomitant peripheral arthritis [48, 50].

The effect of NSAIDs on enthesitis was not specifically evaluated in RCTs of patients with axSpA. The current recommendations suggest that they are effective in a subsample of patients, but that conclusion was extrapolated from studies on psoriatic arthritis or based on expert opinions [57, 58].

Recommendation 3
In patients with active axSpA, we conditionally recommend treatment with NSAIDs over no treatment to alleviate symptoms of peripheral arthritis and enthesitis, since few data have shown moderate efficacy in these clinical manifestations. **Quality of evidence: very low; Degree of agreement: 8.8**

Window of opportunity and treatment strategy

Should NSAIDs be considered first-line treatment in axSpA?

In the INFAST study, 158 patients with axSpA were randomized to receive infliximab + naproxen or placebo + naproxen for 28 weeks. The interesting aspect of this study was that the patients were not refractory to NSAI Ds, as in other immunobiologic RCTs (they were NSAID naïve or used low dose of NSAIDs). At week 28, 62% of the Infliximab + naproxen group had ASAS partial remission versus 35% of the placebo + naproxen group [59]. Later, infliximab was discontinued, and patients who achieved remission were monitored until week 52 under continuous naproxen use or no treatment. A similar percentage maintained remission in both the group using naproxen (47.5%) and the group without any treatment (40%) and independent of the initial therapeutic regimen, despite small sample for the latter analysis. The response rate was higher with anti-TNF, but NSAIDs (with placebo) led to remission in more than 1/3 of the cases [60].

In an open-label follow-up study, 39 of the 40 patients with very early axSpA from the RCT conducted by Barkham *et al* [61] (who had received infliximab or placebo for 16 weeks) were monitored for 5 years. There was no difference in current disease activity or radiographic progression by mSASSS among participants receiving infliximab or placebo in the randomized phase. However, approximately 60% (7/12) of patients who initially received infliximab still needed an anti-TNF after 5 years, while 100% (13/13) of those who received placebo remained on anti-TNF treatment [62].

There are not available data to define whether NSAIDs should remain the first-line treatment in patients with poor prognostic criteria (smokers, with elevated CRP and syndesmophytes on baseline) or whether immunobiologics should be the first choice in these cases. Indeed, the long-term benefit of initiating an immunobiologic agent as first line treatment was not proven, as the data suggesting this benefit originated from a small sample size [62]. In addition, early starting of the NSAID led to a highly significant ASAS partial remission rate (35%) [59].

Considering the low cost, long term experience, and satisfactory response in early disease showed in the INFAST trial [59], the expert panel stated that NSAIDs should still be the first-line treatment in axSpA.

Recommendation 4
In patients with active axSpA, we strongly recommend NSAIDs as the first-line treatment over an immunobiologic agent, considering its low cost and satisfactory efficacy. To date, the benefit of starting an immunobiologic agent in NSAIDs-naïve patients, even in those with poor prognostic criteria, is not proven. **Quality of evidence: low; Degree of agreement: 8.6**

Should NSAIDs be started immediately after the diagnosis of axSpA?

Several studies suggest that the response rates are higher with an earlier onset of treatment [39, 63–65]. In the INFAST study [59], approximately 35% of patients with very early (< 2 years of disease on average) axSpA (AS + nr-axSpA) achieved ASAS partial remission with naproxen versus 9% with placebo (only 15% of patients with AS, with longer disease duration, had achieved this target with etoricoxib in the study by van der Heijde et al) [48]. Barkham et al. achieved 56% ASAS partial remission with infliximab in patients with early axSpA (average of 1 year and 3 months of symptom duration) compared to 22% in the pivotal study of infliximab [61]. Other RCTs found a 70 to 75% ASAS40 response rate after TNF inhibitors in patients with axSpA and disease duration below 3 years, compared to around 40–45% of ASAS40 response rate in those with established AS [59, 66, 67]. Haroon et al. reinforced the importance of early treatment by demonstrating that the delay in the onset of anti-TNF treatment increases the rate of radiographic progression [68]. These results reinforce the idea of a "window of opportunity" during the treatment of axSpA and the importance of effective early onset treatment.

Despite the few available data, the panelists considered important to immediately start an NSAID as soon as the diagnosis of axSpA is confirmed.

Recommendation 5
In patients with active axSpA, we strongly recommend to immediately start an NSAID after the diagnosis, because early treatment may increase the response rate. **Quality of evidence: very low; Degree of agreement: 8.8**

When NSAIDs are prescribed for the treatment of patients with axSpA, should they be used in full dosages or at the lowest possible dosage for symptomatic control?

Six RCTs compared full-dosage versus low-dosage of NSAI Ds in almost 2000 patients with active axial SpA. In two of them the mean disease duration was long (10 to 13 years) [46, 47]. The comparisons were: 1) celecoxib 200 mg x celecoxib 400 mg [44, 49]; 2) ximoprofen 5 mg x ximoprofen 30 mg [47]; 3) meloxicam 15 mg x meloxicam 22.5 mg [46]; 4) etoricoxib 90 mg x etoricoxib 120 mg [48]; and 5) etoricoxib 60 mg x etoricoxib 90 mg [41]. The meta-analyses showed a slight superiority of the higher dosages of NSAIDs in reducing the duration of morning stiffness [SMD: 0.14 (0.02; 0.27)] and the proportion of patients who achieved ASAS 20 [RR: 0.87 (0.77; 0.99)], at the limit of statistical significance. However, there was uncertain risk of bias in four studies [44, 46, 47, 49] and high risk in one study [41]. Regarding the BASDAI and BASFI, the meta-analyses did not demonstrate a significant difference between full- and low-dosage NSAIDs, but the results of the individual studies were consistent in favoring higher dosage. Regarding pain outcomes, including pain VAS and 50% improvement, CRP serum levels and PGA, the data were inconsistent, sometimes favoring high doses and other times favoring lower doses of NSAIDs. ASAS partial remission [48] and BASMI [49] were reported in only one RCT each, with no difference between doses. Also, the results of the RCTs cited above should be interpreted with caution, as the 120 mg dose of etoricoxib and 22.5 mg of meloxicam are not currently in use.

Regarding safety, the meta-analyses showed no differences among NSAIDs dosages on the occurrence of any adverse event, serious adverse event, or adverse events per specific system (cardiovascular, gastrointestinal, neurological, respiratory, or dermatologic). There was also no difference in the proportion of patients who discontinued treatment due to unexpected adverse events. Given the low accuracy of the findings, the results were considered inconclusive.

Recommendation 6

In patients with active axSpA, we strongly recommend to initiate NSAIDs at full dosage over low dosage, because they exhibit a tendency for greater efficacy in achieving ASAS 20, reduction of morning stiffness, BASDAI, pain, patient global assessment of disease activity, and BASFI. We conditionally recommend that the full dosages of NSAIDs should be maintained, with adequate monitoring, until good disease control is achieved. **Quality of evidence: low; Degree of agreement: 9.4**

For how long should we wait for initial response to NSAIDs in axSpA?

The traditional NSAIDs and iCOX2 trials have shown that pain and stiffness measures differed from placebo in the first week and the maximum effect was achieved from 2 to 4 weeks. The majority of the studies had a short duration of 2 to 6 weeks [44–48]. The two trials with an extension phase from 6 to 52 weeks did not show any additional effect size with the use of NSAIDs after 6 weeks [46, 48].

The panelists considered a period of 2 weeks too short to evaluate efficacy and recommended a 4-week period as a reasonable time to change treatment, if no response is observed. Based on the previous guidelines for the treatment of axSpA and the clinical experience, despite lack of evidence, the panel recommended a second NSAID, regardless therapeutic class (selective COX-2 or not), could be used if the first one failed after 4 weeks. The total treatment period with NSAIDs should not exceed 12 weeks, if the predefined target is not achieved [6, 7].

Recommendation 7

In patients with active axSpA, in the absence of a response to the first NSAID at 4 weeks, we conditionally recommend switching to a second traditional NSAID or iCOX2. If the therapeutic target is not reached with the use of NSAIDs for 12 weeks, we strongly recommend to start an immunobiologic agent. **Quality of evidence: low to high; Degree of agreement: 8.6**

Continuous or on-demand use

Is there any significant difference in the reduction of disease activity or safety of NSAIDs when comparing the on-demand versus continuous use for the treatment of axSpA?

Only two RCTs compared continuous and on-demand use of NSAIDs in AS patients. In both studies, the primary outcome was radiographic progression. Wanders et al. [69] evaluated celecoxib continuously or on demand in 215 patients with AS, and disease activity rates were reported as a secondary outcome. After 2 years, there was no significant difference of BASDAI, PGA, overall pain, or C-reactive protein serum levels between two ways of prescribing NSAIDs. More recently, Sieper et al. evaluated 167 patients with AS and compared the continuous or on-demand use of diclofenac. Although not significant, the BASDAI decreased from 4.1 to 2.7, in continuous group, and from 4.2 to 3.2 in on-demand group [70]. Regarding adverse events, there was no difference between continuous and on-demand use in either study.

Despite the lack of evidence, the panel recommended continuous use of NSAIDs in active disease until symptoms relief is achieved, based on the previous guidelines and the clinical experience [6, 7, 71].

Recommendation 8

In patients with active axSpA, we conditionally recommend to start continuous over on-demand NSAIDs until symptoms relief is achieved. After clinical improvement or the clinical target (low disease activity or remission) has been achieved, the treatment regimen can be switched to on-demand strategy. Before prescribing continuous NSAIDs, it is important to take into account patient's opinion, comorbidities and risk factors. **Quality of evidence: very low to moderate; Degree of agreement: 9.4**

Radiographic progression

Is there evidence that NSAIDs can delay or minimize the progression of axial damage in axSpA? Should we switch to an immunobiologic agent in asymptomatic patients with radiographic progression?

Only the two previously cited RCTs had the reduction of radiographic progression through modified Stoke

Ankylosing Spondylitis Spine Score (mSASSS) as the primary outcome. Over a two-year follow-up, Wanders et al. observed higher progression in the on-demand group (+ 1.5 ± 2.5) compared to the continuous-use group (+ 0.4 ± 1.7) (p=0.002) [69]. This result was similarly found in previous retrospective studies [72, 73]. However, a *post-hoc* analysis of the Wanders et al. trial showed a significant difference only in those with elevated CRP, which brought into discussion if celecoxib reduced the radiographic progression due to the reduction of inflammation instead of a specific drug class effect [74].

On the other hand, Sieper et al. did not find any significant difference on radiographic progression between the continuous and on-demand use of diclofenac over 2 years using mSASSS as outcome [70]. Numerically, the progression was higher in continuous group compared to on-demand group (+ 1.3; 95% CI 0.7 to 1.9 vs + 0.8; 95%; CI 0.2 to 1.4, respectively), but there was no statistical significance, even when considering subgroups with the worst prognosis, such as those with higher CRP and previous syndesmophytes. Therefore, the efficacy of NSAIDs in preventing radiographic damage remains an open question. Nowadays, there is growing evidence that immunobiologic agents may reduce long-term radiographic progression, especially after 4 years of treatment. However to date, the benefit of starting an immunobiologic agent in patients with radiographic progression measured by mSASSS, but with a good symptom control with NSAID was not addressed [75–77].

Recommendation 9

Regarding the radiographic progression, we conditionally recommend continuous over on demand use of NSAIDs in patients with active axSpA. Considering controversial results among the studies, we conditionally recommend switching to on demand strategy in inactive disease. We conditionally recommend against switching NSAIDs to immunobiological therapy when there is radiographic progression without evidence of disease activity, because the risk/benefit ratio of starting an immunobiologic agent in this scenario is not clear. **Quality of evidence: very low; Degree of agreement: 8.2**

Comparison among NSAIDs

Is there any difference regarding the efficacy of traditional NSAID versus another traditional NSAID or versus iCOX2 in patients with axSpA? Is there any difference among NSAIDs regarding adverse events in patients with axSpA?

Twenty-six RCTs compared different traditional NSAI Ds in patients with axSpA. A total of 2176 participants aged 35 to 46 years were evaluated. The overall risk of bias in these studies was considered high due to lack of information on randomization, allocation concealment, blinding, and loss to follow-up. Given the data heterogeneity, a meta-analysis was not possible [46, 51–53, 78–95].

Seven trials compared traditional NSAIDs on pain reduction (VAS 0–100 mm) and some statistically significant differences were observed [46, 51, 78, 86, 96–98]: aceclofenac was inferior to indomethacin [SMD: 1.23; (95% CI: 0.98 to 1.47)], piroxicam was superior to naproxen [SMD: – 1.25; (95% CI: – 1.98 to – 0.51)], and diclofenac was superior to sulindac [SMD: – 0.54; (95% CI: – 1.06 to – 0.03). However, no significant difference was observed using a Likert pain scale. Two studies [46, 93, 99] measured the PGA, and only one [93] evaluated the proportion of patients with ≥ 50% pain improvement. However, none of them found significant differences in comparison among traditional NSAIDs (piroxicam vs. meloxicam and ketoprofen vs. phenylbutazone, respectively).

A network meta-analysis, that included 26 RCTs and 3410 patients with AS, did not find any significant difference among 18 different traditional NSAIDs in short-term (between 2 and 12 weeks) [25].

To compare coxibs and nonselective NSAIDs, seven studies were evaluated [38, 40, 41, 44, 45, 48, 49]. Two RCTs used etoricoxib [41, 48], and the others with celecoxib [38, 40, 44, 45, 49]. Three RCTs used diclofenac as comparator, another three used naproxen, and the last used ketoprofen. The meta-analyses did not show significant differences between iCOX2 and traditional NSAIDs for pain VAS 0–100 mm score (Fig. 3), BASDAI, PGA, the proportion of patients who achieved ASAS20, or BASFI. Only the study by van der Heijde et al. found a slight superiority of etoricoxib 90 mg/day over naproxen 1000 mg/day for the outcomes pain VAS 0–100 mm and PGA. This same study found no significant difference regarding BASDAI, BASFI, or ASAS partial remission [48].

In the network meta-analysis by Wang et al., 18 traditional NSAIDs and two iCOX2 agents were compared to each other in treatment of AS. Etoricoxib was superior to celecoxib, ketoprofen, and tenoxicam with regard to pain reduction, but without a significant difference in the duration of morning stiffness. The superiority of etoricoxib should be interpreted with caution because it was based on only one RCT [25, 48].

Regarding any adverse events, there was no significant difference among traditional NSAIDs. In only one of the 19 studies, indomethacin caused more adverse events than oxaprozin [80]. In the analysis by organ system, indomethacin was also associated with a higher rate of neurological adverse events than aceclofenac, oxaprozin, and diclofenac [80, 83, 86]. No difference was observed in adverse events rate (renal, cardiovascular, hepatic, hematological, respiratory, or dermatologic) in patients with axSpA.

In comparison between iCOX2 and traditional NSAIDs, the meta-analysis did not detect differences for any adverse events. In the evaluation by organ system (Fig. 4a and b), there were also no significant differences, except for

	Study or Subgroup	iCOX2 Mean	iCOX2 SD	iCOX2 Total	NSAID Mean	NSAID SD	NSAID Total	Weight	Mean Difference IV, Random, 95% CI
1	Dougados 2001	-27	30	80	-21	26	90	12.3%	-6.00 [-14.49, 2.49]
2	Sieper 2008	38.7	24.9	148	33.8	27.1	154	17.8%	4.90 [-0.97, 10.77]
3	van der Heijde 2005	35.8	21.86	100	43.29	24.62	97	16.3%	-7.49 [-14.00, -0.98]
4	Walker 2016	-25.8	27.9	107	-28.2	26.8	115	14.7%	2.40 [-4.81, 9.61]
5	Balazcz 2016	-31.23	21.24	144	-30.59	21.28	143	20.4%	-0.64 [-5.56, 4.28]
6	Huang 2014	-23.7	20.6	117	-26.7	22.9	115	18.5%	3.00 [-2.61, 8.61]
	Total (95% CI)			**696**			**714**	**100.0%**	**-0.30 [-4.15, 3.54]**

Heterogeneity: Tau² = 12.62; Chi² = 11.28, df = 5 (P = 0.05); I² = 56%
Test for overall effect: Z = 0.15 (P = 0.88)

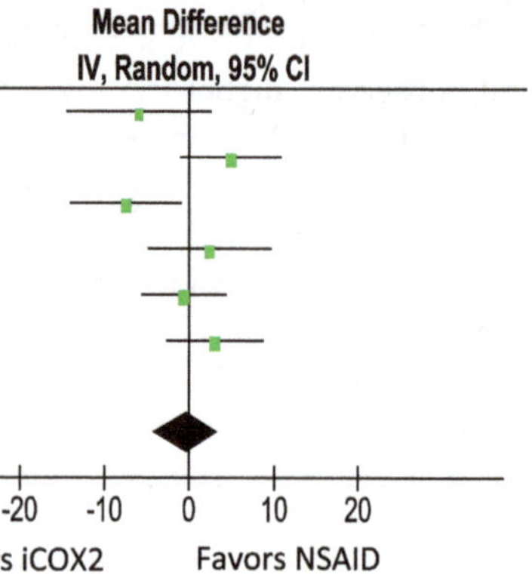

Fig. 3 Spinal pain by visual analog scale (VAS 0–100 mm) comparing traditional NSAIDs versus iCOX2 in patients with ankylosing spondylitis: meta-analysis of six randomized clinical trials. Subtitle: (1) Celecoxib 200 mg vs ketoprofen 200 mg. (2) Celecoxib 400 mg vs diclofenac 75 mg. (3) Etoricoxib 90 mg vs naproxen 1000 mg. (4) Celecoxib 200 mg vs diclofenac 50 mg. (5) Etoricoxib 90 mg vs naproxen 1000 mg. (6) Celecoxib 200 mg vs diclofenac 75 mg

increased hepatic toxicity for iCOX2. However, this finding was highly imprecise and at the limit of statistical significance. Regarding discontinuation of treatment due to adverse events, there were no differences in the comparison of traditional NSAIDs or in the comparison between these and iCOX2. Systematic reviews that included several diseases showed greater gastrointestinal safety of iCOX2 compared to traditional NSAIDs and suggested a greater cardiovascular safety of naproxen compared to other NSAIDs [100, 101]. However, we did not observe any significant difference in the present meta-analysis (see supplementary material).

Recommendation 10
In patients with active axSpA, we conditionally recommend that the choice of a specific NSAID should be based on patient's profile (age, prior toxicity, comorbidities) and on shared decision making. To date, there is no consistent evidence of efficacy and safety differences among the NSAIDs (non-selective or iCOX2) in axSpA. **Quality of evidence: low; Degree of agreement: 9.6**

Safety and adverse reactions

Is there any evidence that NSAIDs carry an increased risk of adverse events in patients with axSpA?

Five studies compared non-selective NSAIDs versus placebo regarding adverse events, totaling 1289 patients evaluated [44–48]. The meta-analysis showed no significant adverse events differences compared to placebo. Furthermore, there was no significant serious adverse events difference or in the discontinuation rate due to adverse events in short-term (6–12 weeks) (Table 3 and Fig. 5). Another 52-week study found no significant adverse event difference among piroxicam 20 mg, meloxicam 15 mg, and meloxicam 22.5 mg compared to placebo in 473 patients with AS (26, 38, 34, and 36%, respectively) [46].

Considering iCOX2, three studies compared the incidence of any adverse events versus placebo in 700 patients with axSpA [44, 45, 48]. Our meta-analysis did not show any significant short-term differences (incidence of any adverse events, serious adverse events, or discontinuation of treatment due to adverse events for iCOX2 compared to placebo) (Table 3 and Fig. 6). In the single RCT with a longer follow-up period (52 weeks), the placebo group was blindly reallocated to receive etoricoxib 90 mg, etoricoxib 120 mg, or naproxen 1000 mg after 6-week follow-up. In the first 6 weeks, the rates of any adverse events were 39.8, 47.6, 48.9, and 41.4% for placebo, etoricoxib 90 mg, etoricoxib 120 mg, and naproxen, respectively. At the end of 1 year, there were no significant differences in any of the adverse events among the three groups (43.5%, 36.1, and 38.5%, respectively), nor in severe adverse events (7.6, 7.2, and 7.7%, respectively) or discontinuation rate due to adverse events (8.7, 4.8, and 7.7%, respectively) [48].

Therefore comparing NSAIDs versus placebo, we did not find statistical differences in the overall incidence of adverse events, which suggests a good safety profile. However, considering specific organ system analyses showed in the following sections, caution is recommended when using NSAIDs, especially regarding gastrointestinal events.

Recommendation 11
Regarding safety, in patients with active axSpA, we strongly recommend treatment with NSAIDs over no treatment, because the available evidence showed an overall good safety profile of these drugs in axSpA. We conditionally recommend that NSAIDS should be used with caution in individuals with risk factors (age > 65 years old, diabetes mellitus, use of aspirin, corticosteroids and other platelet antiaggregants, renal or liver diseases). The risks and benefits of starting them should be shared and individualized according to the patient's risk profile. **Quality of evidence: low, Degree of agreement: 9.0**

Is the use of NSAIDs associated with increased gastrointestinal risk in patients with axSpA?

Five studies compared traditional NSAIDs versus placebo regarding gastrointestinal adverse events in 1289 patients [44–48]. The frequency of gastrointestinal

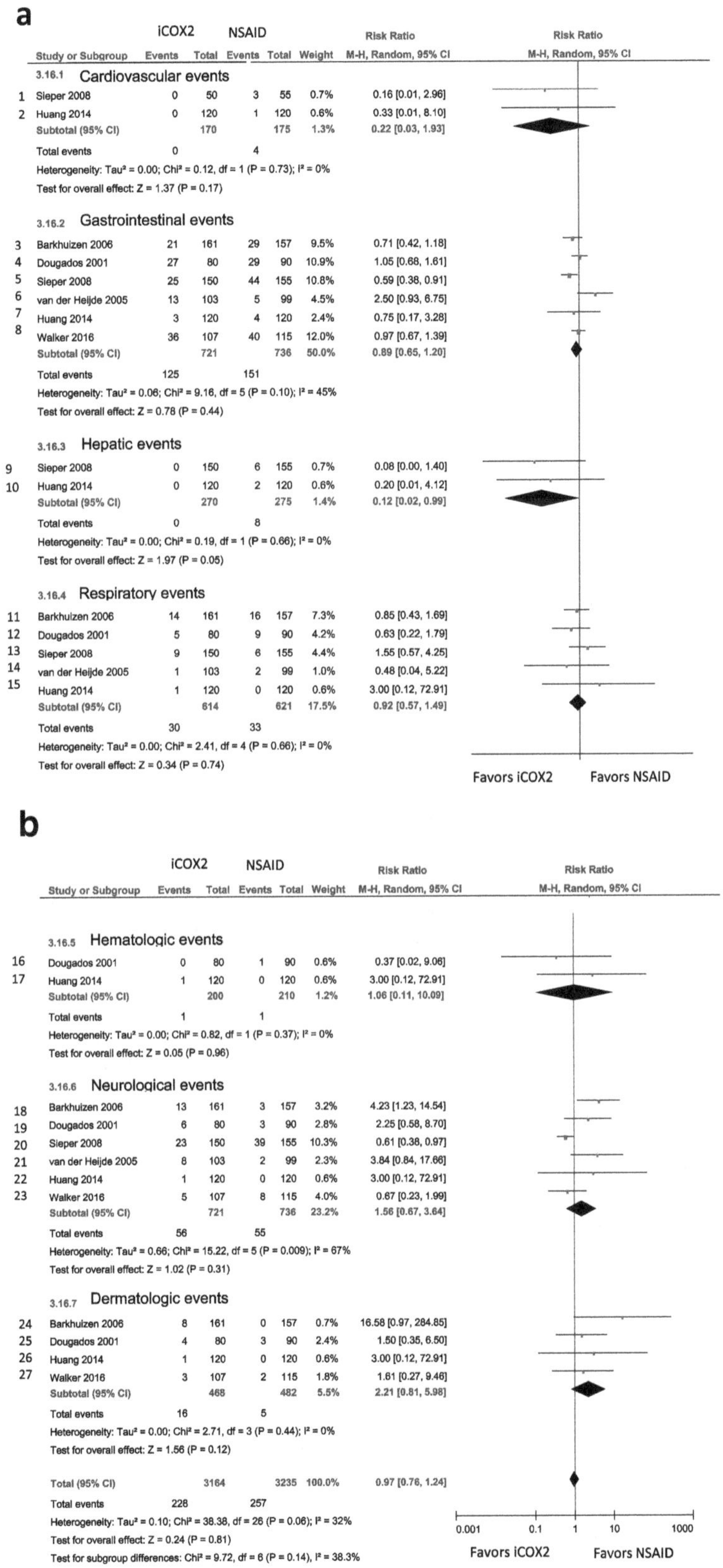

Fig. 4 (See legend on next page.)

(See figure on previous page.)
Fig. 4 a and **b** Incidence of adverse events per organ system in the comparison of COX2 selective inhibitors versus traditional NSAIDs in patients with ankylosing spondylitis: meta-analyses of seven randomized clinical trials. Subtitle: (1) Celecoxib 400 mg vs diclofenac 75 mg. (2) Celecoxib 200 mg vs diclofenac 75 mg (3) Celecoxib 400 mg vs naproxen 500 mg. (4) Celecoxib 200 mg vs ketoprofen 200 mg. (5) Celecoxib 400 mg vs diclofenac 75 mg. (6) Etoricoxib 90 mg vs naproxen 1000 mg. (7) Celecoxib 200 mg vs diclofenac 75 mg. (8) Celecoxib 200 mg vs diclofenac 50 mg (9) Celecoxib 400 mg vs diclofenac 75 mg. (10) Celecoxib 200 mg vs diclofenac 75 mg. (11) Celecoxib 400 mg vs naproxen 500 mg. (12) Celecoxib 200 mg vs ketoprofen 200 mg. (13) Celecoxib 400 mg vs diclofenac 75 mg. (14) Etoricoxib 90 mg vs naproxen 1000 mg. (15) Celecoxib 200 mg vs diclofenac 75 mg (16) Celecoxib 200 mg vs ketoprofen 200 mg. (17) Celecoxib 200 mg vs diclofenac 75 mg. (18) Celecoxib 400 mg vs naproxen 500 mg. (19) Celecoxib 200 mg vs ketoprofen 200 mg. (20) Celecoxib 400 mg vs diclofenac 75 mg. (21) Etoricoxib 90 mg vs naproxen 1000 mg. (22) Celecoxib 200 mg vs diclofenac 75 mg. (23) Celecoxib 200 mg vs diclofenac 50 mg (24) Celecoxib 400 mg vs naproxen 500 mg. (25) Celecoxib 200 mg vs ketoprofen 200 mg (26) Celecoxib 200 mg vs diclofenac 75 mg. (27) Celecoxib 200 mg vs diclofenac 50 mg

events was higher with tranditional NSAIDs than placebo. A similar result was observed with iCOX2 in 769 patients when compared to placebo (Table 3, Figs. 7 and 8) [44, 45, 48]. There was no significant difference in the meta-analysis of six RCTs that compared iCOX2 versus traditional NSAIDs (RR=0.89; 0.65–1.2). Most RCTs were short-term (2–12 weeks) [38, 40, 44, 45, 48, 49].

In the Dougados' study (1999), the extension phase lasted from 6th to 52nd week. In the first 6 weeks, the authors showed 14% gastrointestinal events with traditional NSAIDs versus 7% in placebo group. A total of six (1.7%) individuals from NSAID group had gastroduodenal ulcers, and no patients were diagnosed in placebo group by week 52 [46]. Regarding iCOX2, only the RCT by van der Heijde et al. (2005) analyzed adverse events from week 6 to week 52 in the extension phase, not controlled by placebo. The incidence of pyrosis after 1 year of use was 9.8, 7.2, and 7.7% for etoricoxib 90 mg, etoricoxib 120 mg, and naproxen 1000 mg, respectively. Three (2.4%) patients who received etoricoxib 120 mg and 4 (3.2%) who received naproxen had gastroduodenal ulcers at 1 year of follow-up [48].

Most data on gastrointestinal risk were from studies in other populations (osteoarthritis, rheumatoid arthritis, etc.) and there is no evidence that the risk is different in axSpA. Factors considered high-risk for gastrointestinal complications with NSAIDs are age above 65 years, comorbidities (diabetes, COPD, coronary disease, coagulopathies), alcoholism, concomitant medication (corticosteroids, anticoagulants, aspirin, other antiplatelet aggregation drugs), history of peptic ulcer, and *Helicobacter pylori* infection. An observational study that evaluated 4144 individuals with osteoarthritis (85%), rheumatoid arthritis (11%), or AS (3%) and at least one gastrointestinal risk factor, with a mean follow-up of 6 months, showed an incidence of 0.7 severe events per 100 patients-year after the initiation of NSAIDs. The associated use of gastroprotective drugs, such as proton pump inhibitors, reduced the risk in approximately 30% of patients [100, 102, 103]. Systematic reviews that included several diseases, not restricted to the population with SpA, showed greater gastrointestinal safety of iCOX2 [100, 101], but we did not find any significant difference between iCOX2 and traditional NSAIDs in the present meta-analysis (see Fig. 4a and Supplementary Material).

Recommendation 12
In patients with active axSpA, we conditionally recommend to avoid NSAIDs (non-selective or iCOX2) and to start an immunobiologic agent in those with current or previous peptic ulcer or gastrointestinal bleeding.
We conditionally recommend the use of an iCOX2 agent over a traditional NSAID in patients with gastrointestinal risk factors.
We strongly recommend the use of concomitant gastroprotective drugs in symptomatic or high-risk patients. **Quality of evidence: low; Degree of agreement: 8.9**

Is the use of NSAIDs associated with increased cardiovascular risk in axSpA?

There is growing evidence that SpA is associated with increased mortality, especially for cardiovascular diseases,

Table 3 Incidence of adverse events associated with traditional NSAIDs or iCOX2 compared to placebo in patients with axSpA: meta-analysis of randomized clinical trials

	TRADITIONAL NSAIDs *N*=1289	iCOX2 *N*=669
Adverse events	35.6% vs 36.4% (PbO) RR=1.08 (0.93 to 1.25)	54.6% vs 46.4% (PbO) RR=1.22 (0.93 to 1.62)
Severe adverse events	1% vs 0.6% (PbO) RR=1.71 (0.37 to 8.01)	0.6% vs 0.6% (PbO) RR=0.96 (0.17 to 5.53)
Gastrointestinal adverse events	18% vs 9.5% (PbO) **RR=1.92 (1.41 to 2.61)**	17.7% vs 7.5% (PbO) **RR=2.55 (1.92 to 4.95)**
Discontinuation due to adverse events	5% vs 5.5% (PbO) RR=0.76 (0.48 to 1.22)	4.6% vs 3.4% (PbO) RR=2.14 (0.36 to 12.56)

NSAIDs nonsteroidal anti-inflammatory drugs, *iCOX2* selective cyclooxygenase 2 inhibitors, *PbO* placebo, *RR* relative risk

	Study or Subgroup	NSAID Events	NSAID Total	Placebo Events	Placebo Total	Weight	Risk Ratio M-H, Fixed, 95% CI
1	Barkhuizen 2006	78	157	82	156	39.6%	0.95 [0.76, 1.17]
2	Dougados 1994	11	50	20	95	6.6%	1.04 [0.54, 2.00]
3	Dougados 1999	83	352	26	121	18.6%	1.10 [0.74, 1.62]
4	Dougados 2001	54	90	32	76	16.7%	1.43 [1.04, 1.95]
5	van der Heijde 2005	41	99	37	93	18.4%	1.04 [0.74, 1.47]
	Total (95% CI)		**748**		**541**	**100.0%**	**1.08 [0.93, 1.25]**
	Total events	267		197			

Heterogeneity: $Chi^2 = 4.52$, df = 4 (P = 0.34); $I^2 = 12\%$
Test for overall effect: Z = 1.01 (P = 0.31)

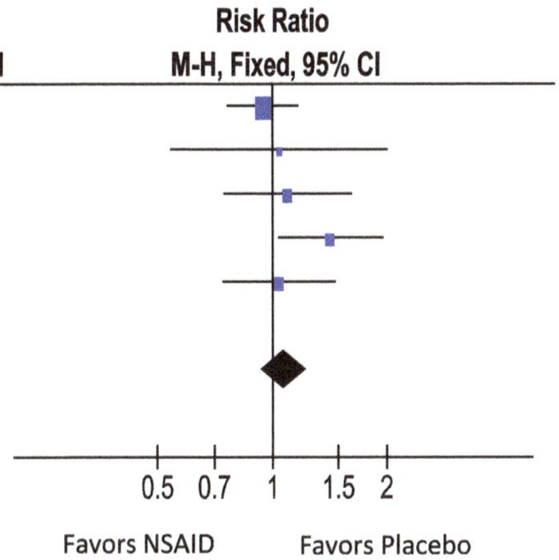

Fig. 5 Incidence of any adverse events in the comparison of traditional NSAIDs versus placebo in patients with ankylosing spondylitis: meta-analysis of five randomized clinical trials. Subtitle: (1) Naproxen 500 mg vs placebo. (2) Ximoprofen 30 mg vs placebo. (3) NSAID (meloxicam 15 mg, meloxicam 22.5 mg, or piroxicam) vs placebo. (4) Ketoprofen 200 mg vs placebo. (5) Naproxen 1000 mg vs placebo

due to multiple factors such as chronic inflammation, associated comorbidities and maybe the drugs used to treat these patients [104–107]. Regarding NSAIDs, large population studies, including a Danish cohort of more than 1 million individuals, suggested 2 to 3-fold increase regarding cardiovascular risk (acute myocardial infarction, stroke, and death from cardiovascular disease) with the chronic use of iCOX2 or nonselective NSAIDs, except for naproxen. Meta-analysis of observational studies estimates an absolute risk of major adverse cardiovascular events (MACE) of approximately 3 per 1000 patients-year with the use of NSAIDs [100, 101, 108, 109]. Furthermore, NSAIDs have been shown to increase mortality in the first 3 to 6 months after acute cardiovascular events [110, 111].

However, in the population with SpA, the relationship of NSAIDs with cardiovascular mortality risk is less clear. Debreuil et al., in a case-control study using a large British database, compared the incidence of acute myocardial infarction (AMI) between a cohort of SpA patients with a cohort of osteoarthritis (OA) patients. Current use of diclofenac (0–180 days prior to index date) compared to remote use (more than 365 days prior to index date) was associated with an increased risk of AMI both in SpA group [adjusted OR=3.32 (95% CI 1.57 to 7.03)] and OA group [(ORa=1.26 (95% CI 1.14 to 1.39)]. Additionally, the risk was different between the two groups [ORa ratio=2.64 (95% CI 1.24 to 5.58, OA as reference)], whereas there was no increased risk of AMI when naproxen was analyzed, either in patients with SpA [(ORa=1.19 (95% CI 0.53 to 2.68)] or in those with OA [112]. Interestingly, other authors have observed a protective effect of NSAIDs against cardiovascular events in patients with axSpA. Haroon et al. studied 21,143 patients with AS compared to 86,606 controls, based on Canadian database, observed a hazard ratio (HR) of 1.36 (95% CI 1.13 to 1.65) for a composite outcome of cardiovascular death. A subgroup analysis of patients older than 65 years demonstrated a protective effect of conventional NSAIDs for

	Study or Subgroup	iCOX2 Events	iCOX2 Total	Placebo Events	Placebo Total	Weight	Risk Ratio M-H, Random, 95% CI
1	Barkhuizen 2006	85	161	82	156	38.8%	1.00 [0.82, 1.24]
2	Dougados 2001	54	80	32	76	31.2%	1.60 [1.18, 2.17]
3	van der Heijde 2005	49	103	37	93	29.9%	1.20 [0.87, 1.65]
	Total (95% CI)		**344**		**325**	**100.0%**	**1.22 [0.93, 1.62]**
	Total events	188		151			

Heterogeneity: $Tau^2 = 0.04$; $Chi^2 = 6.19$, df = 2 (P = 0.05); $I^2 = 68\%$
Test for overall effect: Z = 1.42 (P = 0.16)

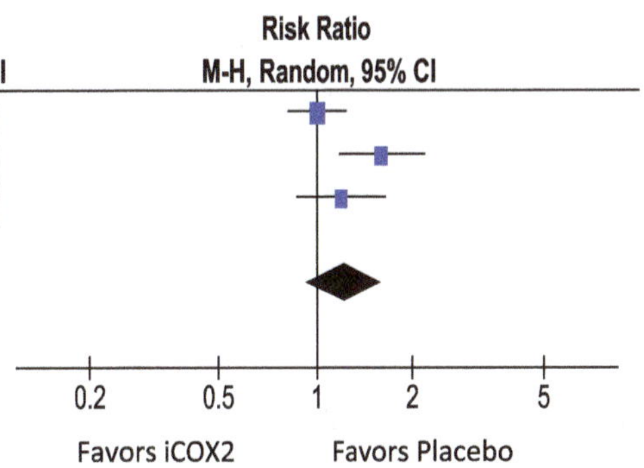

Fig. 6 Incidence of any adverse events in the comparison of selective COX-2 inhibitors versus placebo in patients with ankylosing spondylitis: meta-analysis of three randomized clinical trials. Subtitle: (1) Celecoxib 400 mg vs placebo. (2) Celecoxib 200 mg vs placebo. (3) Etoricoxib 90 mg vs placebo

	Study or Subgroup	NSAID Events	NSAID Total	Placebo Events	Placebo Total	Weight	Risk Ratio M-H, Random, 95% CI
	1.15.1 Gastrointestinal						
1	Barkhuizen 2006	29	157	13	156	10.7%	2.22 [1.20, 4.10]
2	Dougados 1994	11	50	10	95	8.8%	2.09 [0.95, 4.58]
3	Dougados 1999	62	352	10	121	10.5%	2.13 [1.13, 4.02]
4	Dougados 2001	29	90	14	76	11.4%	1.75 [1.00, 3.06]
5	van der Heijde 2005	5	99	5	93	5.4%	0.94 [0.28, 3.14]
	Subtotal (95% CI)		**748**		**541**	**46.9%**	**1.92 [1.41, 2.61]**
	Total events	136		52			
	Heterogeneity: Tau² = 0.00; Chi² = 1.81, df = 4 (P = 0.77); I² = 0%						
	Test for overall effect: Z = 4.16 (P < 0.0001)						
	1.15.2 Respiratory						
6	Barkhuizen 2006	16	157	20	157	10.7%	0.80 [0.43, 1.49]
7	Dougados 1999	1	352	1	121	1.4%	0.34 [0.02, 5.45]
8	Dougados 2001	9	90	9	76	8.0%	0.84 [0.35, 2.02]
9	van der Heijde 2005	2	99	2	93	2.6%	0.94 [0.14, 6.53]
	Subtotal (95% CI)		**698**		**447**	**22.7%**	**0.80 [0.49, 1.30]**
	Total events	28		32			
	Heterogeneity: Tau² = 0.00; Chi² = 0.40, df = 3 (P = 0.94); I² = 0%						
	Test for overall effect: Z = 0.91 (P = 0.36)						
	1.15.3 Hematologic						
10	Dougados 2001	1	90	0	76	1.1%	2.54 [0.10, 61.42]
	Subtotal (95% CI)		**90**		**76**	**1.1%**	**2.54 [0.10, 61.42]**
	Total events	1		0			
	Heterogeneity: Not applicable						
	Test for overall effect: Z = 0.57 (P = 0.57)						
	1.15.4 Neurological						
11	Barkhuizen 2006	3	157	11	156	5.1%	0.27 [0.08, 0.95]
12	Dougados 1999	11	352	7	121	7.5%	0.54 [0.21, 1.36]
13	Dougados 2001	3	90	6	76	4.6%	0.42 [0.11, 1.63]
14	van der Heijde 2005	2	99	3	93	3.1%	0.63 [0.11, 3.66]
	Subtotal (95% CI)		**698**		**446**	**20.3%**	**0.44 [0.24, 0.82]**
	Total events	19		27			
	Heterogeneity: Tau² = 0.00; Chi² = 0.93, df = 3 (P = 0.82); I² = 0%						
	Test for overall effect: Z = 2.60 (P = 0.009)						
	1.15.5 Dermatologic						
15	Barkhuizen 2006	0	157	3	156	1.2%	0.14 [0.01, 2.73]
16	Dougados 1999	10	352	4	121	5.8%	0.86 [0.27, 2.69]
17	Dougados 2001	3	90	1	76	2.0%	2.53 [0.27, 23.86]
	Subtotal (95% CI)		**599**		**353**	**9.1%**	**0.86 [0.27, 2.67]**
	Total events	13		8			
	Heterogeneity: Tau² = 0.19; Chi² = 2.35, df = 2 (P = 0.31); I² = 15%						
	Test for overall effect: Z = 0.27 (P = 0.79)						
	Total (95% CI)		**2833**		**1863**	**100.0%**	**1.07 [0.76, 1.50]**
	Total events	197		119			
	Heterogeneity: Tau² = 0.19; Chi² = 27.93, df = 16 (P = 0.03); I² = 43%						
	Test for overall effect: Z = 0.38 (P = 0.71)						
	Test for subgroup differences: Chi² = 22.34, df = 4 (P = 0.0002), I² = 82.1%						

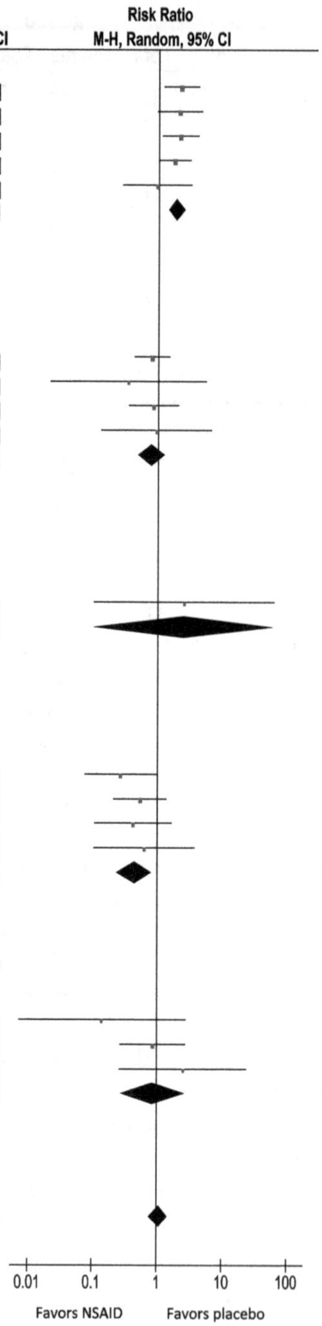

Fig. 7 Incidence of adverse events per organic system in the comparison of traditional NSAIDs versus placebo in patients with ankylosing spondylitis: meta-analyses of five randomized clinical trials. Subtitle: (1) Naproxen 500 mg vs placebo. (2) Ximoprofen 30 mg vs placebo. (3) NSAIDs (meloxicam 15 mg, meloxicam 22.5 mg, or piroxicam) vs placebo. (4) Ketoprofen 200 mg vs placebo. (5) Naproxen 1000 mg vs placebo. (6) Naproxen 500 mg vs placebo. (7) NSAIDs (meloxicam 15 mg, meloxicam 22.5 mg, or piroxicam) vs placebo. (8) Ketoprofen 200 mg vs placebo. (9) Naproxen 1000 mg vs placebo. (10) Ketoprofen 200 mg vs placebo. (11) Naproxen 500 mg vs placebo. (12) NSAIDs (meloxicam 15 mg, meloxicam 22.5 mg or piroxicam) vs placebo. (13) Ketoprofen 200 mg vs placebo. (14) Naproxen 1000 mg vs placebo. (15) Naproxen 500 mg vs placebo. (16) NSAIDs (meloxicam 15 mg, meloxicam 22.5 mg or piroxicam) vs placebo. (17) Ketoprofen 200 mg vs placebo

cardiovascular death [HR=0.1 (95% CI 0.01 to 0.61)] [105]. Tsai et al., using data from the Taiwan Health Insurance, observed a reduced risk of MACE after 12 months in patients with AS who had prolonged use of NSAIDs (> 80% of the observation time) [23]. Another Taiwan case-control study found negative association between the use of celecoxib (versus non-users) and coronary events [OR=0.34 (95% CI 0.13 to 0.89)] in AS patients [26]. Other publications

	Study or Subgroup	iCOX2 Events	iCOX2 Total	Placebo Events	Placebo Total	Weight	Risk Ratio M-H, Random, 95% CI
	2.15.1 Gastrointestinal events						
	Barkhuizen 2006	21	161	13	156	13.1%	1.57 [0.81, 3.02]
1	Dougados 2001	27	80	14	176	13.8%	4.24 [2.35, 7.65]
2	van der Heijde 2005	13	103	5	93	9.7%	2.35 [0.87, 6.33]
3	Subtotal (95% CI)		344		425	36.7%	2.55 [1.32, 4.95]
	Total events	61		32			
	Heterogeneity: Tau² = 0.20; Chi² = 5.01, df = 2 (P = 0.08); I² = 60%						
	Test for overall effect: Z = 2.77 (P = 0.006)						
	2.15.2 Respiratory events						
	Barkhuizen 2006	14	161	20	156	13.2%	0.68 [0.36, 1.29]
4	Dougados 2001	5	80	4	76	7.5%	1.19 [0.33, 4.26]
5	van der Heijde 2005	1	103	3	93	3.4%	0.30 [0.03, 2.84]
6	Subtotal (95% CI)		344		325	24.1%	0.72 [0.41, 1.26]
	Total events	20		27			
	Heterogeneity: Tau² = 0.00; Chi² = 1.20, df = 2 (P = 0.55); I² = 0%						
	Test for overall effect: Z = 1.16 (P = 0.25)						
	2.15.3 Neurological events						
	Barkhuizen 2006	13	161	11	156	11.9%	1.15 [0.53, 2.48]
7	Dougados 2001	6	80	6	76	8.9%	0.95 [0.32, 2.82]
8	van der Heijde 2005	8	103	3	93	7.4%	2.41 [0.66, 8.81]
9	Subtotal (95% CI)		344		325	28.2%	1.25 [0.71, 2.21]
	Total events	27		20			
	Heterogeneity: Tau² = 0.00; Chi² = 1.28, df = 2 (P = 0.53); I² = 0%						
	Test for overall effect: Z = 0.78 (P = 0.43)						
	2.15.4 Dermatologic events						
	Barkhuizen 2006	8	161	3	56	7.4%	0.93 [0.25, 3.37]
10	Dougados 2001	4	80	1	76	3.6%	3.80 [0.43, 33.24]
11	Subtotal (95% CI)		241		132	11.0%	1.43 [0.39, 5.16]
	Total events	12		4			
	Heterogeneity: Tau² = 0.19; Chi² = 1.22, df = 1 (P = 0.27); I² = 18%						
	Test for overall effect: Z = 0.54 (P = 0.59)						
	Total (95% CI)		1273		1207	100.0%	1.46 [0.93, 2.32]
	Total events	120		83			
	Heterogeneity: Tau² = 0.31; Chi² = 23.48, df = 10 (P = 0.009); I² = 57%						
	Test for overall effect: Z = 1.63 (P = 0.10)						
	Test for subgroup differences: Chi² = 8.28, df = 3 (P = 0.04), I² = 63.8%						

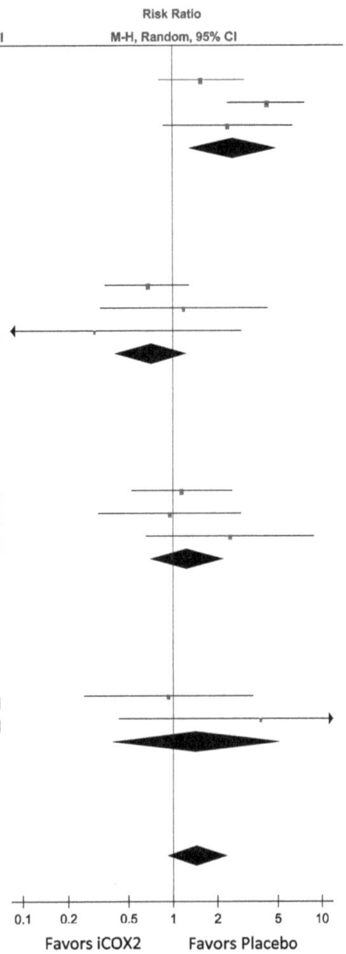

Fig. 8 Incidence of adverse events per organ system in the comparison of selective COX-2 inhibitors versus placebo in patients with ankylosing spondylitis: meta-analysis of three randomized clinical trials. Subtitle: 1) Celecoxib 400 mg vs placebo. (2) Celecoxib 200 mg vs placebo. (3) Etoricoxib 90 mg vs placebo. (4) Celecoxib 400 mg vs placebo. (5) Celecoxib 200 mg vs placebo. (6) Etoricoxib 90 mg vs placebo. (7) Celecoxib 400 mg vs placebo. (8) Celecoxib 200 mg vs placebo. (9) Etoricoxib 90 mg vs placebo. (10) Celecoxib 400 mg vs placebo. (11) Celecoxib 200 mg vs placebo

also suggest the protective effect of NSAIDs against cardiovascular events, but the data should be interpreted with caution because patients with more comorbidities and risk factors tend to be less exposed to NSAIDs [17, 106]. In summary, it is still controversial whether the beneficial effect of reducing inflammation would outweigh the negative effects of NSAIDs per se regarding cardiovascular risk.

The present systematic review, which included only RCTs and not observational studies, did not find higher cardiovascular risk when comparing traditional NSAIDs or iCOX2 versus placebo. Two RCTs compared traditional NSAIDs versus iCOX2 on cardiovascular events incidence [2% (4/175) and 0% (0/170), respectively] and no significant difference in meta-analysis [RR=0.22 (95% CI 0.03 to 1.93)] was observed [38, 49].

Furthermore, the panel decided to conditionally recommend caution when prescribing NSAIDs in patients with cardiovascular risks factors, specially in those with a recent myocardial infarction or stroke.

Recommendation 13
In patients with active axSpA, we conditionally recommend to avoid NSAID therapy and to start an immunobiologic agent in those with cardiovascular risk factors, mainly in those with previous acute myocardial infarction or stroke, especially if recent (past 12 months).
Quality of evidence: very low; Degree of agreement: 8.4

Are NSAIDs associated with increased renal risk in patients with axSpA?

The RCTs selected for this systematic review did not report renal toxicity from NSAIDs in patients with axSpA. Similarly to the cardiovascular toxicity, the renal adverse events evidences were obtained from data including other populations. A large cohort study (183,

446 patients; 80% women; mean age of 78 years) found an incidence of 0.5% (1 in 200 new treatments) of acute kidney injury (AKI), requiring hospitalization, in a period of up to 45 days after the onset of NSAIDs [113]. A meta-analysis evaluated 28,992 patients and demonstrated a RR of AKI associated with NSAIDs ranging from 1.25 to 2.21 that was statistically significant for several NSAIDs [114]. Regarding the possibility of progression to chronic kidney disease, a prospective study with 10,184 patients (57% women; mean age 76 years) found RR=1.26 (95% CI 1.04 to 1.53) for a reduction of glomerular filtration rate of at least 15 ml/min/1.73 m^2 among NSAID users when compared with non-users during a median follow-up of 2.75 years [115].

Does the use of NSAIDs increase the risk of adverse events in other organs/systems in axSpA?

Considering five RCTs of non-selective NSAIDs versus placebo and three of iCOX2 versus placebo, neither the meta-analysis nor individual studies found an increase in respiratory, hematological, dermatologic, or neurological adverse events [44–48]. Additionally, no significant differences were found in the comparison of iCOX2 versus traditional NSAIDs [38, 40, 44, 45, 48, 49]. In the comparison of NSAIDs with other NSAIDs, selective or not for COX-2, only indomethacin was associated with a greater number of neurological adverse events [80, 83, 86]. Despite data from general population have suggested some hepatotoxic effect of NSAIDs, no specific RCTs were found for NSAIDs versus placebo in patients with axSpA [116]. The current meta-analysis found greater hepatic toxicity for iCOX2 compared to non-selective NSAIDs, but with high imprecision data and at the limit of statistical significance (Figs. 7 and 8).

Recommendation 14

In patients with active axSpA, we conditionally recommend to avoid NSAIDs and to start an immunobiologic agent in thoses with increased risk of renal adverse events. The decision should be individualized and risk/benefits shared with the patient.

We strongly recommend caution and regular monitoring of renal function, especially in high-risk individuals (elderly, hypertension, diabetes, kidney dysfunction). **Quality of evidence: very low; Degree of agreement: 9.4**

Conclusions

The most recently published guidelines for the management of axSpA recommended NSAIDs as the first line treatment, but none of them has addressed specifically the current role of NSAIDs in the treatment of patients with axSpA regarding efficacy, safety and therapeutic strategy [6, 7, 71]. The present systematic review and critical analysis of the available evidences have confirmed that NSAIDs are still the basis for the treatment of patients with axSpA, as they are effective in most part of those patients.

There is no doubt that the immunobiologic agents are quite effective and brought great benefit for the management of axSpA, but they carry a high cost which demands the best rationale for prescribing them. Our recommendations, in consonance with the most important guidelines, strengthen the statement that NSAIDs are the first line treatment in patients with axSpA and they should be started as soon as the diagnosis is confirmed.

The benefit of NSAIDs in delaying radiographic progression in axSpA and if immunobiologics should be the first line treatment in patients with poor prognostic criteria (elevated CRP, smokers and those with previous syndesmophytes) remain an open question.

This review has also shown that NSAIDs have a good safety profile and are usually well tolerated for the long-term use. The concerns about the cardiovascular and renal side effects are based mostly in data from other populations, but not in patients with axSpA that are usually younger and have less comorbidities and risk factors than other NSAID's long-term or frequently users, like patients with osteoarthritis for example.

One possible limitation of these recommendations is that we did not include a patient representative in the voting panel. This strategy could be used in future guidelines.

The purpose of these guidelines was to provide recommendations elaborated by a panel of rheumatologists with expertise in the field of SpA, mainly to support clinician's decision making, without taking out his/her autonomy to choose the best therapeutic option for an individual patient.

Abbreviations

AxSpA: Axial Spondyloarthritis; AS: Ankylosing Spondylitis; PsA: Psoriatic Arthritis; ASAS: Ankylosing Spondylitis Assessment Study Group; RCT: Randomized Clinical Trial; TNFi: Tumor Necrosis Factor inhibitor; IL17i: Interleukin-17 inhibitor; NSAID: Nonsteroidal Anti-inflammatory Drug; iCOX2: Specific Cycloxigenase-2 inhibitor; BASDAI: Bath Ankylosing Spondylitis Disease Activity Index; ASDAS: Ankylosing Spondylitis Disease Activity Score; BASFI: Bath Ankylosing Spondylitis Disease Functional Index; PAIN50%: ≥ 50% improvement in pain; MD: Mean Difference; SMD: Standard Mean Difference; CRP: C Reactive Protein; ESR: Erythrocyte Sedimentation Rate; PAIN-VAS: Pain by Visual Analogue Scale; PGA: Patient Global Assessment of disease activity; ASAS20: At least 20% improvement according to ASAS response criteria; ASAS40: At least 40% improvement according to ASAS response criteria; mSASSS: modified Stoke Ankylosing Spondylitis Spine Score

Acknowledgements

We thank Haliton Alves de Oliveira Junior and Anna Maria Buehler for technical support in the systematic review, statistical assistance and for performing the meta-analyses.

Authors' contributions

All authors made contributions to the acquisition of data, have been involved in drafting the manuscript or revising it critically for important intellectual content, participated in the voting rounds, gave final approval of the version to be published and have participated sufficiently in the work to take public responsibility for appropriate portions of the content.

Competing interests

Ricardo da Cruz Lage received lecture fees from Abbvie, Pfizer and Novartis; sponsorship for events from Janssen, Novartis, Pfizer and Abbvie; research payments from Abbvie.
Cláudia Diniz Lopes Marques received lecture fees from Abbvie, Janssen, Pfizer and Novartis; advisory board from Novartis and Abbvie; sponsorship for events from Abbvie, Janssen, Pfizer, Novartis, and Lilly.
Thauana Luíza Oliveira received lecturer fees from Abbvie, Novartis and Janssen; support to congresses from Abbvie and Janssen.
Gustavo Gomes Resende received lecture fees from Abbvie, Janssen, Novartis, Pfizer, and UCB; advisory board from Abbvie, Janssen, and Novartis; Research support from Brazilian Society of Rheumatology, FAPEMIG and UCB; clinical research payments from Abbvie and Pfizer; sponsorship for scientific events from Abbvie, Janssen, Lilly, Novartis, Pfizer, and UCB.
Charles Lubianca Kohen received financial support for advisory board participation from Novartis; speaker fee from Janssen, Abbvie, Novartis, Pfizer, UCB; support to events from Janssen, Abbvie, Roche, Astra-Zeneca, Novartis.
Carla Gonçalves Saad has no conflicts of interest.
Antônio Carlos Ximenes received payments for participation in clinical research from Abbvvie, Pfizer, Roche, BMS, and Amgen; on scientific board of Pfizer, and Abbivie; as a lecturer from AbbVie, Pfizer, and Abbott.
Célio Roberto Gonçalves has no conflicts of interest.
Washington Alves Bianchi has no conflicts of interest.
Eduardo de Souza Meirelles received payments as a speaker from Novartis, Abbvie, Abbott and Marjan; research grants from Novartis and Pfizer; support for conferences and courses from Aché, Pfizer, Novartis, Janssen, Abbvie, Roche, and Lilly; Advisory board fee from Novartis and Marjan.
Mauro Waldemar Keiserman received financial support for lectures, advisory bord and clinical research from Abbvie, Actelion, Biogen, Bristol, Celltrion, Lilly, Human Genome Sceiences, Janssen, Pfizer, Novartis, Roche, Sanofi, and UCB.
Adriano Chiereghin received honoraria as a speaker from Janssen, Novartis, UCB, and Pfizer; support to courses and congresses from Abbvie, Janssen, Novartis, UCB, and Pfizer; advisory board from Novartis and Janssen.
Cristiano Barbosa Campanholo received financial support for advisory board participation from Janssen, Abbvie, Bristol, Lilly, Novartis, Pfizer, UCB; speaker fee from Janssen, Abbvie, Lilly, Novartis, and Pfizer, UCB; support to events from Janssen, Abbvie, Bristol, Novartis, and Pfizer.
Andre Marun Lyrio received payments from Speaker of Janssen and UCB; support to courses/congresses from Janssen, Abbvie, Pfizer, UBC, Novartis, and Lily.
Cláudia Goldenstein Schainberg has participated in the pharmaceutical advisory board of AbbVie, Janssen, Lilly, Novartis, and Pfizer; is a speaker invited by AbbVie, Janssen, Lilly, Novartis, Pfizer; has no stock of these pharmaceutical industries.

Lenise Brandao Pieruccetti has no conflicts of interest.
Michel Alexandre Yazbek received financial support from Abbvie, UCB, Novartis and Lilly.
Penelope Esther Palominos has no conflicts of interest.
Rafaela Silva Guimarães Goncalves received fees for lectures from Janssen, Novertis, Abbvie, Apsen, Bristol, and Pfizer; advisory board from Janssen.
Rodrigo Luppino Assad received fees for lectures and advisory board from Abbvie, Novartis, Janssen, UCB, Lilly, and Bristol; research support from Abbvie and UCB.
Rubens Bonfiglioli received financial support for clinical research from Roche, Pfizer, Amgen, and Novartis; for scientific advisory from Lilly, Abbvie, Roche, and UCB; for support to events from Roche, Pfizer, Abbvie and Novartis; for symposia and sponsored meetings from Roche, Pfizer, and Janssen.
Sônia Maria Alvarenga Anti received financial support from Abbvie, Jansen, Novartis, Lilly, and UCB.

Sueli Coelho da Silva Carneiro received honorary speaker from Abbvie, Janssen, Lilly, Novartis and Pfizer; support to research from CNPq and FAPE RJ; support for congresses from Abbvie, Janssen, Novartis, Pfizer, CNPq and FAPERJ; advisory board from Janssen, Lilly, and Novartis.
Valderílio Feijó Azevedo is GRAPPA member; Medical diretor of Edumed Biotech; received for clinical research from Pfizer, Roche, Janssen, Bristol, Abbvie, Medimmune, Boehringer, GSK, USB, Sanofi, Takeda, Bird Rock Bio, and NovoNordisk; financial support to events and lectures from Pfizer, Hospira, Roche, MSD, BMS, Merck Senoro, Janssen, Novertis, Celltrion, UCB, and AztraZeneca.
Cleandro Pires Albuquerque has no conflicts of interest.
Wanderley Marques Bernardo has no conflicts of interest.
Percival Degrava Sampaio-Barros received for participation in lectures, boards or scientific events from laboratories Abbvie, Janssen, Novartis, Pfizer and UCB.
Marcelo de Medeiros Pinheiro received financial support for advisory board from Novartis and Janssen; by lectures from Novartis, Janssen, Abbvie.

Author details

[1]Universidade Federal de Minas Gerais (UFMG), Alameda Álvaro Celso 175, Ambulatório Bias Fortes, 2° andar, Belo Horizonte, MG 30150-260, Brazil. [2]Universidade Federal de Pernambuco (UFPE), Recife, PE, Brazil. [3]Universidade Federal de São Paulo (UNIFESP/ EPM), São Paulo, SP, Brazil. [4]Universidade Federal do Rio Grande do Sul (UFRGS), Porto Alegre, Brazil. [5]Universidade de São Paulo (USP), São Paulo, SP, Brazil. [6]Hospital Estadual Geral de Goiania (HGG), Goiânia, Brazil. [7]Santa Casa de Misericórdia (SCM) do Rio de Janeiro, Rio de Janeiro, RJ, Brazil. [8]Pontifícia Universidade Católica (PUC) de Porto Alegre, Porto Alegre, RS, Brazil. [9]Pontifícia Universidade Católica (PUC) de Sorocaba, Sorocaba, SP, Brazil. [10]Santa Casa de Misericórdia (SCM) de São Paulo, São Paulo, SP, Brazil. [11]Pontifícia Universidade Católica (PUC) de Campinas, Campinas, SP, Brazil. [12]Hospital Heliópolis, São Paulo, SP, Brazil. [13]Universidade Estadual de Campinas (UNICAMP), Campinas, SP, Brazil. [14]Ribeirão Preto, Ribeirão Preto, Brazil. [15]Hospital do Servidor Público do Estado de São Paulo, São Paulo, SP, Brazil. [16]Universidade Federal do Rio De Janeiro (UFRJ), Rio de Janeiro, RJ, Brazil. [17]Universidade Federal do Paraná (UFPR), Curitiba, PR, Brazil. [18]Universidade de Brasília (UnB), Brasília, DF, Brazil.

References

1. Rudwaleit M, Landewe R, van der Heijde D, Listing J, Brandt J, Braun J, et al. The development of Assessment of SpondyloArthritis international Society classification criteria for axial spondyloarthritis (part I): classification of paper patients by expert opinion including uncertainty appraisal. Ann Rheum Dis. 2009;68(6):770–6.
2. Rudwaleit M, van der Heijde D, Landewe R, Akkoc N, Brandt J, Chou CT, et al. The Assessment of SpondyloArthritis International Society classification criteria for peripheral spondyloarthritis and for spondyloarthritis in general. Ann Rheum Dis. 2011;70(1):25–31.
3. Rudwaleit M, van der Heijde D, Landewe R, Listing J, Akkoc N, Brandt J, et al. The development of Assessment of SpondyloArthritis international Society classification criteria for axial spondyloarthritis (part II): validation and final selection. Ann Rheum Dis. 2009;68(6):777–83.
4. van der Linden S, Valkenburg HA, Cats A. Evaluation of diagnostic criteria for ankylosing spondylitis. A proposal for modification of the New York criteria. Arthritis Rheum. 1984;27(4):361–8.
5. Sieper J, van der Heijde D. Review: Nonradiographic axial spondyloarthritis: new definition of an old disease? Arthritis Rheum. 2013;65(3):543–51.
6. van der Heijde D, Ramiro S, Landewe R, Baraliakos X, Van den Bosch F, Sepriano A, et al. 2016 update of the ASAS-EULAR management recommendations for axial spondyloarthritis. Ann Rheum Dis. 2017;76(6): 978–91.
7. Resende GG, Meirelles ES, Marques CDL, Chiereghin A, Lyrio AM, Ximenes AC, et al. The Brazilian Society of Rheumatology guidelines for axial spondyloarthritis - 2019. Adv Rheumatol. 2020;60(1):19.
8. FPB K, der Burg LRA v, Ramiro S, RBM L, Buchbinder R, Falzon L, et al. Non-steroidal anti-inflammatory drugs (NSAIDs) for axial spondyloarthritis (ankylosing spondylitis and non-radiographic axial spondyloarthritis). Cochrane Database Syst Rev. 2015;17(7):CD010952-CD.
9. Baraliakos X, Kiltz U, Peters S, Appel H, Dybowski F, Igelmann M, et al. Efficiency of treatment with non-steroidal anti-inflammatory drugs according to current recommendations in patients with radiographic and non-radiographic axial spondyloarthritis. Rheumatology (Oxford). 2017;56(1): 95–102.
10. Bhuvanesh M, Balaji C, Saranya C, Ramesh R, Tamilselvam T, Rajeswari S.

Serum levels of tumor necrosis factor-alpha and vascular endothelial growth factor as markers of disease activity in patients with axial spondyloarthritis. Indian J Rheumatol. 2018;13(1):9–13.

11. Essers I, Stolwijk C, Boonen A, De Bruin ML, Bazelier MT, de Vries F, et al. Ankylosing spondylitis and risk of ischaemic heart disease: a population-based cohort study. Ann Rheum Dis. 2016;75(1):203–9.
12. Gaydukova IZ, Gamayunova Cyrillic A cKA, Dorogoykina KD, Rebrov AP. Efficiency of different celecoxib regimens in patients with active axial spondyloarthritis: Results of the 4-week pilot open-label comparative single-center study 'AIM'. Ter Arkh. 2017;89(6):78–83.
13. Gaydukova IZ, Rebrov AP. Efficiency and safety of different etoricoxib regimens in patients with axial spondyloarthritis, including ankylosing spondylitis. Ter Arkh. 2015;87(3):77–82.
14. Gratacos J, Moreno Martinez-Losa M, Font P, Montilla C, Fernandez-Espartero C, Linares LF, et al. Etoricoxib in ankylosing spondylitis: is there a role for active patients refractory to traditional NSAIDs? Clin Exp Rheumatol. 2016;34(1):94–9.
15. Guellec D, Nocturne G, Tatar Z, Pham T, Sellam J, Cantagrel A, et al. Should non-steroidal anti-inflammatory drugs be used continuously in ankylosing spondylitis? Joint Bone Spine. 2014;81(4):308–12.
16. Karateev A, Chernikhova E, Erdes S. AB0735 Upper Gastrointestinal Tract Pathology in Patients with Ankylosing Spondylitis. Ann Rheum Dis. 2015; 74(Suppl 2):1144 LP.
17. Kristensen LE, Jakobsen AK, Askling J, Nilsson F, Jacobsson LTH. Safety of Etoricoxib, Celecoxib, and Nonselective Nonsteroidal Antiinflammatory Drugs in Ankylosing Spondylitis and Other Spondyloarthritis Patients: A Swedish National Population-Based Cohort Study. Arthritis Care Res. 2015; 67(8):1137–49.
18. Maas F, Spoorenberg A, van der Slik BPG, van der Veer E, Brouwer E, Bootsma H, et al. Clinical Risk Factors for the Presence and Development of Vertebral Fractures in Patients With Ankylosing Spondylitis. Arthritis Care Res. 2017;69(5):694–702.
19. Molto A, Granger B, Wendling D, Dougados M, Gossec L. Use of nonsteroidal anti-inflammatory drugs in early axial spondyloarthritis in daily practice: Data from the DESIR cohort. Joint Bone Spine. 2017;84(1):79–82.
20. Regel A, Sepriano A, Baraliakos X, van der Heijde D, Braun J, Landewe R, et al. Efficacy and safety of non-pharmacological and non-biological pharmacological treatment: a systematic literature review informing the 2016 update of the ASAS/EULAR recommendations for the management of axial spondyloarthritis. RMD Open. 2017;3(1):e000397-e.
21. Tam H-W, Yeo K-J, Leong P-Y, Chen C-H, Li Y-C, Ma C-M, et al. Sulfasalazine might reduce risk of cardiovascular diseases in patients with ankylosing spondylitis: A nationwide population-based retrospective cohort study. Int J Rheum Dis. 2017;20(3):363–70.
22. Tang M, Xue L, Shen Y, Bo L, Yang R, Wen J, et al. Efficacy of long-term nonsteroidal antiinflammatory drug treatment on magnetic resonance imaging-determined bone marrow oedema in early, active axial spondyloarthritis patients. Clin Rheumatol. 2018;37(1):245–50.
23. Tsai W-C, Ou T-T, Yen J-H, Wu C-C, Tung Y-C. Long-term frequent use of non-steroidal anti-inflammatory drugs might protect patients with ankylosing spondylitis from cardiovascular diseases: a nationwide case-control study. PLoS One. 2015;10(5):e0126347-e.
24. Varkas G, Jans L, Cypers H, Van Praet L, Carron P, Elewaut D, et al. Brief Report: Six-Week Treatment of Axial Spondyloarthritis Patients With an Optimal Dose of Nonsteroidal Antiinflammatory Drugs: Early Response to Treatment in Signal Intensity on Magnetic Resonance Imaging of the Sacroiliac Joints. Arthritis Rheumatol (Hoboken, NJ). 2016;68(3):672–8.
25. Wang R, Dasgupta A, Ward MM. Comparative efficacy of non-steroidal anti-inflammatory drugs in ankylosing spondylitis: a Bayesian network meta-analysis of clinical trials. Ann Rheum Dis. 2016;75(6):1152–60.
26. Wu L-C, Leong P-Y, Yeo K-J, Li T-Y, Wang Y-H, Chiou J-Y, et al. Celecoxib and sulfasalazine had negative association with coronary artery diseases in patients with ankylosing spondylitis: A nation-wide, population-based case-control study. Medicine. 2016;95(36):e4792-e.
27. Couderc M, Pereira B, Molto A, Tiple A, Soubrier M, Dougados M. The Prevalence of Renal Impairment in Patients with Spondyloarthritis: Results from the International ASAS-COMOSPA Study. J Rheumatol. 2018;45(6):795–801.
28. Dregan A, Chowienczyk P, Molokhia M. Cardiovascular and type 2 diabetes morbidity and all-cause mortality among diverse chronic inflammatory disorders. Heart (British Cardiac Society). 2017;103(23):1867–73.
29. Fattahi MJ, Jamshidi AR, Mahmoudi M, Vojdanian M, Yekaninejad MS, Jafarnezhad-Ansariha F, et al. Evaluation of the efficacy and safety of beta-d-mannuronic acid in patients with ankylosing spondylitis: A 12-week randomized, placebo-controlled, phase I/II clinical trial. Int Immunopharmacol. 2018;54:112–7.
30. Gao G, Lu L, Li Z, Li Y. THU0367 The influences of non-steroidal anti-inflammatory drugs on serum VEGF and BMP-2 levels in patients with axial spondyloarthritis. Ann Rheum Dis. 2017;76(Suppl 2):344 LP.
31. Gao G-M, Li Y-M, Zheng X-L, Jiang D-B, Zhang L-L, Xu P-H, et al. The Efficacy of Imrecoxib and Celecoxib in Axial Spondyloarthritis and Their Influence on Serum Dickopff-Related Protein 1 (DKK-1) Levels. Med Sci Monit. 2017;23: 2985–92.
32. Jafarnezhad-Ansariha F, Yekaninejad MS, Jamshidi A-R, Mansouri R, Vojdanian M, Mahmoudi M, et al. The effects of beta-D-mannuronic acid (M2000), as a novel NSAID, on COX1 and COX2 activities and gene expression in ankylosing spondylitis patients and the murine monocyte/macrophage, J774 cell line. Inflammopharmacology. 2018;26(2):375–84.
33. Bedaiwi M, Thavaneswaran A, Haroon N, Anton A, Inman R. Profiling ankylosing spondylitis patients likely to respond to NSAID treatment; 2014.
34. Zengin O, Kısacık B, Kimyon G, Uyar N, Onat AM. AB0751 Treatment Response in Spondylitis Without Sacroiliitis to Nonsteroidal Antiinflammatory Drugs is More Difficult than Axial Spondyloarthritis. Ann Rheum Dis. 2015;74(Suppl 2):1150.1.
35. Sánchez MD, Montilla-Morales CA, Gómez-Castro S, Hidalgo-Calleja C, Carranco-Medina T, Calero-Paniagua I, et al. AB0705 Nonsteroidal Antiinflammatory Drugs and Bone Mineral Density and Fractures in Patients with Ankylosing Spondylitis. Ann Rheum Dis. 2014;73(Suppl 2):1037 LP.
36. Shukla A, Rai MK, Prasad N, Agarwal V. Short-term non-steroid anti-inflammatory drug use in spondyloarthritis patients induces subclinical acute kidney injury: biomarkers study. Nephron. 2017;135(4):277–86.
37. Bedaiwi MK, Sari I, Wallis D, O'Shea FD, Salonen D, Haroon N, et al. Clinical efficacy of celecoxib compared to acetaminophen in chronic nonspecific low back pain: results of a randomized controlled trial. Arthritis Care Res. 2016;68(6):845–52.
38. Huang F, Gu J, Liu Y, Zhu P, Zheng Y, Fu J, et al. Efficacy and safety of celecoxib in chinese patients with ankylosing spondylitis: a 6-week randomized, double-blinded study with 6-week open-label extension treatment. Curr Ther Res Clin Exp. 2014;76:126–33.
39. Sieper J, van der Heijde D, Dougados M, Mease PJ, Maksymowych WP, Brown MA, et al. Efficacy and safety of adalimumab in patients with non-radiographic axial spondyloarthritis: results of a randomised placebo-controlled trial (ABILITY-1). Ann Rheum Dis. 2013;72(6):815–22.
40. Walker C, Essex MN, Li C, Park PW. Celecoxib versus diclofenac for the treatment of ankylosing spondylitis: 12-week randomized study in Norwegian patients. J Int Med Res. 2016;44(3):483–95.
41. Balazcs E, Sieper J, Bickham K, Mehta A, Frontera N, Stryszak P, et al. A randomized, clinical trial to assess the relative efficacy and tolerability of two doses of etoricoxib versus naproxen in patients with ankylosing spondylitis. BMC Musculoskelet Disord. 2016;17(1):426.
42. Guyatt G, Oxman AD, Akl EA, Kunz R, Vist G, Brozek J, et al. GRADE guidelines: 1. Introduction-GRADE evidence profiles and summary of findings tables. J Clin Epidemiol. 2011;64(4):383–94.
43. Guyatt GH, Oxman AD, Kunz R, Falck-Ytter Y, Vist GE, Liberati A, et al. Going from evidence to recommendations. Bmj. 2008;336(7652):1049–51.
44. Barkhuizen A, Steinfeld S, Robbins J, West C, Coombs J, Zwillich S. Celecoxib is efficacious and well tolerated in treating signs and symptoms of ankylosing spondylitis. J Rheumatol. 2006;33(9):1805–12.
45. Dougados M, Behier JM, Jolchine I, Calin A, van der Heijde D, Olivieri I, et al. Efficacy of celecoxib, a cyclooxygenase 2-specific inhibitor, in the treatment of ankylosing spondylitis: a six-week controlled study with comparison against placebo and against a conventional nonsteroidal antiinflammatory drug. Arthritis Rheum. 2001;44(1):180–5.
46. Dougados M, Gueguen A, Nakache JP, Velicitat P, Veys EM, Zeidler H, et al. Ankylosing spondylitis: what is the optimum duration of a clinical study? A one year versus a 6 weeks non-steroidal anti-inflammatory drug trial. Rheumatology (Oxford). 1999;38(3):235–44.
47. Dougados M, Nguyen M, Caporal R, Legeais J, Bouxin-Sauzet A, Pellegri-Guegnault B, et al. Ximoprofen in ankylosing spondylitis. A double blind placebo controlled dose ranging study. Scand J Rheumatol. 1994;23(5):243–8.
48. van der Heijde D, Baraf HSB, Ramos-Remus C, Calin A, Weaver AL, Schiff M, et al. Evaluation of the efficacy of etoricoxib in ankylosing spondylitis: results

of a fifty-two-week, randomized, controlled study. Arthritis Rheum. 2005; 52(4):1205–15.

49. Sieper J, Klopsch T, Richter M, Kapelle A, Rudwaleit M, Schwank S, et al. Comparison of two different dosages of celecoxib with diclofenac for the treatment of active ankylosing spondylitis: results of a 12-week randomised, double-blind, controlled study. Ann Rheum Dis. 2008;67(3):323–9.
50. Gossec L, van der Heijde D, Melian A, Krupa DA, James MK, Cavanaugh PF, et al. Efficacy of cyclo-oxygenase-2 inhibition by etoricoxib and naproxen on the axial manifestations of ankylosing spondylitis in the presence of peripheral arthritis. Ann Rheum Dis. 2005;64(11):1563–7.
51. Villa Alcazar LF, de Buergo M, Rico Lenza H, Montull Fruitos E. Aceclofenac is as safe and effective as tenoxicam in the treatment of ankylosing spondylitis: a 3 month multicenter comparative trial. Spanish Study Group on Aceclofenac in Ankylosing Spondylitis. J Rheumatol. 1996;23(7):1194–9.
52. Ebner W, Poal Ballarin JM, Boussina I. Meclofenamate sodium in the treatment of ankylosing spondylitis. Report of a European double-blind controlled multicenter study. Arzneimittel-Forschung. 1983;33(4A):660–3.
53. Good A, Mena H. Treatment of ankylosing spondylitis with flurbiprofen and indomethacin. Curr Med Res Opin. 1977;5(1):117–21.
54. Zochling J, Bohl-Buhler MH, Baraliakos X, Feldtkeller E, Braun J. Nonsteroidal anti-inflammatory drug use in ankylosing spondylitis--a population-based survey. Clin Rheumatol. 2006;25(6):794–800.
55. Carbo MJG, Spoorenberg A, Maas F, Brouwer E, Bos R, Bootsma H, et al. Ankylosing spondylitis disease activity score is related to NSAID use, especially in patients treated with TNF-alpha inhibitors. PLoS One. 2018; 13(4):e0196.
56. Zochling J, van der Heijde D, Dougados M, Braun J. Current evidence for the management of ankylosing spondylitis: a systematic literature review for the ASAS/EULAR management recommendations in ankylosing spondylitis. Ann Rheum Dis. 2006;65(4):423–32.
57. Coates LC, Kavanaugh A, Mease PJ, Soriano ER, Laura Acosta-Felquer M, Armstrong AW, et al. Group for Research and Assessment of Psoriasis and Psoriatic Arthritis 2015 Treatment Recommendations for Psoriatic Arthritis. Arthritis Rheum. 2016;68(5):1060–71.
58. Gossec L, Smolen JS, Ramiro S, de Wit M, Cutolo M, Dougados M, et al. European League Against Rheumatism (EULAR) recommendations for the management of psoriatic arthritis with pharmacological therapies: 2015 update. Ann Rheum Dis. 2016;75(3):499–510.
59. Sieper J, Lenaerts J, Wollenhaupt J, Rudwaleit M, Mazurov VI, Myasoutova L, et al. Efficacy and safety of infliximab plus naproxen versus naproxen alone in patients with early, active axial spondyloarthritis: results from the double-blind, placebo-controlled INFAST study, Part 1. Ann Rheum Dis. 2014;73(1):101–7.
60. Sieper J, Lenaerts J, Wollenhaupt J, Rudwaleit M, Mazurov VI, Myasoutova L, et al. Maintenance of biologic-free remission with naproxen or no treatment in patients with early, active axial spondyloarthritis: results from a 6-month, randomised, open-label follow-up study, INFAST Part 2. Ann Rheum Dis. 2014;73(1):108–13.
61. Barkham N, Keen HI, Coates LC, O'Connor P, Hensor E, Fraser AD, et al. Clinical and imaging efficacy of infliximab in HLA-B27-Positive patients with magnetic resonance imaging-determined early sacroiliitis. Arthritis Rheum. 2009;60(4):946–54.
62. Ash Z, Barkham N, McGonagle D, Hensor E, Emery P, Marzo-Ortega H. Induction approach to early axial spondyloarthritis: still looking for the window of opportunity. Arthritis Rheum. 2011;63:1285.
63. Baraliakos X, Koenig AS, Jones H, Szumski A, Collier D, Bananis E. Predictors of clinical remission under anti-tumor necrosis factor treatment in patients with ankylosing spondylitis: pooled analysis from large randomized clinical trials. J Rheumatol. 2015;42(8):1418–26.
64. Robinson PC, Brown MA. The window of opportunity: a relevant concept for axial spondyloarthritis. Arthritis Res Ther. 2014;16(3):109.
65. Rudwaleit M, Listing J, Brandt J, Braun J, Sieper J. Prediction of a major clinical response (BASDAI 50) to tumour necrosis factor alpha blockers in ankylosing spondylitis. Ann Rheum Dis. 2004;63(6):665–70.
66. Song IH, Hermann K, Haibel H, Althoff CE, Listing J, Burmester G, et al. Effects of etanercept versus sulfasalazine in early axial spondyloarthritis on active inflammatory lesions as detected by whole-body MRI (ESTHER): a 48-week randomised controlled trial. Ann Rheum Dis. 2011;70(4):590–6.
67. Song IH, Hermann KG, Haibel H, Althoff CE, Poddubnyy D, Listing J, et al. Consistently good clinical response in patients with early axial spondyloarthritis after 3 years of continuous treatment with etanercept: longterm data of the ESTHER trial. J Rheumatol. 2014;41(10):2034–40.
68. Haroon N, Inman RD, Learch TJ, Weisman MH, Lee M, Rahbar MH, et al. The impact of tumor necrosis factor alpha inhibitors on radiographic progression in ankylosing spondylitis. Arthritis Rheum. 2013;65(10):2645–54.
69. Wanders A, Heijde D, Landewe R, Behier JM, Calin A, Olivieri I, et al. Nonsteroidal antiinflammatory drugs reduce radiographic progression in patients with ankylosing spondylitis: a randomized clinical trial. Arthritis Rheum. 2005;52(6):1756–65.
70. Sieper J, Listing J, Poddubnyy D, Song I-H, Hermann K-G, Callhoff J, et al. Effect of continuous versus on-demand treatment of ankylosing spondylitis with diclofenac over 2 years on radiographic progression of the spine: results from a randomised multicentre trial (ENRADAS). Ann Rheum Dis. 2016;75(8):1438–43.
71. Ward MM, Deodhar A, Akl EA, Lui A, Ermann J, Gensler LS, et al. American College of Rheumatology/Spondylitis Association of America/ Spondyloarthritis Research and Treatment Network 2015 recommendations for the treatment of ankylosing spondylitis and nonradiographic axial spondyloarthritis. Arthritis Rheumatol (Hoboken, NJ). 2016;68(2):282–98.
72. Boersma JW. Retardation of ossification of the lumbar vertebral column in ankylosing spondylitis by means of phenylbutazone. Scand J Rheumatol. 1976;5(1):60–4.
73. Poddubnyy D, Rudwaleit M, Haibel H, Listing J, Marker-Hermann E, Zeidler H, et al. Effect of non-steroidal anti-inflammatory drugs on radiographic spinal progression in patients with axial spondyloarthritis: results from the German Spondyloarthritis Inception Cohort. Ann Rheum Dis. 2012;71(10): 1616–22.
74. Kroon F, Landewe R, Dougados M, van der Heijde D. Continuous NSAID use reverts the effects of inflammation on radiographic progression in patients with ankylosing spondylitis. Ann Rheum Dis. 2012;71(10):1623–9.
75. Jeong H, Eun YH, Kim IY, Park EJ, Kim H, Lee J, et al. Effect of tumor necrosis factor alpha inhibitors on spinal radiographic progression in patients with ankylosing spondylitis. Int J Rheum Dis. 2018;21(5):1098–105.
76. Molnar C, Scherer A, Baraliakos X, de Hooge M, Micheroli R, Exer P, et al. TNF blockers inhibit spinal radiographic progression in ankylosing spondylitis by reducing disease activity: results from the Swiss Clinical Quality Management cohort. Ann Rheum Dis. 2018;77(1):63–9.
77. Louie GH, Ward MM. Measurement and treatment of radiographic progression in ankylosing spondylitis: lessons learned from observational studies and clinical trials. Curr Opin Rheumatol. 2014;26(2):145–50.
78. Tannenbaum H, DeCoteau WE, Esdaile JM. A double blind multicenter trial comparing piroxicam and indomethacin in ankylosing spondylitis with long-term follow-up. Curr Therapeut Res - Clin Exp. 1984;36(3):426–35.
79. Astorga G. Double-blind, parallel clinical trial of tenoxicam (Ro 12–0068) versus piroxicam in patients with ankylosing spondylitis. Eur J Rheumatol Inflamm. 1987;9(2):70–3.
80. Caldwell JR, Altman RD, Burch FX, Calin A. Treatment of ankylosing spondylitis with oxaprozin: a comparison with indomethacin. Semin Arthritis Rheum. 1986;15(3, Supplement 2):95–100.
81. Calin A, Britton M. Sulindac in ankylosing spondylitis. Double-blind evaluation of sulindac and indomethacin. JAMA. 1979;242(17):1885–6.
82. Heinrichs KK. Treatment of spondylitis ankylosans: controlled comparative study with tiaprofenic acid and diclofenac. Med Klin. 1985;80(21):597–601.
83. Khan MA. Diclofenac in the treatment of ankylosing spondylitis: review of worldwide clinical experience and report of a double-blind comparison with indomethacin. Semin Arthritis Rheum. 1985;15(2 Suppl 1):80–4.
84. Lomen PL, Turner LF, Lamborn KR, Brinn EL. Flurbiprofen in the treatment of ankylosing spondylitis. a comparison with indomethacin. Am J Med. 1986; 80(3A):127–32.
85. Lomen PL, Turner LF, Lamborn KR, Brinn EL, Sattler LP. Flurbiprofen in the treatment of ankylosing spondylitis. A comparison with phenylbutazone. Am J Med. 1986;80(3A):120–6.
86. Batlle-Gualda E, Figueroa M, Ivorra J, Raber A. The efficacy and tolerability of aceclofenac in the treatment of patients with ankylosing spondylitis: a multicenter controlled clinical trial. Aceclofenac Indomethacin Study Group. J Rheumatol. 1996;23(7):1200–6.
87. Mena HR, Good AE. Management of ankylosing spondylitis with flurbiprofen or indomethacin. South Med J. 1977;70(8):945–7.
88. Nissila M, Kajander A. Proquazone (Biarison) and indomethacin (Indocid) in the treatment of ankylosing spondylitis. Two comparative, clinical, double-blind studies. Scand J Rheumatol Suppl. 1978;7(21):36–9.
89. Palferman TG, Webley M. A comparative study of nabumetone and indomethacin in ankylosing spondylitis. Eur J Rheumatol Inflamm. 1991; 11(2):23 9.

90. Pasero G, Ruju G, Marcolongo R, Senesi M, Seni U, Mannoni A, Mannoni A, et al. Aceclofenac versus naproxen in the treatment of ankylosing spondylitis: A double-blind, controlled study. Curr Therapeut Res - Clin Exp. 1994;55(7):833–42.
91. Rejholec V, Vapaatalo H, Tokola O, Gothoni G. Tolfenamic acid in ankylosing spondylarthritis: a double-blind comparison to indomethacin. Scand J Rheumatol Suppl. 1980;36:1–7.
92. Franssen MJ, Gribnau FW, van de Putte LB. A comparison of diflunisal and phenylbutazone in the treatment of ankylosing spondylitis. Clin Rheumatol. 1986;5(2):210–20.
93. Jessop JD. Double-blind study of ketoprofen and phenylbutazone in ankylosing spondylitis. Rheumatol Rehabil. 1976;15(Suppl 5):37–42.
94. Schwarzer AC, Cohen M, Arnold MH, Kelly D, McNaught P, Brooks PM. Tenoxicam compared with diclofenac in patients with ankylosing spondylitis. Curr Med Res Opin. 1990;11(10):648–53.
95. Simpson MR, Simpson NR, Scott BO, Beatty DC. A controlled study of flufenamic acid in ankylosing spondylitis. A preliminary report. Ann Phys Med. 1966;8(Suppl 1):126–8.
96. Myklebust G. Comparison of naproxen and piroxicam in rheumatoid arthritis and Bechterew's syndrome. A double-blind parallel multicenter study. Tidsskr Nor Laegeforen. 1986;106(17–18):1485–7.
97. Nahir AM, Scharf Y. A comparative study of diclofenac and sulindac in ankylosing spondylitis. Rheumatol Rehabil. 1980;19(3):193–8.
98. Santo JE, Queiroz MV. Oxaprozin versus diclofenac sodium in the treatment of ankylosing spondylitis. J Int Med Res. 1988;16(2):150–6.
99. Ansell BM. A comparative study of Butacote and naproxen in ankylosing spondylitis. J Int Med Res. 1977;5(Suppl 2):95.
100. Coxib, traditional NTC, Bhala N, Emberson J, Merhi A, Abramson S, et al. Vascular and upper gastrointestinal effects of non-steroidal anti-inflammatory drugs: meta-analyses of individual participant data from randomised trials. Lancet. 2013;382(9894):769–79.
101. Kearney PM, Baigent C, Godwin J, Halls H, Emberson JR, Patrono C. Do selective cyclo-oxygenase-2 inhibitors and traditional non-steroidal anti-inflammatory drugs increase the risk of atherothrombosis? Meta-analysis of randomised trials. Bmj. 2006;332(7553):1302–8.
102. Lanas A, Boers M, Nuevo J. Gastrointestinal events in at-risk patients starting non-steroidal anti-inflammatory drugs (NSAIDs) for rheumatic diseases: the EVIDENCE study of European routine practice. Ann Rheum Dis. 2015;74(4): 675–81.
103. Poddubnyy D, van der Heijde D. Therapeutic controversies in spondyloarthritis: nonsteroidal anti-inflammatory drugs. Rheum Dis Clin North Am. 2012;38(3):601–11.
104. Bakland G, Gran JT, Nossent JC. Increased mortality in ankylosing spondylitis is related to disease activity. Ann Rheum Dis. 2011;70(11):1921–5.
105. Haroon NN, Paterson JM, Li P, Inman RD, Haroon N. Patients with ankylosing spondylitis have increased cardiovascular and cerebrovascular mortality: a population-based study. Ann Intern Med. 2015;163(6):409–16.
106. Lehtinen K. Mortality and causes of death in 398 patients admitted to hospital with ankylosing spondylitis. Ann Rheum Dis. 1993;52(3):174–6.
107. Liew JW, Ramiro S, Gensler LS. Cardiovascular morbidity and mortality in ankylosing spondylitis and psoriatic arthritis. Best Pract Res Clin Rheumatol. 2018;32(3):369–89.
108. Fosbol EL, Gislason GH, Jacobsen S, Folke F, Hansen ML, Schramm TK, et al. Risk of myocardial infarction and death associated with the use of nonsteroidal anti-inflammatory drugs (NSAIDs) among healthy individuals: a nationwide cohort study. Clin Pharmacol Ther. 2009;85(2):190–7.
109. Trelle S, Reichenbach S, Wandel S, Hildebrand P, Tschannen B, Villiger PM, et al. Cardiovascular safety of non-steroidal anti-inflammatory drugs: network meta-analysis. Bmj. 2011;342:c7086.
110. Gislason GH, Jacobsen S, Rasmussen JN, Rasmussen S, Buch P, Friberg J, et al. Risk of death or reinfarction associated with the use of selective cyclooxygenase-2 inhibitors and nonselective nonsteroidal antiinflammatory drugs after acute myocardial infarction. Circulation. 2006;113(25):2906–13.
111. Nussmeier NA, Whelton AA, Brown MT, Langford RM, Hoeft A, Parlow JL, et al. Complications of the COX-2 inhibitors parecoxib and valdecoxib after cardiac surgery. N Engl J Med. 2005;352(11):1081–91.
112. Dubreuil M, Louie-Gao Q, Peloquin CE, Choi HK, Zhang Y, Neogi T. Risk of myocardial infarction with use of selected non-steroidal anti-inflammatory drugs in patients with spondyloarthritis and osteoarthritis. Ann Rheum Dis. 2018;77(8):1137–42.
113. Winkelmayer WC, Waikar SS, Mogun H, Solomon DH. Nonselective and cyclooxygenase-2-selective NSAIDs and acute kidney injury. Am J Med. 2008;121(12):1092–8.
114. Ungprasert P, Cheungpasitporn W, Crowson CS, Matteson EL. Individual non-steroidal anti-inflammatory drugs and risk of acute kidney injury: A systematic review and meta-analysis of observational studies. Eur J Intern Med. 2015;26(4):285–91.
115. Gooch K, Culleton BF, Manns BJ, Zhang J, Alfonso H, Tonelli M, et al. NSAID use and progression of chronic kidney disease. Am J Med. 2007;120(3):280 e1–7.
116. Cao YL, Tian ZG, Wang F, Li WG, Cheng DY, Yang YF, et al. Characteristics and clinical outcome of nonsteroidal anti-inflammatory drug-induced acute hepato-nephrotoxicity among Chinese patients. World J Gastroenterol. 2014; 20(38):13956–65.

6

Treatment of knee osteoarthritis with a new formulation of a fixed-dose combination of glucosamine sulfate and bovine chondroitin: A multicenter, randomized, single-blind, non-inferiority clinical trial

Andrea Barranjard Vannucci Lomonte[1*], Emerson Gimenez[2], Antônio Carlos da Silva[3], Sebastião Cezar Radominski[4], Morton Aaron Scheinberg[5], Antônio Carlos Ximenes[6] and Cristiano Augusto de Freitas Zerbini[1]

Abstract

Objectives: To compare the efficacy and safety of a new formulation of a fixed dose combination of glucosamine sulfate (GS; 1500 mg) and bovine chondroitin sulfate (CS; 1200 mg) versus the reference product (RP) in patients with knee osteoarthritis (OA).

Methods: In this multicenter, randomized, single-blind trial, 627 patients with knee osteoarthritis (OA)—Kellgren-Lawrence grades 2 or 3 and mean score ≥ 40 mm in the WOMAC pain subscale—were randomized to receive GS/CS or the RP for 24 weeks. The primary efficacy endpoint was the absolute change in WOMAC pain subscale score. The secondary endpoints included the following: WOMAC total and subscale scores, overall assessment of the disease by the patient and the investigator, SF-12 score, OMERACT-OARSI response rate to the treatment, and rescue medication use.

Results: Mean reductions of WOMAC pain score were – 35.1 (sd = 23.2) mm in the GS/CS group and – 36.5 (sd = 24.9) mm in the RP group. The difference between the adjusted means of both treatments confirmed the non-inferiority of GS/CS versus the RP. Improvement was observed in pain, stiffness, physical function and total WOMAC score, as well as in overall OA assessment by the patient and the investigator for both groups. No improvement was observed in SF-12. The rate of OMERACT-OARSI responders was 89.4% in GS/CS group and 87.9% in the RP group. Headache and changes in glucose tolerance were the most frequent treatment-related adverse events.

(Continued on next page)

* Correspondence: andrea.lomonte@cepic.com.br
[1]Centro Paulista de Investigação Clínica (CEPIC), Rua Moreira e Costa, 342 – Ipiranga, São Paulo, SP 04266-010, Brazil

(Continued from previous page)

Conclusions: The new formulation of a fixed-dose combination of glucosamine sulfate and bovine chondroitin sulfate was non-inferior to the RP in symptomatic treatment of knee OA, with a high responder rate and good tolerability profile.

Trial registration: ClinicalTrials.gov; Registration number NCT02830919; Date of registration: July 13, 2016; First randomization date: December 05, 2016).

Keywords: Glucosamine, Chondroitin, Osteoarthritis, Knee, Pain

Introduction

Osteoarthritis (OA) is an important cause of morbidity and functional impairment [1]. An increase of 31.4% in disability-adjusted life-years (DALYs) was observed for musculoskeletal diseases, including OA, from 2007 to 2017 [2]. The functional impairment caused by this disease has a significant socioeconomic impact: a review of studies published between 2006 and 2016 addressing the economic impact of OA showed that the average per patient direct costs of the disease in the United States ranged from US$ 1442 to US$ 21,335 per year [3].

Symptomatic knee OA is a highly prevalent disease, affecting nearly 14 million people in the United States [4]. A continuous growth in disease incidence is expected, due to increased life expectancy and the prevalence of obesity, which is a known risk factor for OA [4, 5].

Therefore, it is important to investigate therapies which can promote symptomatic relief without risks of severe adverse events. The current treatment algorithm of the European Society for Clinical and Economic Aspects of Osteoporosis, Osteoarthritis and Musculoskeletal Diseases (ESCEO) proposes the early introduction of symptomatic slow-acting drugs for OA (SYSADOAs), among which glucosamine sulfate and chondroitin sulfate are included [6].

Glucosamine is an aminosaccharide which corresponds to the main component of the glycosaminoglycans that form the matrix of connective tissue. Glucosamine acts by increasing the synthesis of proteoglycans, and by inhibiting enzymes that degrade the cartilage, such as collagenase, phospholipase A2 and lysosomal enzymes [7, 8]. Furthermore, glucosamine inhibits several pro-inflammatory mediators, such as nitric oxide, cyclooxygenase-2 and metalloproteinases [9].

Chondroitin sulfate consists of repeated chains of sulfate glycosaminoglycans, which are important components of the extracellular matrix of connective tissue. Its main functions include: granting resistance and elasticity to articular cartilage, inhibiting the synthesis of inflammatory mediators and catabolic enzymes, stimulating the synthesis of cartilage matrix components, and reducing chondrocyte apoptosis [10, 11]. Chondroitin sulfate may have different origins and may be obtained from different animal species. Currently, medicinal products which are extracted from avian, bovine, porcine, and marine (shark) sources are available worldwide. Randomized clinical trials with chondroitin sulfate from these different origins have already been conducted [10, 12].

In Brazil, a product containing glucosamine sulfate and chondroitin sulfate of shark origin, Ártico® (Eurofarma Laboratórios S.A., São Paulo, S.P., Brazil), is commercially available. However, due to increasing scarcity of many shark species, replacing sharks with another animal species as a source of raw material for chondroitin production has become necessary. This led to the search for other source of chondroitin sulfate for this product.

The purpose of this study was to evaluate the efficacy and safety of a new formulation for Ártico® using a fixed-dose combination of glucosamine sulfate (1500 mg) and chondroitin sulfate (1200 mg) of bovine origin provided in sachets for the treatment of knee OA and establishing its non-inferiority compared to the reference product (RP), Condroflex® (Zodiac Laboratórios S.A., São Paulo, S.P., Brazil). The choice of the comparator, which also contains chondroitin of bovine origin, was a requirement of the Brazilian food and drug regulatory agency (Agência Nacional de Vigilância Sanitária, ANVI SA) for this clinical trial.

Patients and methods

Study design. This phase III, multicenter, randomized, single-blind, non-inferiority, parallel-group, active-controlled clinical trial was conducted from December 2016 to November 2018 at six Brazilian sites.

During the screening period, routine laboratory tests, knee x-rays, and physical exams were performed, and clinical histories and information on ongoing medications were collected. Radiographs were read at each study site, to determine the Kellgren-Lawrence grade of knee OA. All pharmacological treatments for OA were discontinued, and only paracetamol (500 mg up to 4 times daily) was allowed for residual pain. A specific washout period between screening and randomization visits was defined for each non-steroidal anti-inflammatory drug (NSAID) for patients undergoing such treatment.

The randomization visit (RV) was performed up to 15 days after the screening visit (SV). Clinical visits were scheduled 1 week (visit 1 – V1), 6 weeks (visit 2 – V2), 12 weeks (visit 3 – V3), 18 weeks (visit 4 – V4), and 24 weeks (final visit – FV) after the RV. Efficacy evaluations were performed at visits V2, V3, and FV. Both treatments were administered throughout the study, with a maximum treatment duration of 171 days.

Ethics, consent, and permissions

The study was conducted under international and local ethical standards and regulations, in accordance with the principles of the Declaration of Helsinki. It was approved by the Research Ethics Committee (RECs) of each participating institution before its beginning, with the following RECs and their respective sites: Faculdade de Medicina do ABC/ Fundação do ABC (Centro Paulista de Investigação Clínica and Instituto de Pesquisa Clínica e Medicina Avançada), Comitê Permanente de Ética em Pesquisa com Seres Humanos - COPEP (Clínica Clinilive), Comitê de Ética em Pesquisa em Seres Humanos do Hospital de Clínicas da Universidade Federal do Paraná (Centro de Estudos em Terapias Inovadoras), Comitê de Ética em Pesquisa da Associação de Assistência à Criança Deficiente (Associação de Assistência à Criança Deficiente), and Comitê de Ética em Pesquisa do Hospital Alberto Rassi – CEPHGG (Centro Internacional de Pesquisa).

Patients

Eligible patients met the following criteria:

1. ≥40 years old;
2. Diagnosed with knee OA as per the American College of Rheumatology (ACR) criteria;
3. Graded 2 or 3 by the Kellgren-Lawrence imaging classification;
4. Presented with pain in the target knee within 3 months prior to study screening;
5. Scored ≥40 mm in the visual analogue scale (VAS – 0 to 100 mm) for pain assessment (at the SV, and mean score ≥ 40 mm in the pain subscale of the Western Ontario and McMaster Universities (WOMAC) questionnaire at the randomization visit);
6. ACR functional status I to III.

All subjects gave written informed consent before inclusion in the study.

The main exclusion criteria included:

1. Diagnosis of other diseases of the knee;
2. Serious knee misalignment;
3. Serious trauma or surgery in the target knee within 6 months prior to enrollment,
4. Symptomatic OA of the ipsilateral hip;
5. Use of NSAIDs, dipyrone and opioid analgesics or narcotics from the SV, or washout period for these drugs shorter than defined by the protocol;
6. Use of oral, intravenous, or intramuscular corticosteroids within 30 days prior to the SV;
7. Intra-articular injection of corticosteroids and/or hyaluronic acid in the target knee within 6 months prior to the SV;
8. Use of diacerein, chloroquine, or soybean and avocado unsaponifiable extracts within the last 3 months; duloxetine hydrochloride over the last 30 days; glucosamine sulfate and/or chondroitin sulfate and strontium ranelate in the past 6 months;
9. Body mass index (BMI) ≥ 40 kg/m [2];
10. Fasting blood glucose > 110 mg/dL or glycated hemoglobin (HbA1c) > 6.5%.

In case of bilateral knee OA, a target knee was defined as the knee with the most severe pain symptoms according to medical evaluation.

Treatment and randomization

Eligible patients were randomized at a 1:1 ratio to one of the following study groups: [1] a group treated with the new formulation of a fixed-dose combination of glucosamine sulfate (1500 mg) and bovine chondroitin sulfate (1200 mg) (GS/CS group, Eurofarma Laboratórios S.A. São Paulo, S.P., Brazil) or [2] a group treated with the RP of glucosamine sulfate (1500 mg) and bovine chondroitin sulfate (1200 mg) (Condroflex®, Zodiac Laboratórios S.A., São Paulo, S.P., Brazil). In both groups, the drug was supplied in sachets, and a daily dosage of one sachet was administered. Randomization was made through an interactive web response system (IWRV) integrated to the electronic case report form (eCRF), by which a code was informed to identify the product to be dispensed to each subject. Since the organoleptic properties (powder, color, and flavor) are different in both study treatments, the study was single-blinded, and only the patient and the study pharmacist were unblinded to the assigned treatment. The investigator and all other members of the study team were kept blind to the study treatment. Patients were instructed not to reveal the characteristic of the product in use to the investigator throughout the study. The sachet package (primary package) given to both groups had a similar characteristic, and identical labels were stuck to the sachets of both products to hide all available information and differences in the original packaging. The single-blind nature of the study was kept by using boxes (secondary package) with similar appearance and form for both study treatments.

Efficacy and safety evaluations

The following efficacy evaluations were performed:

- Primary endpoint:
    - Absolute change in pain subscale score on WOMAC questionnaire (normalized for 0 to 100 mm) at week 24 versus baseline score.
- Secondary endpoints:
    - Absolute change in pain, stiffness, and function subscale scores on WOMAC questionnaire (normalized for 0 to 100 mm) throughout the treatment in relation to baseline score;
    - Absolute change in overall assessment of the disease by the patient and investigator throughout the treatment, using the visual analogue scale (VAS) (0 to 100 mm), in relation to baseline assessment;
    - Absolute change in score of physical and mental components of Short Form-12 (SF-12) questionnaire at week 24 versus baseline score;
    - Treatment response rate throughout the study, according to the Outcome Measures in Rheumatology Clinical Trials and Osteoarthritis Research Society International (OMERACT-OARSI) criteria;
    - Number of tablets of rescue medication administered during treatment.

The WOMAC questionnaire was administered by a professional duly trained for such a purpose in each study site, and patients were instructed to give answers only considering symptoms in the target knee within the previous 48 h.

Rescue medication consisted of paracetamol (500 mg). Up to 4 tablets/day was allowed for no more than 5 consecutive days. Patients were instructed not to use paracetamol within 12 h before visits in which efficacy analyses were scheduled.

Safety evaluation outcomes included:

- Incidence and profile of adverse events (AEs);
- Frequency of discontinuations due to AEs and laboratory abnormalities.

Statistical analysis

Sample size calculations were based on the evaluation of a non-inferiority hypothesis of GS/CS compared to the reference product, established in terms of the primary efficacy variable. It was considered the one-sided means test for two independent samples (significance level = 2.5), the difference between the treatment means equal to zero, a standard deviation of 98 mm, and a non-inferiority margin of 35 mm for the pain subscale of the WOMAC score (ranging from 0 to 500 mm, or equivalent to 7 mm in a normalized scale from 0 to 100 mm). We determined that 250 patients (125 in each study group) would give 80% of power to demonstrate the non-inferiority of the investigational product compared to the reference product. The estimated rate of patient withdrawal from the per protocol population (PP) was 20%, with randomization of 314 subjects planned.

In order to update the standard deviation sample size estimations, a blinded interim analysis was conducted after 214 patients completed the study. The estimated standard deviation value was 134.6 mm and the adjusted sample size was 468 patients. Considering a withdrawal rate from the PP population of 20%, it was established that 586 patients would be enrolled in the study.

The efficacy evaluations were performed in the intention to treat (ITT) population and in the PP population. The ITT population was defined as all randomized study subjects that received at least one dose of the study drug and that had at least one primary assessment of efficacy. The PP population was composed of all subjects of the ITT population that completed the study, that had a drug adherence between 80 and 120% and that were compliant with all study requirements. The safety evaluations were conducted to all randomized study subjects that received at least one dose of the study drug.

A covariance analysis model was adjusted for assessment of the primary efficacy variable, with the treatment group as a fixed factor and the site and baseline WOMAC pain subscale score as covariates. The evaluation of non-inferiority of GS/CS versus the reference product was conducted based on the two-sided confidence interval (95%) for the difference between the means of absolute changes of the WOMAC pain subscale score between study groups, with the non-inferiority of GS/CS combination versus the reference product being stated if the upper limit of the confidence interval was lower than the non-inferiority margin of 7 mm.

For all secondary efficacy variables, a two-sided confidence interval (95%) was established for the difference between the groups. Covariance models and analysis of variance models for repeated measures were adjusted for group comparisons.

Patient distribution according to OMERACT-OARSI treatment response criteria was evaluated through a generalized linear model for repeated measures, considering the binomial response, treatment, and week as factors, and treatment*week interaction, and site as covariates.

The mixed-effects Poisson regression model was used in the analysis of the number of tablets of rescue medication administered per week, pre- and post-treatment.

Safety analyses were performed through descriptive statistics and confidence intervals (95%).

Results

Demographics and baseline clinical characteristics

A total of 858 patients were screened for the study, 627 of which fulfilled the eligibility criteria and were randomized. A total of 314 patients were assigned to the GS/CS group and 313 patients were assigned to the RP group. All patients received the treatment to which they were randomized, except for a patient who was randomized to the GS/CS group but received the reference drug at V3. This patient was discontinued at V4. Among randomized patients, 489 (78%) completed the study (251 (79.9%) in the GS/CS group and 238 (76%) in the reference group). The most frequent reasons for early treatment

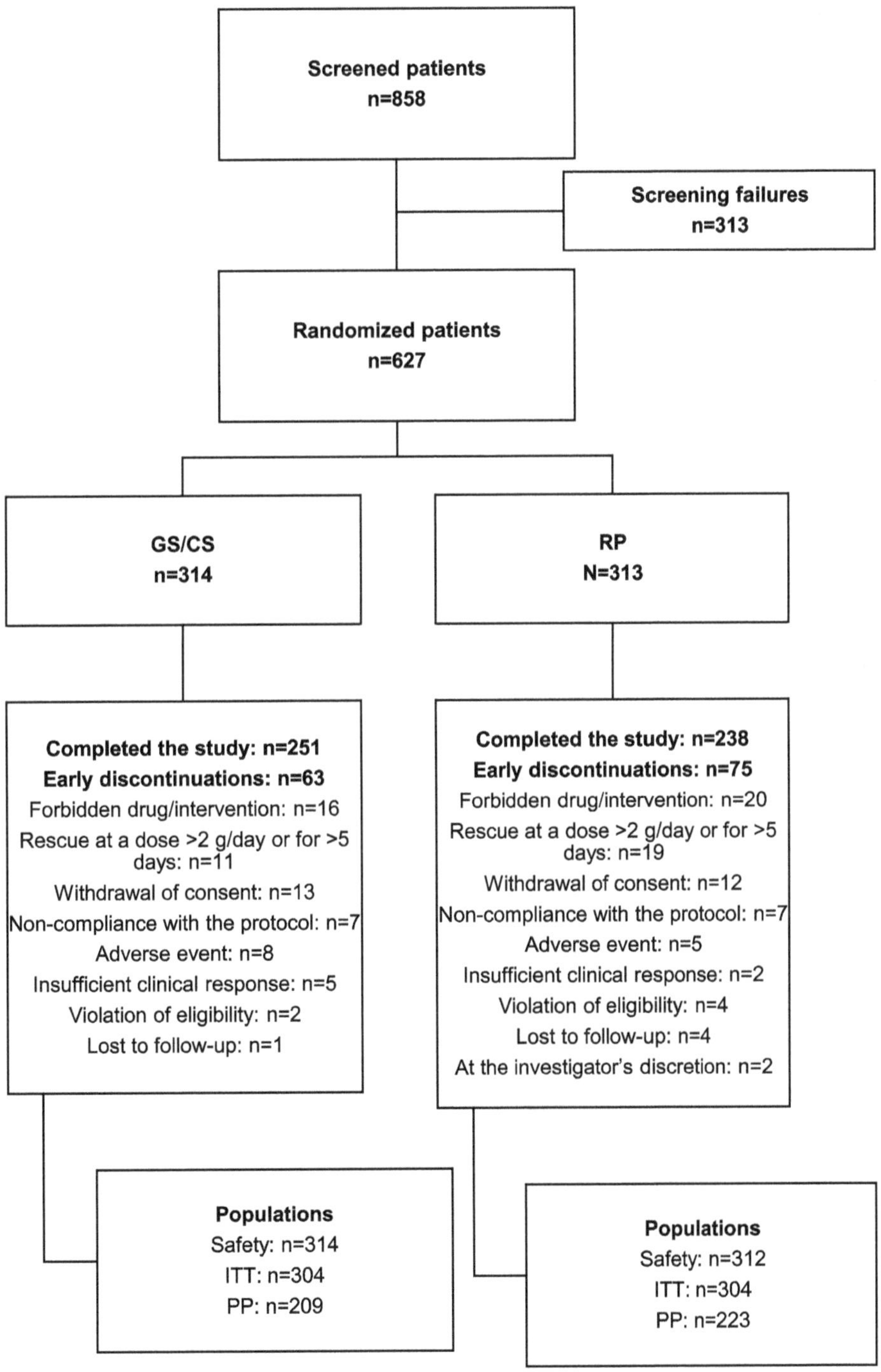

Fig 1 Disposition of study patients

discontinuation were use of forbidden medications, inadequate use of rescue therapy, and withdrawal of consent. Figure 1 shows patients' disposition in both study groups and populations.

Demographics and baseline clinical characteristics of the studied population are presented in Table 1. Most patients were female and Caucasian, with a median BMI of 30.6 kg/m^2, indicating obesity grade I. Patients' age ranged from 40 to 86 years, predominantly over 60 (65.9%). Mean OA duration was around 7 years in both groups. Most patients were Kellgren-Lawrence grade 2 on the target knee (67% in both groups). The mean value (standard deviation, sd) of the WOMAC questionnaire pain subscale score was approximately 67.2 (sd = 13.4) mm for the studied population. Systemic arterial hypertension was the most frequent comorbidity in both groups. Demographics and clinical characteristics of the PP population were similar to the ITT population, and treatment groups were homogeneous for these characteristics.

Table 1 Baseline clinical and demographic characteristics in PP population

Baseline characteristics	GS/CS (*N* = 209)	RP (*N* = 223)
Female, n (%)	184 (88)	193 (86.6)
Age, mean (sd), years	62.8 (8.9)	63 (8)
Caucasian, n (%)	133 (63.6)	133 (59.6)
Osteoarthritis duration, mean (sd), years	7.7 (6.9)	7.4 (5.7)
BMI, mean (sd), kg/m^2	30.4 (4.7)	30.7 (4.4)
Kellgren-Lawrence grading, n (%)		
II	146 (69.9)	151 (67.7)
III	63 (30.1)	72 (32.3)
Overall assessment of OA by the patient, mean (sd), VAS 0-100 mm	66.7 (18.1)	65 (19.2)
Overall assessment of OA by the physician, mean (sd), VAS 0-100 mm	61.8 (12.5)	62.9 (14.1)
WOMAC, mean (sd), mm		
Pain subscale	66.3 (13.2)	68.1 (13.5)
Stiffness subscale	64.9 (21.1)	65.4 (20.9)
Physical function subscale	65.7 (13.7)	65.4 (14.6)
Total score	196.9 (39.9)	198.9 (41.7)
SF-12, mean (sd)		
Physical component	34.9 (7.4)	35.7 (7.5)
Mental component	49 (10.6)	46.9 (11.3)
Comorbidities (reported by ≥ 5% of patients), n (%)		
Back pain	56 (25.8)	61 (27.4)
Musculoskeletal pain / Arthralgia / Pain in the extremities	46 (22)	46 (20.6)
Osteoporosis/ Osteopenia	34 (16.3)	30 (13.5)
Dyslipidemia / Hypercholesterolemia	69 (33)	70 (31.4)
Impaired glucose tolerance	33 (15.8)	40 (17.9)
Headache / Migraine	60 (28.7)	77 (34.5)
Hypothyroidism	40 (19.1)	39 (17.5)
Gastritis	26 (12.4)	30 (13.5)
Gastroesophageal reflux disease	9 (4.3)	14 (6.3)
Depression	13 (6.2)	17 (7.6)
Insomnia	11 (5.3)	15 (6.7)
Systemic arterial hypertension	128 (61.2)	130 (58.3)
Lower limbs varices	44 (21.1)	69 (30.9)

P < 0,05 between groups for all characteristics. *BMI* body mass index, *kg/m^2* kilogram per square meter, *GS/CS* glucosamine sulfate/ chondroitin sulfate, *n (%)* number and percentage of patients in relation to the total number of patients in PP population, *OA* osteoarthritis, *PP* per protocol, *RP* reference product, *sd* standard deviation, *SF-12* short-form 12 questionnaire, *VAS* visual analogue scale, *WOMAC* Western Ontario and McMaster Universities index

The mean value of treatment adherence in the PP population was 97.1 (sd = 4) % in the GS/CS group and 96.1 (sd = 4.8) % in the reference group, with no statistically significant difference between the groups.

Efficacy Outcomes

Primary efficacy analysis

The mean value of the pain subscale score at baseline was 66.3 (sd = ±13.2) mm in GS/CS group and 68.1 (sd = 13.5) mm in the reference group. Mean reductions of the WOMAC pain subscale score on week 24 compared to baseline in the PP population was − 35.1 (sd = 23.2) mm (a 53% reduction) in the GS/CS group and − 36.5 (sd = 24.9) mm (a 53.7% reduction) in the reference group, with a between-treatments difference of 1.4 mm (CI = 95%: − 3.2 mm; 6 mm). Adjusted estimates obtained from a covariance analysis model showed a reduction in pain score at the end of the study of − 30.9 (±2) mm in GS/CS group and − 31.8 (±2) mm in the reference group, with a between-treatments difference of adjusted means of 0.9 (±2.1) mm and respective CI (95%) equal to (− 3.21 mm; 4.99 mm). In the ITT population, adjusted estimates showed a mean reduction of the WOMAC pain subscale of − 29.5 (sd = 1.7) mm in the GS/CS group and − 28.9 (sd = 1,7) mm in the RP group on week 24 compared to baseline, with a between-treatments difference of − 0.5 (CI 95%: − 4.2 mm; 3.1 mm). In both PP and ITT population, the upper limit of the confidence interval of the difference between the adjusted mean of both treatments for the pain subscale was lower than the non-inferiority margin of 7 mm established prior to the study, confirming the non-inferiority of the new GS/CS fixed-dose combination versus the RP.

Secondary efficacy analyses

Table 2 shows the changes in the WOMAC score and Table 3 shows the results for the other secondary efficacy endpoints. No statistically significant difference between the groups was observed for secondary efficacy evaluations conducted in all timepoints throughout the study, both in PP and in ITT populations. These data support the non-inferiority of the new GS/CS formulation versus the reference product.

Improvements were observed in both treatment groups in pain, stiffness, physical function and total WOMAC score 6, 12, and 24 weeks after treatment initiation. A statistically significant improvement was also observed in the VAS for overall OA assessment, both by the patient and the investigator. These outcomes are represented in Fig. 2.

No statistically significant effects of treatment related to physical ($p = 0.369$) and mental ($p = 0.089$) components of the SF-12 questionnaire were observed 24 weeks after treatment initiation, with no difference between groups.

A progressive increase in the response rate to treatment according to OMERACT-OARSI criteria was

Table 2 Changes in the WOMAC score during the treatment in PP population[a]

WOMAC	GS/ CS (N = 209)	RP (N = 223)	Difference between the treatments	CI (95%)
Absolute change in score of WOMAC "pain" subscale, mm, mean (se)				
Week 6	- 18.2 (1.7)	- 20.2 (1.72)	1.98 (2)	(− 1.95; 5.9)
Week 12	- 23.3 (1.7)	- 24.7 (1.7)	1.3 (2)	(− 2.6; 5.3)
Week 24	- 32.8 (1.8)	−33.3 (1.7)	0.54 (2)	(− 3.5; 4.5)
Absolute change in score of WOMAC "stiffness" subscale, mm, mean (se)				
Week 6	- 15.4 (2)	- 17 (2)	1.6 (2.3)	(− 3; 6.1)
Week 12	- 19.1 (2)	- 22.5 (2)	3.4 (2.3)	(− 1.1; 8)
Week 24	- 28.6 (2)	- 30.1 (2)	1.4 (2.4)	(− 3.2; 6.1)
Absolute change in score of WOMAC "function" subscale, mm, mean (se)				
Week 6	- 14.2 (1.7)	- 15.1 (1.7)	0.9 (2)	(− 2.94; 4.78)
Week 12	- 19.6 (1.7)	- 21.4 (1.7)	1.8 (2)	(− 2.1; 5.7)
Week 24	- 28.9 (1.8)	- 29.5 (1.7)	0.6 (2)	(− 3.3; 4.5)
Absolute change in WOMAC total score, mm, mean (se)				
Week 6	- 48.1 (5.1)	- 52.83 (5)	4.8 (5.8)	(− 6.6; 16.1)
Week 12	- 62.3 (5.1)	- 69.1 (5)	6.9 (5.8)	(− 4.6; 18.3)
Week 24	- 90.6 (5.1)	- 93.4 (5.1)	2.9 (5.9)	(−8.7; 14.4)

[a]Estimates of the mixed model for repeated measures adjusted per baseline score and site. *CI (95%)* two-sided confidence interval for change mean, with confidence coefficient of 95%, *GS/CS* glucosamine sulfate/ chondroitin sulfate, *PP* per protocol, *RP* Reference Product, *se* standard estimate, *WOMAC* Western Ontario and McMaster Universities questionnaire (score normalized at the scale from 0 to 100 mm)

Table 3 Secondary efficacy analyses during the treatment in PP population[a]

Efficacy endpoint	GS/ CS (N = 209)	RP (N = 223)	Difference between the treatments[b]	CI (95%)
Absolute change in overall OA assessment by the patient (VAS), mm, mean (se)				
Week 6	- 20.2 (1.9)	- 18.8 (1.9)	- 1.37 (2.2)	(− 5.72; 3)
Week 12	- 24.4 (1.9)	- 24.5 (1.9)	0.2 (2.2)	(− 4.2; 4.5)
Week 24	- 35. 5 (1.9)	- 32.6 (1.9)	- 2.9 (2.3)	(−7.3; 1.5)
Absolute change in overall OA assessment by the physician (VAS), mm, mean (se)				
Week 6	- 20 (1.5)	- 21.6 (1.4)	1.6 (1.7)	(− 1.7; 5)
Week 12	- 27.1 (1.5)	- 28.5 (1.5)	1.4 (1.7)	(− 1.9; 4.8)
Week 24	- 37.6 (1.5)	- 36.7 (1.5)	- 0.9 (1.7)	(− 4.3; 2.5)
Absolute change in SF-12 physical component, points, mean (se)				
Week 24	5 (0.7)	5.7 (0.7)	- 0.7 (0.7)	(−2.1; 0.8)
Absolute change in SF-12 mental component, points, mean (se)				
Week 24	2.7 (0.9)	1.12 (0.9)	1. 6 (0.9)	(− 0.2; 3.4)
Treatment response rate by OMERACT-OARSI criteria, n (%)				
Week 6	130 (62.5)	137 (61.4)	1.1	(− 8.1; 10.2)
Week 12	143 (69.8)	155 (69.8)	- 0.1	(− 8.8; 8.7)
Week 24	166 (83.4)	172 (80.4)	3	(− 4.4; 10.5)
Number of tablets of rescue medication administered per week, mean (se)				
SV to RV	3.8 (4.8)	3.7 (4.7)		
RV to V2	1.4 (2.2)	1.3 (2)		
V2 to V3	0.9 (1.8)	0.9 (1.7)		
V3 to V4	0.8 (1.7)	0.8 (1.7)		
V4 to FV	0.7 (1.6)	0.8 (1.5)		

[a]Estimates of the mixed model for repeated measures adjusted per baseline score and site. [b] Difference between the treatments evaluated by the mean (se) for VAS and SF-12 variables, and as percentage of responders to the treatment for OMERACT-OARSI criteria. *CI (95%)* two-sided confidence interval for change mean, with confidence coefficient of 95%, *GS/ CS* glucosamine sulfate/ chondroitin sulfate, *OA* osteoarthritis; se: standard estimate, *OMERACT-OARSI* Outcome Measures in Rheumatology Clinical Trials and Osteoarthritis Research Society International, *PP* per protocol, *RP* reference product, *SF-12* Short Form 12 questionnaire, *VAS* visual analogue scale

observed throughout the study (Table 3). The overall response rate was 89.4% in the GS/CS group and 87.9% in the reference group, with a between-groups difference of 1.5 (CI 95%: – 4.5%; 7.5%).

The median number of tablets of rescue medication used for pain in the knees during the total treatment period was 12 tablets in the GS/CS group and 13 tablets in the reference group. Table 2 shows the number of tablets of rescue treatment used at each study visit.

Safety

A total of 1076 AEs were reported during the study, of which 504 occurred in the GS/CS group and 572 in the reference group (most of mild intensity). The number of AEs considered related to the study treatment were 116 (23%) in the GS/CS group and 160 (28%) in the reference group.

The most frequent treatment-related AE was headache, reported by 12.7% of the patients in the GS/CS group and 14.4% of the patients in the reference group, followed by impaired glucose tolerance, reported by 2.9% of patients in the GS/CS group and 5.5% of patients in the reference group. A summary of the AEs with incidence ≥5% in the safety population is described in Table 4.

Five serious adverse events (SAEs) were reported by 3 patients from the GS/CS group (intestinal obstruction and abdominal hernia repair; nephrolithiasis and urinary tract infection; and amyotrophic lateral sclerosis), and 2 SAEs were reported by 2 patients in the reference group (road traffic accident and cholecystitis); none of the reported SAEs were assessed as related to the study treatment. No deaths occurred during the study.

Discussion

Both formulations of a fixed-dose combination of glucosamine sulfate and bovine chondroitin sulfate provided in sachets provided clinically relevant improvement of pain and physical function in patients with primary OA of the knee, establishing proof of non-inferiority between the two products. An improvement in overall OA assessment was reported both by patients and investigators, and a progressive increase was observed in the rate of treatment responders according to OMERACT-OARSI criteria

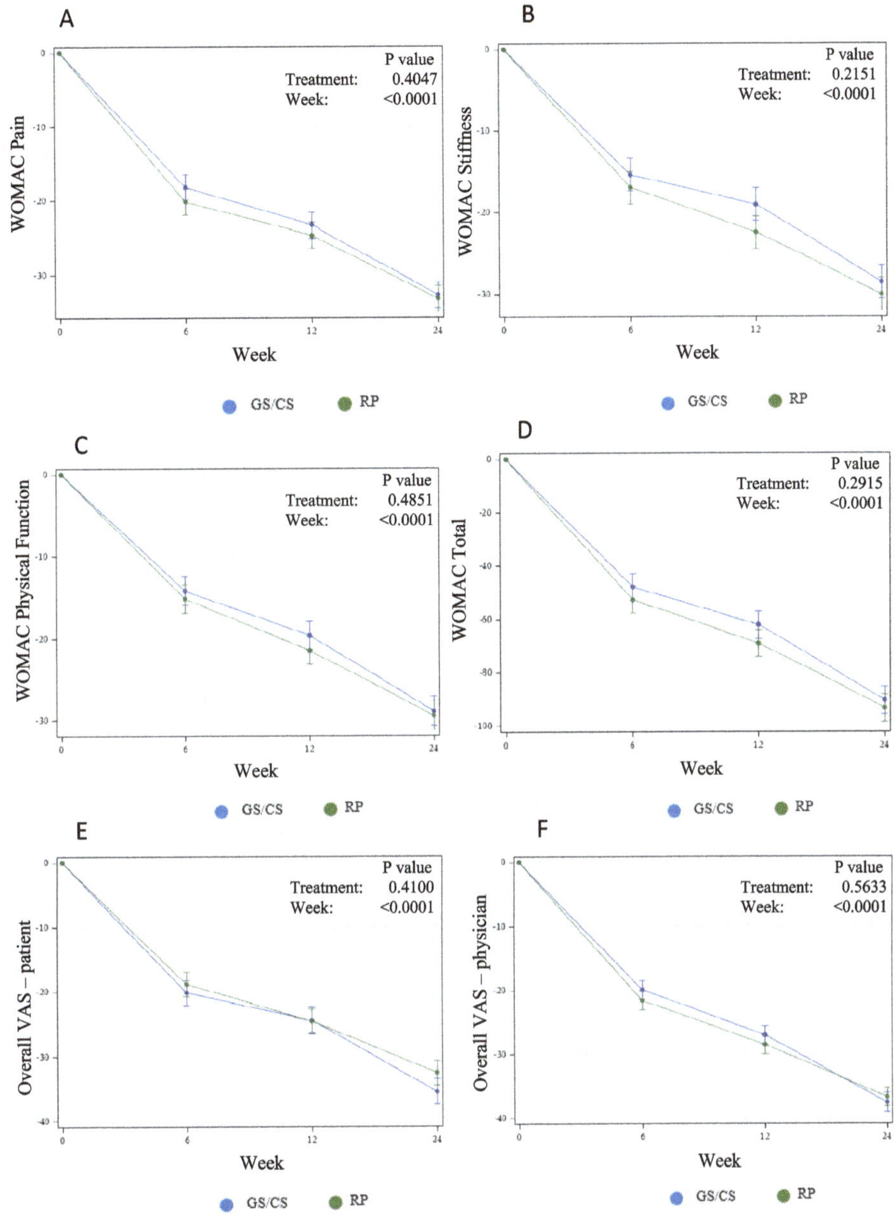

Fig. 2 WOMAC **a** "pain" subscale, **b** "stiffness" subscale, **c** "physical function" subscale and **d** total score; **e** VAS overall assessment of OA by the patient; **f** VAS overall assessment of OA by the physician. Adjusted estimates and two-sided CI (95%) of absolute ranges for each variable in PP population. P value indicates the differences between the treatment groups and between week 24 visit and baseline assessment. OA: osteoarthritis; RP: reference product; VAS: visual analogue scale; WOMAC: Western Ontario and McMaster Osteoarthritis questionnaire

throughout the study, with over 80% of responders in each study group at the end of the 6-month treatment. On the other hand, no significant improvement in quality of life was observed in either group, as assessed by the SF-12 questionnaire.

The large number (> 600) of randomized patients is one of the strengths of this study. The study was conducted in several research sites, with evaluations performed during 24 weeks of treatment. Different endpoints were used, including a WOMAC questionnaire, VAS for overall disease assessment by the patient and the investigator, an SF-12 questionnaire, and treatment response rate evaluation as per OMERACT-OARSI criteria. The choice of comparator was a requirement of the Brazilian food and drug regulatory agency (Agência Nacional de Vigilância Sanitária, ANVISA), since the chondroitin sulfate substrate of the reference product is of bovine origin. The blinding strategy of the study treatments enabled keeping the single-blind nature of the study, despite drugs having different organoleptic characteristics.

Table 4 Adverse events observed in the safety population

Adverse events	GS/CS ($N = 314$)	RP ($N = 312$)
Patients reporting at least one AE, n (%)	195 (62.1)	202 (64.7)
Total AEs reported, n	504	572
Incidence of AEs considered related to the treatment, n (%)	67 (21.3)	85 (27.2)
Incidence of serious AEs, n (%)	3 (0.96)	2 (0.6)
Total of serious AEs, n	5	2
Incidence of AEs leading to treatment discontinuation, n (%)	9 (2.9)	8 (2.6)
AEs with incidence ≥ 5%		
Arthralgia, n (%)	15 (4.8)	19 (6.1)
Myalgia, n (%)	10 (3.2)	18 (5.8)
Back pain, n (%)	30 (9.6)	27 (8.7)
Pain in the extremity, n (%)	20 (6.4)	23 (7.4)
Impaired glucose tolerance, n (%)	12 (3.8)	20 (6.4)
Headache, n (%)	45 (14.3)	49 (15.7)
Upper respiratory tract infection, n (%)	24 (7.6)	21 (6.7)
Nasopharyngitis, n (%)	13 (4.1)	19 (6.1)
Flu, n (%)	13 (4.1)	21 (6.7)

$P < 0.05$ between groups for all descriptions. AE(s): adverse event(s); GS/CS: glucosamine sulfate/ chondroitin sulfate; n (%): number and percentage of patients with at least one AE reported in relation to the total number of patients in the safety population; RP: reference product

The need for replacing the raw material for chondroitin manufacturing has led to the development of a new formulation and, therefore, is the initiative for this clinical trial. A fixed-dose combination of glucosamine sulfate and chondroitin sulfate obtained from shark cartilage (Ártico®, Eurofarma Laboratórios S.A., São Paulo, S.P., Brazil), is currently marketed in Brazil as a prescription product approved for medical use by ANVI SA, based on the demonstration of its efficacy and safety in previous clinical trials [13, 14]. However, due to the need to protect increasingly endangered shark species whose populations have exponentially decreased over the last five decades, with no signs of a satisfactory recovery [15, 16], a new source of raw material for chondroitin has become necessary. The option of using bovine cartilage as a substrate for the new formulation was based on the wide availability of this raw material in the Brazilian territory, as well as on evidence of bovine chondroitin efficacy available in the medical literature.

Our findings support the efficacy and safety of the glucosamine sulfate and chondroitin sulfate combination. However, there is still much discussion in the scientific literature about the role of this combination in knee OA, due to controversial results from previous clinical trials. In a randomized, double-blind trial conducted in Spain, the glucosamine sulfate and chondroitin sulfate combination was not observed to be superior to a placebo during a 6-month treatment trial [17].

On the other hand, our results are similar to those from the MOVES study, in which the efficacy of the glucosamine hydrochloride and chondroitin sulfate combination was compared to celecoxib. Despite the differences in the methodologies between the studies, the high OMERACT-OARSI response rate (79% both for the glucosamine/chondroitin sulfate combination and for celecoxib) observed in the MOVES study was similar to the response rate found in our study [18]. The improvement in pain and physical function by the WOMAC questionnaire during 6 months of follow-up was also observed in both studies.

The safety profile of the new formulation was similar to the comparator drug. Headaches and changes in glucose tolerance were the most frequent treatment-related AEs. Different results regarding the effect of glucosamine on glucose metabolism are found in the literature [19]. No SAEs related to the study treatment were reported during the study. This data is supported by a systematic review and meta-analysis about safety of symptomatic slow-acting drugs for OA, which did not show any increase in the risk of SAEs or severe AEs compared to placebo [20].

One factor that could impact our study results was the use of paracetamol as a rescue therapy for OA residual pain. However, the use of the rescue therapy was low in both groups, and it would not be ethical to forbid the use of a pain relief medication during the study. Aiming to reduce the influence of the pain relief medication in questionnaire responses, its use was forbidden within 12 h prior to efficacy evaluations performed in the study. The Kellgren-Lawrence grade of knee OA was evaluated by a physician at each study site. The lack of a central reading system of the radiographs could introduce greater variability in the imaging interpretation and was another limitation. Another point to be mentioned is the proportion of over 60% of Caucasian people in this Brazilian study. According to the Brazilian Institute of Geography and Statistics (IBGE, Instituto Brasileiro de Geografia e Estatística), the self-reported race is white for about 40% of the Brazilian population [21], but we have seen more than 60% of white people in our sample. This could be explained by a larger number of patients who came from centers in São Paulo and Paraná, where there is a higher proportion of whites compared to other regions of the country. Finally, the high drop-out rate of over 20% is also a limitation of the present study, but a per protocol analysis did not show group differences.

Conclusion

In conclusion, this clinical study showed that the new formulation of a fixed-dose combination of glucosamine sulfate and chondroitin sulfate of bovine origin is not inferior to the reference product. The new combination showed a good safety profile in this large population studied. New controlled clinical studies with a large number of patients and evaluating treatment response rate with the combination of glucosamine sulfate and chondroitin sulfate are warranted.

Acknowledgements

The authors thank the trial subjects and the study team from each one of the sites involved in the clinical trial.

Authors' contributions

Dr. Andrea B. V. Lomonte contributed in the clinical trial conception, design, data acquisition, data analysis and interpretation, article writing. Dr. Emerson Gimenez, Dr. Antônio C. da Silva, Dr. Sebastião C. Radominski, Dr. Morton A. Scheinberg, Dr. Antônio C. Ximenes and Dr. Cristiano A. F. Zerbini contributed to data acquistion, study conduction, and article review. The authors read and approved the final manuscript.

Author details

[1]Centro Paulista de Investigação Clínica (CEPIC), Rua Moreira e Costa, 342 – Ipiranga, São Paulo, SP 04266-010, Brazil. [2]Instituto de Pesquisa Clínica e Medicina Avançada (IMA Brasil), São Paulo, Brazil. [3]Clínica Clinilive, Maringá, Brazil. [4]Centro de Estudos em Terapias Inovadoras (CETI), Curitiba, Brazil. [5]Associação de Assistência à Criança Deficiente (AACD), São Paulo, Brazil. [6]Centro Internacional de Pesquisa, Goiânia, Brazil.

References

1. Vina ER, Kwoh CK. Epidemiology of osteoarthritis: literature update. Curr Opin Rheumatol. 2018;30(2):160–7.
2. GBD 2017 DALYs and HALE collaborators. Global, regional, and national disability-adjusted life-years (DALYs) for 359 diseases and injuries and healthy life expectancy (HALE) for 195 countries and territories, 1990–2017: a systematic analysis for the Global Burden of Disease Study 2017. Lancet. 2018;392:1859–922.
3. Xie F, Kovic B, Jin X, He X, Wang M, Silvestre C. Economic and humanistic burden of osteoarthritis: a systematic review of large sample studies. Pharmacoeconomics. 2016;34(11):1087 100.
4. Deshpande BR, Katz JN, Solomon DH, et al. Number of persons with symptomatic knee osteoarthritis in the US: impact of race and ethnicity, age, sex, and obesity. Arthritis Care Res (Hoboken). 2016;68(12):1743–50.
5. Bijlsma JW, Berenbaum F, Lafeber FP. Osteoarthritis: an update with relevance for clinical practice. Lancet. 2011;377(9783):2115–26.
6. Bruyère O, Honvo G, Veronese N, et al. An updated algorithm recommendation for the management of knee osteoarthritis from the European Society for Clinical and Economic Aspects of osteoporosis, osteoarthritis and musculoskeletal diseases (ESCEO). Semin Arthritis Rheum. 2019;49(3):337–50.
7. Towheed TE, Anastassiades T. Glucosamine therapy for osteoarthritis: an update. J Rheumatol. 2007;34(9):1787–90.
8. Piperno M, Reboul P, Hellio Le Graverand MP, Peschard MJ, et al. Glucosamine sulfate modulates dysregulated activities of human osteoarthritic chondrocytes in vitro. Osteoarthr Cartil. 2000;8(3):207–12.
9. Aghazadeh-Habashi A, Jamali F. The glucosamine controversy: a pharmacokinetic issue. J Pharm Sci. 2011;14(2):264–73.
10. Henrotin Y, Mathy M, Sanchez C, Lambert C. Chondroitin sulfate in the treatment of osteoarthritis: from in vitro studies to clinical recommendations. Ther Adv Musculoskelet Dis. 2010;2(6):335–48.
11. Hardingham T. Chondroitin sulfate and joint disease. Osteoarthritis Cartilage. 1998;6(Suppl A):3–5.
12. Fardellone P, Zaim M, Saurel AS, Maheu E. Comparative efficacy and safety study of two chondroitin sulfate preparations from different origin (avian and bovine) in symptomatic osteoarthritis of the knee. Open Rheumatol J. 2013;7:1–12.
13. Brandão GC, Korukian M, Brandão DC, Mainine S, Souza Júnior AP. Association of glucosamine sulfate and chondroitin sulfate for patients with osteoarthritis of the knee. Rev Bras Med. 2009;66(11):405–8.
14. Lomonte ABV, Mendonça JA, de Castro BG, Castro ML. Multicenter, randomized, double-blind clinical trial to evaluate efficacy and safety of combined glucosamine sulfate and chondroitin sulfate capsules for treating knee osteoarthritis. Adv Rheumatol. 2018;58(1):41.
15. Roff G, Brown CJ, Priest MA, Mumby PJ. Decline of coastal apex shark populations over the past half century. Commun Biol. 2018;1:223.
16. Ferretti F, Curnick D, Liu K, Romanov EV, Block BA. Shark baselines and the conservation role of remote coral reef ecosystems. Science Advances. 2018; 4(3):eaaq0333. https://doi.org/10.1126/sciadv.aaq0333.
17. Roman-Blas JA, Castañeda S, Sánchez-Pernaute O, Largo R, Herrero-Beaumont G. CS/GS combined therapy study group. Combined treatment with chondroitin sulfate and glucosamine sulfate shows no superiority over placebo for reduction of joint pain and functional impairment in patients with knee osteoarthritis: a six-month multicenter, randomized, double-blind, placebo-controlled clinical trial. Arthritis Rheumatol. 2017;69(1):77–85.
18. Hochberg MC, Martel-Pelletier J, Monfort J, et al. Combined chondroitin sulfate and glucosamine for painful knee osteoarthritis: a multicentre, randomised, double-blind, non-inferiority trial versus celecoxib. Ann Rheum Dis. 2016;75(1):37–44.
19. Dostrovsky NR, Towheed TE, Hudson RW, Anastassiades TP. The effect of glucosamine on glucose metabolism in humans: a systematic review of the literature. Osteoarthr Cartil. 2011;19(4):375–80.
20. Honvo G, Reginster JY, Rabenda V, et al. Safety of symptomatic slow-acting drugs for osteoarthritis: outcomes of a systematic review and meta-analysis. Drugs Aging. 2019;36(Suppl 1):65–99.
21. IBGE. Pesquisa Nacional por Amostra de Domicílios Contínua Trimestral 2017–2020. http://www.sidra.ibge.gov.br/tabela/6403#resultado. Accessed 22 Nov 2020.

7

Associations between serum calcium, 25(OH)D level and bone mineral density in adolescents

Kaiyu Pan[1], Rongliang Tu[2], Xiaocong Yao[3] and Zhongxin Zhu[3,4*]

Abstract

Backgrounds: It is important to improve our understanding of the roles of calcium and vitamin D in bone health for preventing osteoporosis. We aimed at exploring the associations between serum calcium, vitamin D level, and bone mineral density (BMD) in adolescents included in the National Health and Nutrition Examination Survey (NHANES) 2001–2006.

Methods: Weighted multivariate linear regression models were used to estimate the associations of serum calcium, 25(OH)D level with total BMD. Smooth curve fitting was used to explore the potential non-linear relationship.

Results: A total of 5990 individuals aged between 12 and 19 years were included in this study. The fully-adjusted model showed serum calcium positively correlated with total BMD. However, an inverted U-shaped relationship was found when we performed the smooth curve fitting method, and the inflection point was calculated at 9.6 mg/dL using the two-piecewise linear regression model. In contrast, there was a positive correlation between serum 25(OH)D and total BMD after adjusting for potential confounders.

Conclusions: The present study revealed a positive correlation between serum 25(OH)D level and total BMD, and an inverted U-shaped relationship between serum calcium and total BMD.

Keywords: Calcium, Vitamin D, Bone health, Adolescent, NHANES

Introduction

Osteoporosis is a global health problem that is reported to originate during childhood or adolescence [1]. Adolescence is a critical period of skeletal development and peak bone mass (PBM) may be reached in late adolescence [2]. Evidence indicates that when PBM increases by 5% during childhood and adolescence, the risk of osteoporotic fracture reduces by 40%, while when PBM increases by 10%, this risk decreases by 50% [3, 4]. Therefore, increased bone mass accumulation during this period is an effective way to maintain bone health in adulthood and prevent osteoporosis in older age [5].

Calcium is an essential nutrient for skeletal development and maintenance [6]. Calcium supplementation is recommended for improving bone health in older adults. However, the effect of calcium supplementation on bone mineral density (BMD) remains controversial [7], and it is uncertain whether an elevated serum calcium level is beneficial to bone health [8, 9]. Moreover, vitamin D is known to play an essential role in maintaining normocalcaemia, thus permitting normal skeletal mineralization [10]. In individuals with a low BMD or those at a high risk of osteoporotic fractures, calcium and vitamin D supplementation are suggested as adjuncts to osteoporosis therapies [11]. However, their effect on fracture risk is

* Correspondence: orthozzx@163.com
[3]Department of Osteoporosis Care and Control, Xiaoshan Affiliated Hospital of Wenzhou Medical University, Hangzhou 311200, Zhejiang, China
[4]Clinical Research Center, Xiaoshan Affiliated Hospital of Wenzhou Medical University, Hangzhou 311200, Zhejiang, China

unclear [12]. Furthermore, whether serum calcium, and vitamin D independently correlate with BMD in the general population or certain population groups remains unclear [13, 14]. To the best of our knowledge, no large-sample study has been performed in adolescents. Moreover, the beneficial effect of vitamin D on bone health was reported to be associated with serum 25(OH)D level and not (1,25(OH)2D) [15], and serum 25(OH)D level has been used to assess vitamin D status [16, 17]. Therefore, in this study, we examined the associations of serum calcium, and 25(OH)D level with total BMD among US adolescents using samples from a database of a multiracial population.

Methods

Study population

As a nationally representative survey, the National Health and Nutrition Examination Survey (NHANES) collected health examination data from the non-institutionalized US population [18]. These data are released on a two-year cycle. We used the data from three cycles of NHANES 2001–2006 in this study. A total of 5990 individuals aged 12–19 years with available data on serum calcium, and 25(OH)D levels, and total BMD were included. The NHANES protocols were approved by the Institutional Review Board of the National Center for Health Statistics, and participants or their proxies (< 18 years) provided informed consent [19].

Variables

In this study, the dependent variable was total BMD, and the independent variables were serum calcium and 25(OH)D levels. All subjects included in the present study received dual-energy X-ray absorptiometry (DXA) total body scans. For the 2001–2006 cycles, total BMD was measured using the DXA scans obtained from a QDR-4500A fanbeam densitometer (Hologic, Inc., Bedford, Massachusetts) by trained and certified radiologic technologists. The Beckman Synchron LX20 (Beckman Coulter, Brea, CA) was used to determine serum calcium, and a radioimmunoassay kit (DiaSorin, Stillwater, Minnesota, USA) was used to determine serum 25(OH)D for the 2001–2006 cycles.

The following variables were selected as potential confounders: age, gender, race/ethnicity, physical activity

Table 1 Participant characteristics

Characteristic	Boys ($n = 3086$)	Girls ($n = 2904$)	*P* value
Age, mean ± SD (years)	15.46 ± 2.26	15.35 ± 2.23	0.0551
Race/Ethnicity (%)			0.9754
Non-Hispanic White	62.87	63.15	
Non-Hispanic Black	14.47	14.48	
Mexican American	11.50	11.13	
Other race/ethnicity	11.16	11.25	
BMI, mean ± SD (kg/m^2)	23.31 ± 5.50	23.55 ± 5.78	0.1073
Income to poverty ratio, mean ± SD	2.64 ± 1.62	2.57 ± 1.62	0.0912
Physical activity (%)			< 0.0001
Sedentary	2.95	4.85	
Low	7.72	11.63	
Moderate	6.51	8.47	
High	22.05	16.20	
Not recorded	60.77	58.85	
Calcium supplementation (%)			< 0.0001
Not use	87.21	83.80	
< 0.4 g/d	10.94	12.99	
≥ 0.4 g/d	1.84	3.21	
Serum calcium, mean ± SD (mg/dL)	9.80 ± 0.30	9.64 ± 0.30	< 0.0001
Serum vitamin D, mean ± SD (ng/mL)	24.23 ± 8.63	23.32 ± 10.02	0.0002
Total BMD, mean ± SD (g/cm^2)	1.10 ± 0.14	1.06 ± 0.10	< 0.0001

Mean ± SD for continuous variables: *P* value was calculated by weighted linear regression model
% for categorical variables: *P* value was calculated by weighted chi-square test
Abbreviation: *BMI*, body mass index, *BMD* bone mineral density

Table 2 Associations of serum calcium, 25(OH)D with total bone mineral density

	Model 1 β (95% CI)	Model 2 β (95% CI)	Model 3 β (95% CI)
Serum calcium	−0.0157 (−0.0257, −0.0058)	−0.0003 (− 0.0083, 0.0077)	0.0084 (0.0007, 0.0160)
Serum calcium (quartile)			
Q1	Reference	Reference	Reference
Q2	−0.0065 (− 0.0163, 0.0033)	0.0072 (− 0.0003, 0.0148)	0.0088 (0.0017, 0.0160)
Q3	0.0008 (−0.0087, 0.0103)	0.0136 (0.0062, 0.0211)	0.0141 (0.0070, 0.0212)
Q4	−0.0144 (− 0.0233, − 0.0055)	0.0032 (− 0.0040, 0.0103)	0.0098 (0.0030, 0.0166)
P for trend	0.004	0.484	0.008
Serum 25(OH)D	−0.0005 (− 0.0009, − 0.0002)	0.0001 (− 0.0003, 0.0003)	0.0006 (0.0003, 0.0008)
Serum 25(OH)D (quartile)			
Q1	Reference	Reference	Reference
Q2	−0.0415 (− 0.0532, − 0.0298)	−0.0051 (− 0.0145, 0.0044)	0.0050 (− 0.0040, 0.0139)
Q3	−0.0475 (− 0.0581, − 0.0369)	0.0046 (− 0.0046, 0.0138)	0.0166 (0.0079, 0.0254)
Q4	−0.0384 (− 0.0483, − 0.0284)	0.0030 (− 0.0062, 0.0122)	0.0202 (0.0113, 0.0291)
P for trend	< 0.001	0.181	< 0.001

Model 1: no covariates were adjusted
Model 2: age, gender, race/ethnicity were adjusted
Model 3: age, gender, race/ethnicity, body mass index, income to poverty ratio, physical activity, and calcium supplementation use were adjusted

(based on suggested metabolic equivalent rank) [20], income to poverty ratio, body mass index, and calcium supplementation use. Detailed information on serum calcium, and 25(OH)D levels, total BMD, and other variables can be found at www.cdc.gov/nchs/nhanes/.

Statistical analysis

We used sample weights in all analyses according to the stratified, multistage probability sampling design. The *P*-value was calculated using the weighted chi-square test for categorical variables, and the weighted linear regression model for continuous variables. The weighted multivariate linear regression model was used to investigate whether serum calcium and 25(OH)D levels independently correlated with total BMD. We used generalized additive models and smooth curve fitting to explore potential non-linear relationships. We further calculated the inflection points using the two-piecewise linear regression model. All analyses were conducted using

Table 3 Total bone mineral density by quartiles of serum calcium, stratified by race/ethnicity and age

Quartiles of serum calcium	White	Black	Mexican American	Other race
	Total BMD g/cm^2 (95% Confidence Interval)			
12 to 15 years				
Lowest quartile	1.012 (0.994, 1.029)	1.069 (1.055, 1.083)	1.015 (1.000, 1.031)	1.015 (0.983, 1.047)
2nd	1.011 (0.996, 1.026)	1.068 (1.055, 1.081)	1.008 (0.995, 1.021)	1.024 (1.000, 1.048)
3rd	1.011 (0.998, 1.025)	1.065 (1.052, 1.077)	1.010 (0.998, 1.023)	1.027 (1.002, 1.052)
Highest quartile	1.006 (0.995, 1.017)	1.062 (1.052, 1.072)	0.994 (0.983, 1.005)	0.998 (0.978, 1.018)
P for trend	0.540	0.383	0.031	0.200
16 to 19 years				
Lowest quartile	1.132 (1.118, 1.146)	1.207 (1.195, 1.220)	1.120 (1.109, 1.131)	1.139 (1.116, 1.162)
2nd	1.137 (1.124, 1.151)	1.203 (1.190, 1.216)	1.117 (1.105, 1.128)	1.164 (1.139, 1.189)
3rd	1.140 (1.127, 1.152)	1.214 (1.202, 1.225)	1.117 (1.105, 1.129)	1.132 (1.108, 1.156)
Highest quartile	1.137 (1.126, 1.148)	1.207 (1.196, 1.219)	1.113 (1.102, 1.125)	1.152 (1.127, 1.176)
P for trend	0.598	0.722	0.485	0.883

Gender, body mass index, income poverty ratio, physical activity, and calcium supplement use were adjusted

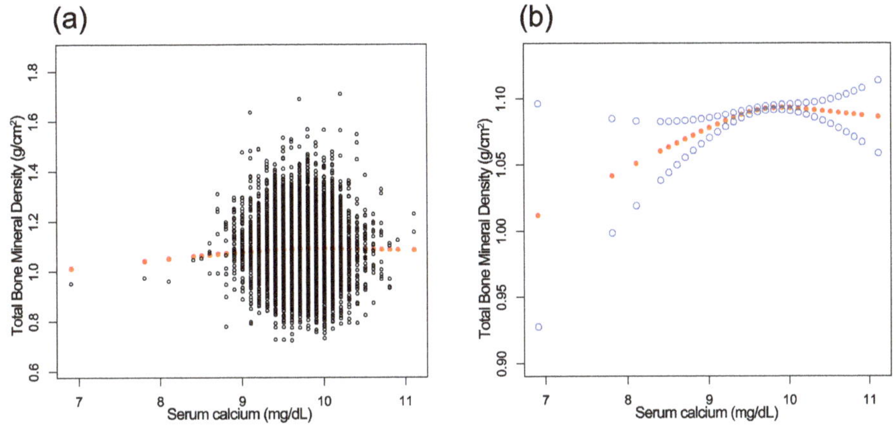

Fig. 1 The association between serum calcium and total bone mineral density. **a** Each black point represents a sample. **b** Solid rad line represents the smooth curve fit between variables. Blue bands represent the 95% of confidence interval from the fit. Adjusted for age, gender, race/ethnicity, income to poverty ratio, education, physical activity, body mass index, calcium supplementation use

R (version 3.5.3) and EmpowerStats software (http://www.empowerstats.com). P-value < 0.05 was considered statistically significant.

Results

The weighted characteristics of the study population according to gender are presented in Table 1. Most of the participants were racially/ethnically classified as "non-Hispanic white". A total of 3086 boys and 2904 girls were included in this study: For boys and girls, respectively, the mean age was 15.46 ± 2.26 and 15.35 ± 2.23 years, mean serum calcium was 9.80 ± 0.30 mg/dL and 9.64 ± 0.30 mg/dL, mean serum 25(OH)D was 24.23 ± 8.63 ng/mL and 23.32 ± 10.02 ng/mL, and mean total BMD was 1.10 ± 0.14 g/cm^2 and 1.06 ± 0.10 g/cm^2.

Association between serum calcium level and total BMD

There was a negative correlation between the serum calcium level and total BMD in the unadjusted model [− 0.0157 (− 0.0257, − 0.0058)] (Table 2), while after adjusting for all potential confounders, a positive correlation was found [0.0084 (0.0007, 0.0160)]. Compared to participants with the lowest serum calcium level in Q1, participants in other groups had a higher total BMD. The results of total BMD by quartiles of the serum calcium level, stratified by race/ethnicity and age, are shown in Table 3. Furthermore, we found an inverted U-shaped relationship between the serum calcium level and total BMD using the smooth curve fitting method (Fig. 1). We subsequently calculated that the inflection point was 9.6 mg/dL using the two-piecewise linear regression model (Table 4). In the subgroup analysis stratified by gender and race/ethnicity, this inverted U-shaped relationship existed in boys, Whites and Blacks (Figs. 3 and 4), whereas the serum calcium level positively correlated with total BMD in girls, Mexican Americans and other race/ethnicity. In addition, we calculated that the inflection points were 9.6 mg/dL in boys and Whites, and 9.2 mg/dL in Blacks.

Association between serum 25(OH)D level and total BMD

The serum 25(OH)D level negatively correlated with total BMD in the unadjusted model [0.0005 (− 0.0009, − 0.0002)] (Table 2). This association became positive after adjusting for all potential confounders [0.0006 (0.0003, 0.0008)] (Table 2, Fig. 2). Compared to participants with the lowest serum 25(OH)D level in Q1, participants in the other groups had a higher total BMD. The trend test remained significant ($P < 0.001$). The results of total BMD by quartiles of serum 25(OH)D, stratified by race/ethnicity and age. Are shown in Table 5. In the subgroup analysis stratified by gender and race/ethnicity, we found a U-shaped relationship in boys, and an inverted U-shaped relationship in girls and Whites (Figs. 3 and 4). The results of the inflection points are shown in Table 4.

Discussion

The aim of this study was to explore whether there are independent correlations between serum calcium, and 25(OH)D levels and total BMD among adolescents aged 12–19 years. The results showed that serum 25(OH)D was positively correlated with total BMD, and the relationship of serum calcium with total BMD assumed an inverted U-shaped (inflection point: 9.6 mg/dL).

Calcium plays an important role in many biological systems, most notably in bones. Thus, it is essential to

Table 4 Threshold effect analysis of serum calcium and 25(OH)D on total bone mineral density by using two-piecewise linear regression

	Adjusted ß (95% CI), *p*-value
Serum calcium	
Total	
Fitting by standard linear model	0.0084 (0.0007, 0.0160) 0.0317
Fitting by two-piecewise linear model	
Inflection point	9.6
Serum calcium < 9.6 (mg/dL)	0.0348 (0.0165, 0.0530) 0.0002
Serum calcium > 9.6 (mg/dL)	−0.0051 (− 0.0164, 0.0063) 0.3824
Log likelihood ratio	0.002
Boy	
Fitting by standard linear model	0.0034 (−0.0076, 0.0143) 0.5446
Fitting by two-piecewise linear model	
Inflection point	9.6
Serum calcium < 9.6 (mg/dL)	0.0447 (0.0128, 0.0765) 0.0060
Serum calcium > 9.6 (mg/dL)	−0.0109 (− 0.0260, 0.0042) 0.1564
Log likelihood ratio	0.007
White	
Fitting by standard linear model	0.0129 (−0.0017, 0.0276) 0.0843
Fitting by two-piecewise linear model	
Inflection point	9.6
Serum calcium < 9.6 (mg/dL)	0.0465 (0.0091, 0.0839) 0.0148
Serum calcium > 9.6 (mg/dL)	−0.0025 (− 0.0240, 0.0191) 0.8218
Log likelihood ratio	0.055
Black	
Fitting by standard linear model	0.0053 (−0.0080, 0.0187) 0.4353
Fitting by two-piecewise linear model	
Inflection point	9.2
Serum calcium < 9.2 (mg/dL)	0.1074 (0.0200, 0.1949) 0.0161
Serum calcium > 9.2 (mg/dL)	−0.0011 (− 0.0155, 0.0133) 0.8780
Log likelihood ratio	0.020
Serum 25(OH)D	
Boy	
Fitting by standard linear model	0.0013 (0.0009, 0.0018) < 0.0001
Fitting by two-piecewise linear model	
Inflection point	24
Serum 25(OH)D < 24(ng/mL)	0.0024 (0.0015, 0.0034) < 0.0001
Serum 25(OH)D > 24(ng/mL)	0.0007 (0.0000, 0.0014) 0.0400
Log likelihood ratio	0.008
Girl	
Fitting by standard linear model	0.0003 (−0.0000, 0.0007) 0.0565
Fitting by two-piecewise linear model	
Inflection point	26
Serum 25(OH)D < 26(ng/mL)	0.0011 (0.0005, 0.0018) 0.0006
Serum 25(OH)D > 26(ng/mL)	−0.0003 (− 0.0008, 0.0003) 0.3218

Table 4 Threshold effect analysis of serum calcium and 25(OH)D on total bone mineral density by using two-piecewise linear regression *(Continued)*

	Adjusted ß (95% CI), *p*-value
Log likelihood ratio	0.004
White	
Fitting by standard linear model	0.0003 (−0.0002, 0.0009) 0.1945
Fitting by two-piecewise linear model	
Inflection point	23
Serum 25(OH)D < 23(ng/mL)	0.0035 (0.0018, 0.0052) < 0.0001
Serum 25(OH)D > 23(ng/mL)	−0.0005 (− 0.0011, 0.0002) 0.1629
Log likelihood ratio	< 0.001

age, gender, race/ethnicity, body mass index, income to poverty ratio, physical activity, and calcium supplementation use were adjusted
In the analysis for boy/girl, white/black, the model is not adjusted for gender or race/ethnicity, respectively

ensure adequate calcium intake throughout life for building and maintaining bones [21]. However, a lower-than-recommended calcium intake has been reported for European and Brazilian populations [22, 23]. Several trials have suggested that supplementing by oral calcium salts is notably associated with bone attenuation [24, 25]. Some recent studies showed either no significant correlation or a negative association between serum calcium level with BMD [8, 9, 13]; our results suggested an inverted U-shaped relationship in adolescents aged 12–19 years. There are some biological explanations for the findings of this study. It was found that a high calcium intake or an intake exceeding the optimal level, could reduce osteoblast differentiation and mineralization in vitro [26, 27] and in some animals [28]. Thus, there may be a narrow range of optimal calcium levels that promote bone growth, whereas elevated calcium levels may have deleterious effects on bone. The above evidence suggested that calcium intake is required to improve BMD in subjects with low serum calcium levels.

It has been shown that a low serum 25(OH)D level has an adverse effect on bone health [29]. Several cross-sectional studies reported a positive association between serum 25(OH)D level and BMD in adults [30–32]. Vitamin D deficiency has been a global health problem in the general population, with a distinct lack of data in children and adolescents [33]. Recent studies showed that hypovitaminosis D is a common disease in children, and studies in an adult population regarding the aetiology of osteoporosis have somewhat linked the evidence to vitamin D deficiency during childhood and adolescence [34]. The results of a cross-sectional study of 100 Indian healthy school-age children showed that the serum 25(OH)D level positively related to BMD [35].

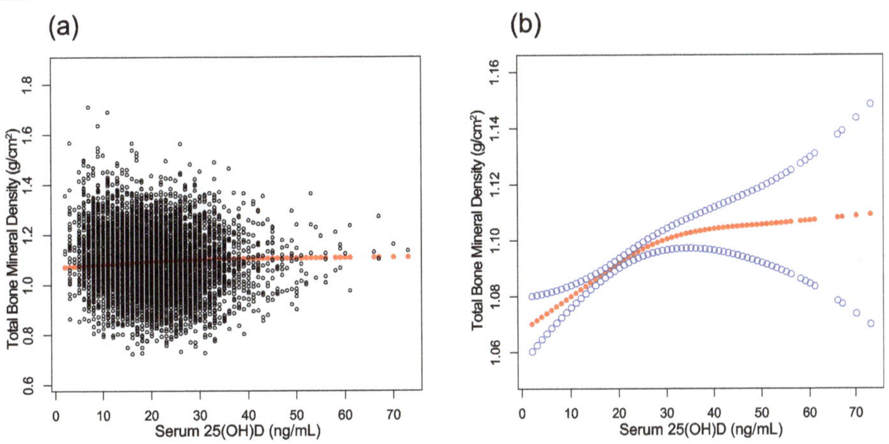

Fig. 2 The association between serum 25(OH)D level and total bone mineral density. **a** Each black point represents a sample. **b** Solid rad line represents the smooth curve fit between variables. Blue bands represent the 95% of confidence interval from the fit. Adjusted for age, gender, race/ethnicity, income to poverty ratio, education, physical activity, body mass index, calcium supplementation use

Table 5 Total bone mineral density by quartiles of serum 25(OH)D level, stratified by race/ethnicity and age

Quartiles of 25(OH)D level	White	Black	Mexican American	Other race
	Total BMD g/cm^2 (95% Confidence Interval)			
12 to 15 years				
Lowest quartile	0.975 (0.929, 1.022)	1.064 (1.054, 1.074)	0.996 (0.979, 1.013)	1.027 (0.996, 1.058)
2nd	0.994 (0.973, 1.015)	1.068 (1.056, 1.079)	0.994 (0.982, 1.007)	0.993 (0.970, 1.016)
3rd	1.013 (1.001, 1.025)	1.061 (1.048, 1.075)	1.012 (1.002, 1.023)	1.000 (0.981, 1.020)
Highest quartile	1.011 (1.002, 1.020)	1.071 (1.052, 1.090)	1.014 (1.000, 1.027)	1.050 (1.026, 1.074)
P for trend	0.134	0.780	0.024	0.079
16 to 19 years				
Lowest quartile	1.106 (1.073, 1.139)	1.212 (1.204, 1.220)	1.107 (1.094, 1.120)	1.135 (1.107, 1.162)
2nd	1.126 (1.106, 1.146)	1.203 (1.191, 1.215)	1.109 (1.098, 1.119)	1.153 (1.128, 1.178)
3rd	1.127 (1.115, 1.140)	1.198 (1.182, 1.215)	1.115 (1.104, 1.125)	1.136 (1.115, 1.157)
Highest quartile	1.144 (1.136, 1.152)	1.210 (1.188, 1.232)	1.140 (1.128, 1.152)	1.160 (1.136, 1.185)
P for trend	0.003	0.262	< 0.001	0.347

Gender, body mass index, income poverty ratio, physical activity, and calcium supplement use were adjusted

Our results also showed a positive association between the serum 25(OH)D level and total BMD. We performed subgroup analyses to describe the data in more detail following the STROBE guidelines [36]. A non-linear relationship between the 25(OH)D level and total BMD was found, and the inflection points were detected. These findings suggest a potentially optimal serum vitamin D level for BMD, while elevated 25(OH)D levels (beyond the turning point) may lead to a lower BMD in girls and Whites. The heterogeneity among these studies, including differences in participant selection, study size, study design, and controlled confounders, may provide a possible explanation for these conflicting conclusions.

To the best of our knowledge, this is the largest study investigating the relationships between serum calcium, and 25(OH)D levels and BMD in adolescents, and this representative sample of a multiracial population may be used as a general investigation of the whole population. Some limitations are worth noting. First, accurate data on puberty status were not included in our study. Although age was adjusted as a covariate in this study, the possible bias related to the unmeasured puberty status remained a limitation. Second, due to its cross-sectional design, this research had less power regarding the determination of causal relationships between serum calcium, and 25(OH)D levels and BMD.

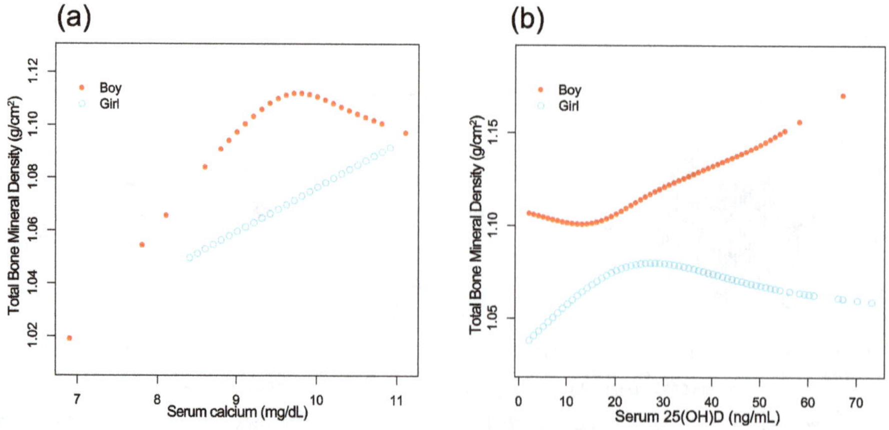

Fig. 3 The associations between serum calcium (**a**), serum 25(OH)D (**b**) and total bone mineral density stratified by gender. Adjusted for age, race/ethnicity, income to poverty ratio, education, physical activity, body mass index, calcium supplementation use

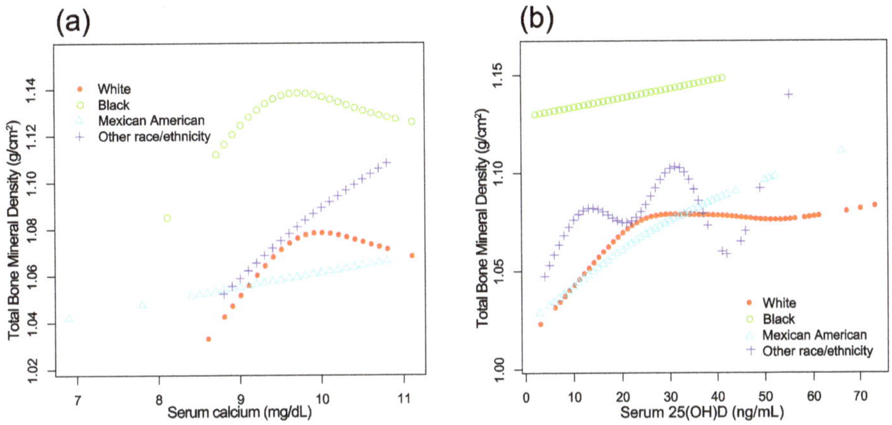

Fig. 4 The associations between serum calcium (**a**), serum 25(OH)D (**b**) and total bone mineral density stratified by race/ethnicity. Adjusted for age, gender, income to poverty ratio, education, physical activity, body mass index, calcium supplementation use

Conclusions

We found that serum calcium level had an inverted U-shaped relationship with total BMD, while serum 25(OH)D level positively correlated with total BMD. Further studies are needed to assess whether increased serum 25 (OH) D or calcium levels may have a beneficial effect on BMD in adolescents with low serum 25 (OH) D or calcium levels.

Acknowledgements

The authors appreciate the time and effort given by participants during the data collection phase of the NHANES project.

Authors' contributions

KYP, RLT, and XYC contributed to data collection, analysis and writing of the manuscript. ZXZ contributed to study design and writing of the manuscript. The authors read and approved the final manuscript.

Author details

[1]Department of Paediatrics, Xiaoshan Affiliated Hospital of Wenzhou Medical University, Hangzhou 311200, Zhejiang, China. [2]Department of Paediatrics, Zhejiang Xiaoshan Hospital, Hangzhou 311200, Zhejiang, China. [3]Department of Osteoporosis Care and Control, Xiaoshan Affiliated Hospital of Wenzhou Medical University, Hangzhou 311200, Zhejiang, China. [4]Clinical Research Center, Xiaoshan Affiliated Hospital of Wenzhou Medical University, Hangzhou 311200, Zhejiang, China.

References

1. Yang X, Zhai Y, Zhang J, Chen JY, Liu D, Zhao WH. Combined effects of physical activity and calcium on bone health in children and adolescents: a systematic review of randomized controlled trials. WJP. 2020;16(4):356-65.
2. Baxter-Jones AD, Faulkner RA, Forwood MR, Mirwald RL, Bailey DA. Bone mineral accrual from 8 to 30 years of age: an estimation of peak bone mass. J Bone Miner Res. 2011;26(8):1729–39.
3. van der Sluis IM, de Muinck Keizer-Schrama SM. Osteoporosis in childhood: bone density of children in health and disease. J Pediatr Endocrinol Metab. 2001;14(7):817–32.
4. Goulding A, Jones IE, Taylor RW, Manning PJ, Williams SM. More broken bones: a 4-year double cohort study of young girls with and without distal forearm fractures. J Bone Miner Res. 2000;15(10):2011–8.
5. Rizzoli R, Bianchi ML, Garabedian M, McKay HA, Moreno LA. Maximizing bone mineral mass gain during growth for the prevention of fractures in the adolescents and the elderly. Bone. 2010;46(2):294–305.
6. Rooney MR, Michos ED, Hootman KC, Harnack L, Lutsey PL. Trends in calcium supplementation, National Health and nutrition examination survey (NHANES) 1999-2014. Bone. 2018;111:23–7.
7. Tai V, Leung W, Grey A, Reid IR, Bolland MJ. Calcium intake and bone mineral density: systematic review and meta-analysis. BMJ (Clinical research ed). 2015;h4183:351.
8. Cerani A, Zhou S, Forgetta V, Morris JA, Trajanoska K, Rivadeneira F, Larsson SC, Michaelsson K, Richards JB. Genetic predisposition to increased serum calcium, bone mineral density, and fracture risk in individuals with normal calcium levels: mendelian randomisation study. BMJ (Clinical research ed). 2019;l4410:366.
9. Dalemo S, Eggertsen R, Hjerpe P, Almqvist EG, Bostrom KB. Bone mineral density in primary care patients related to serum calcium concentrations: a longitudinal cohort study from Sweden. Scand J Prim Health Care. 2018; 36(2):198–206.
10. Reid IR, Vitamin D. Effect on bone mineral density and fractures. Endocrinol Metab Clin N Am. 2017;46(4):935–45.
11. Shoback D, Rosen CJ, Black DM, Cheung AM, Murad MH, Eastell R. Pharmacological management of osteoporosis in postmenopausal women: an endocrine society guideline update. J Clin Endocrinol Metab. 2020;105(3).
12. Hauk L. Treatment of low BMD and osteoporosis to prevent fractures: updated guideline from the ACP. Am Fam Physician. 2018;97(5):352–3.
13. Liu M, Yao X, Zhu Z. Associations between serum calcium, 25(OH)D level and bone mineral density in older adults. J Orthop Surg Res. 2019;14(1):458.
14. Li GH, Robinson-Cohen C, Sahni S, Au PC, Tan KC, Kung AW, Cheung CL. Association of genetic variants related to serum calcium levels with reduced bone mineral density. J Clin Endocrinol Metab. 2020;105(3):e328-36.
15. Sharma DK, Sawyer RK, Robertson TS, Stamenkov R, Solomon LB, Atkins GJ, Clifton PM, Morris HA, Anderson PH. Elevated serum 25-Hydroxyvitamin D levels are associated with improved bone formation and micro-structural measures in elderly hip fracture patients. J Clin Med. 2019;8(11).
16. Holick MF. Vitamin D deficiency. N Engl J Med. 2007;357(3):266–81.
17. Vieth R. Vitamin D supplementation, 25-hydroxyvitamin D concentrations, and safety. Am J Clin Nutr. 1999;69(5):842–56.
18. Curtin LR, Mohadjer LK, Dohrmann SM, Montaquila JM, Kruszan-Moran D, Mirel LB, Carroll MD, Hirsch R, Schober S, Johnson CL. The National Health and Nutrition Examination Survey: Sample Design, 1999-2006. Vital Health Stat Ser 2 Data Eval Methods Res. 2012;(155):1–39.
19. Zipf G, Chiappa M, Porter KS, Ostchega Y, Lewis BG, Dostal J. National health and nutrition examination survey: plan and operations, 1999-2010. Vital Health Stat Ser 1 Programs Collection Proced. 2013;(56):1 37.

20. Patel CJ, Pho N, McDuffie M, Easton-Marks J, Kothari C, Kohane IS, Avillach P. A database of human exposomes and phenomes from the US National Health and nutrition examination survey. Sci Data. 2016;3: 160096.
21. Hodges JK, Cao S, Cladis DP, Weaver CM. Lactose intolerance and bone health: the challenge of ensuring adequate calcium intake. Nutrients. 2019; 11(4).
22. Mensink GB, Fletcher R, Gurinovic M, Huybrechts I, Lafay L, Serra-Majem L, Szponar L, Tetens I, Verkaik-Kloosterman J, Baka A, et al. Mapping low intake of micronutrients across Europe. Br J Nutr. 2013;110(4):755–73.
23. Pinheiro MM, Schuch NJ, Genaro PS, Ciconelli RM, Ferraz MB, Martini LA. Nutrient intakes related to osteoporotic fractures in men and women--the Brazilian osteoporosis study (BRAZOS). Nutr J. 2009;8:6.
24. Asmus HG, Braun J, Krause R, Brunkhorst R, Holzer H, Schulz W, Neumayer HH, Raggi P, Bommer J. Two year comparison of sevelamer and calcium carbonate effects on cardiovascular calcification and bone density. Nephrol Dial Transplant. 2005;20(8):1653–61.
25. Raggi P, James G, Burke SK, Bommer J, Chasan-Taber S, Holzer H, Braun J, Chertow GM. Decrease in thoracic vertebral bone attenuation with calcium-based phosphate binders in hemodialysis. J Bone Miner Res. 2005;20(5):764–72.
26. Eklou-Kalonji E, Denis I, Lieberherr M, Pointillart A. Effects of extracellular calcium on the proliferation and differentiation of porcine osteoblasts in vitro. Cell Tissue Res. 1998;292(1):163–71.
27. Dvorak MM, Siddiqua A, Ward DT, Carter DH, Dallas SL, Nemeth EF, Riccardi D. Physiological changes in extracellular calcium concentration directly control osteoblast function in the absence of calciotropic hormones. Proc Natl Acad Sci U S A. 2004;101(14):5140–5.
28. Al-Dujaili SA, Koh AJ, Dang M, Mi X, Chang W, Ma PX, McCauley LK. Calcium sensing receptor function supports osteoblast survival and acts as a co-factor in PTH anabolic actions in bone. J Cell Biochem. 2016;117(7):1556–67.
29. Christakos S, Li S, DeLa Cruz J, Verlinden L, Carmeliet G. Vitamin D and bone. Handb Exp Pharmacol. 2020;262:47-63.
30. von Muhlen DG, Greendale GA, Garland CF, Wan L, Barrett-Connor E, Vitamin D. Parathyroid hormone levels and bone mineral density in community-dwelling older women: the rancho Bernardo study. Osteoporos Int. 2005;16(12):1721–6.
31. Bischoff-Ferrari HA, Dietrich T, Orav EJ, Dawson-Hughes B. Positive association between 25-hydroxy vitamin D levels and bone mineral density: a population-based study of younger and older adults. Am J Med. 2004; 116(9):634–9.
32. Collins D, Jasani C, Fogelman I, Swaminathan R. Vitamin D and bone mineral density. Osteoporos Int. 1998;8(2):110–4.
33. White Z, White S, Dalvie T, Kruger MC, Van Zyl A, Becker P. Bone health, body composition, and vitamin D status of black preadolescent children in South Africa. Nutrients. 2019;11(6).
34. Guillemant J, Taupin P, Le HT, Taright N, Allemandou A, Peres G, Guillemant S. Vitamin D status during puberty in French healthy male adolescents. Osteoporos Int. 1999;10(3):222–5.
35. Sharawat IK, Dawman L. Bone mineral density and its correlation with vitamin D status in healthy school-going children of Western India. Arch Osteoporos. 2019; 14(1):13.
36. von Elm E, Altman DG, Egger M, Pocock SJ, Gotzsche PC, Vandenbroucke JP. The strengthening the reporting of observational studies in epidemiology (STROBE) statement: guidelines for reporting observational studies. Lancet (London, England). 2007;370(9596):1453–7.

8

Functional index for hand osteoarthritis (FIHOA) is associated with pain, muscle strength and EQ-5D in hand osteoarthritis

Seong-Kyu Kim*, Ui Hong Jung and Jung-Yoon Choe

Abstract

Background: This study identified whether Functional Index for Hand Osteoarthritis (FIHOA) is associated with pain, hand muscle strength, health-related quality of life, and radiographic severity in hand osteoarthritis (OA).

Methods: We consecutively recruited 95 patients with hand OA. The FIHOA was used to assess questionnaire-based physical function in hand OA. Health-related quality of life was evaluated using EuroQol-5 dimension (EQ-5D). Radiographic changes of hand joints were measured by Kellgren-Lawrence (K-L) grade, which was determined based on total radiographic severity score and number of affected joints. Other measures included patient's visual analogue scale (VAS) score for pain and performance-based function indexes such as grip and pinch strength. Statistical analysis was performed using Mann-Whitney U test, Spearman's correlation analysis, and multivariate logistic regression analysis.

Results: FIHOA score was negatively associated with grip and pinch hand strength and EQ-5D and positively correlated to VAS pain ($p < 0.05$ for all). There were significant differences of grip and pinch strength, VAS pain, EQ-5D index, and EQ-VAS between two FIHOA groups (≤ 4 vs. > 4) ($p < 0.05$ for all). Multivariate logistic regression analysis showed that higher FIHOA score (FIHOA > 4) was related with increased VAS pain and with lower EQ-5D index ($p = 0.008$ and $p = 0.013$, respectively). There was no association between FIHOA score and measures of total radiographic severity score and number of affected joints.

Conclusion: This study observes that FIHOA score is associated with patient-reported VAS pain, hand muscle strength indexes, and EQ-5D but not radiographic severity in hand OA.

Keywords: Osteoarthritis, Hand, FIHOA, EQ-5D, VAS, Kellgren-Lawrence grade

Background

Hand osteoarthritis (OA) is a prevalent degenerative disease that leads to pain, joint deformity, functional disability, and impaired quality of life [1, 2]. The clinical phenotypes of hand OA seem to be heterogeneous according to number and pattern of joint involvement. The Outcome Measures in Rheumatology (OMERACT) and the Osteoarthritis Research Society International (OARSI) Task Force on Clinical Trials Guidelines have been frequently used in clinical trials [3, 4]. For assessment of physical function based on a questionnaire for hand OA, outcome measures from the pain subscale of the Australian/Canadian (AUSCAN) Index [5], the Cochin hand functional disability scale [6], and the Functional Index for Hand Osteoarthritis (FIHOA) [7] have been used in clinical trials and have been shown to be valid, reliable, and relevant.

The FIHOA is a unidimensional questionnaire that is structurally different from the AUSCAN index, which measures pain, stiffness, and function dimensions [7, 8]. A case-control study revealed that FIHOA score was gradually increased as the severity of hand OA increased [9].

* Correspondence: kimsk714@cu.ac.kr
Division of Rheumatology, Department of Internal Medicine, Catholic University of Daegu School of Medicine, 33, Duryugongwon-ro 17-gil, Nam-gu, Daegu 42472, Republic of Korea

In a study that analyzed 18 patients with hand OA, FIHOA score was found to be correlated with the degree of radiological damage, but not synovial inflammation based on magnetic resonance image (MRI) [10]. Compatible with previous studies [7, 8], Koutroumpas et al. confirmed significant association between FIHOA and clinical assessment for erosive hand OA [11]. In addition, FIHOA was noted to related with MRI-defined bone attrition in 77 female patients with hand OA [12]. However, there is a lack of research data regarding FIHOA score and hand muscle strength or quality of life in hand OA. The main aim of this study is to determine association of FIHOA-based functional status with pain, grip and pinch strength, quality of life, and radiographic severity in hand OA.

Subjects and methods

Study population

A total of 95 patients with Korean hand OA that met the American College of Rheumatology (ACR) classification criteria was recruited from the Rheumatology Clinic and enrolled in this study from February 2019 to January 2020 [13]. All patients showed radiographic changes at more than one of both hand joints assessed according to the Kellgren-Lawrence (K-L) grading system [14]. This study excluded patients diagnosed with rheumatoid arthritis, systemic lupus erythematosus, psoriatic arthritis, and gouty arthritis.

Clinical information

Demographic data were age (years), sex, body mass index (BMI, kg/m^2), systolic blood pressure (SBP, mmHg), diastolic blood pressure (DBP, mmHg), and symptom duration (months) at time of enrollment. Acute phase reactants, such as erythrocyte sediment rate (ESR) and C-reactive protein (CRP), were measured. Pain was scored using a 100 mm Visual Analogue Scale (VAS). The Functional Index for Hand Osteoarthritis (FIHOA) questionnaire was assessed for hand physical function scores from 0 to 30 and was composed of 10 doctor-administered questions with semi-quantitative assessment on a 4-point Likert scale ranging from 0 to 3 [7, 8]. This study used a Korean version of the FIHOA, which was validated in Korean patients with hand OA [15]. FIHOA scores were divided into two groups based on four points (FIHOA ≤4 vs. FIHOA > 4) according to classification by an earlier study [7].

EuroQol-5 dimension (EQ-5D) measurement

The Korean version of EQ-5D is a tool to measure health-related quality of life (HRQOL) [16]. The EQ-5D consists of the EQ-5D index and the EQ-VAS. The EQ-5D index consists of five questions that ask about the current state of health as mobility, self-care, usual activities, pain/discomfort, and anxiety/depression.

Radiological assessment

Total radiographic severity scores were the sum of Kellgren-Lawrence (K-L) grade scores at a total of 20 joints such as 2nd – 5th distal interphalangeal (DIP) joints, 2nd – 5th proximal interphalangeal (PIP) joints, thumb interphalangeal (IP) joint, and first carpometacarpal joint of both hands, which ranged from grade 0 to grade 80. The number of affected joints with any kind of radiologic change was calculated for each subject according to the K-L grading system. A single rheumatologist completing a training program (UH Jung) provided radiographic digital images of hand joints from the Korean College of Rheumatology.

Muscle strength measurement

Measurement for grip strength in both hands was performed with arms and elbows at right angles using a dynamometer (Jamar Hydraulic Hand Dynamometer, Nottinghamshire, UK). Pinch strength for the first and second fingers was measured by a pinch gauge (B&L Engineering, Tustin, CA, USA). The mean values for grip strength and pinch strength were presented after measurements on both hands.

Statistical analysis

Data are described as median (interquartile range [IQR]) for continuous variables and number (percentage [%]) for nominal variables. The Shapiro-Wilk test was applied to test normality and showed a non-normal distribution. The correlations between FIHOA score and clinical and radiographic variables were measured by Spearman's correlation coefficient. The differences of variables between FIHOA ≤4 and FIHOA > 4 were calculated by Mann-Whitney U test. Multivariate logistic regression analysis was performed to identify clinical and radiographic variables related to higher FIHOA score > 4 along with the odds ratio (OR) and 95% confidence interval (CI). A P value less than 0.5 was considered statistically significant. Statistical analyses were performed by IBM SPSS Statistics 19.0 (IBM Corp., Armonk, NY, USA).

Results

Baseline characteristics

Baseline characteristics of enrolled subjects are described in Table 1. The median age was 60.0 years (IQR 54.0–66.0), and most subjects were female (n = 90, 94.7%). The average values of grip strength and pinch strength were 20.0 (IQR 16.5–24.5) and 5.7 (IQR 4.8–6.5), respectively, and the median score of FIHOA was 65.0 (IQR 50.0–80.0). Radiographic changes were measured as 6.0 (IQR 2.0–18.0) for total radiographic severity score and 5.0 (IQR 2.0 9.0) for affected joint count.

Table 1 Baseline characteristics of enrolled subjects

Variables	Results
Age (year)	60.0 (54.0–66.0)
Sex, female (n, %)	90 (94.7)
Symptom duration (month)	6.0 (1.0–73.0)
BMI (kg/m^2)	23.4 (21.5–24.9)
SBP (mmHg)	127.0 (115.0–135.0)
DBP (mmHg)	74.0 (69.0–80.0)
ESR (mm/hr)	14.0 (9.0–32.0)
CRP (mg/L)	0.6 (0.6–0.8)
Past history	
Hypertension (n, %)	24 (25.3)
Diabetes mellitus (n, %)	10 (10.5)
Grip strength	
Mean[a]	20.0 (16.5–24.5)
Right	20.0 (16.0–25.0)
Left	22.0 (16.0–25.0)
Pinch strength	
Mean[a]	5.7 (4.8–6.5)
Right	6.0 (5.0–6.8)
Left	5.5 (4.8–6.5)
VAS pain	34.0 (20.0–52.0)
FIHOA	65.0 (50.0–80.0)
EQ-5D index	0.82 (0.77–0.87)
EQ-VAS	65.0 (50.0–80.0)
Total radiographic severity scores (0–80) [b]	6.0 (2.0–18.0)
Number of affected joints (0–20) [b]	5.0 (2.0–9.0)

Data were described as median (Interquartile range) or number (%)
Abbreviation: *BMI* body mass index; *SBP* systolic blood pressure; *DBP* diastolic blood pressure; *ESR* erythrocyte sedimentation rate; *CRP* C-reactive protein; *VAS* visual analogue scale; *FIHOA* Functional Index for Hand Osteoarthritis; *EQ-5D* EuroQol-5 dimension
[a]Average value of the sum of right and left hand scores
[b]Based on Kellgren-Lawrence grade

Comparison of variables according to FIHOA group

There were no differences in age, sex, symptom duration, BMI, SBP, DBP, ESR, CRP, total radiographic severity score, and number of affected joints between the high and low FIHOA groups ($p > 0.05$ for all) (Table 2). Subjects with high FIHOA score had lower grip and pinch hand strength, higher patient VAS pain score, and lower EQ-5D index and EQ-VAS scores ($p < 0.05$ for all).

Associations between FIHOA score and variables

Analysis for variables related with FIHOA score showed that the score was negatively associated with mean grip and pinch hand muscle strengths, EQ-5D index, and EQ-VAS (Fig. 1). In contrast, FIHOA score was positively related with patient VAS pain. However, there were no relationships between FIHOA score and age, sex, symptom duration, BMI, SBP, DBP, ESR, CRP, total radiographic severity score, or number of affected joints.

Variables associated with high FIHOA score

Mean grip and pinch strength, patient VAS pain, EQ-5D index, and EQ-VAS were associated with high FIHOA score in univariate regression analysis (Table 3). Multivariate regression analysis after adjusting for confounding factors of age, sex, and symptom duration revealed that high FIHOA score was significantly linked to patient VAS pain and EQ-5D index ($p = 0.008$ and $p = 0.013$, respectively).

Discussion

This study assessed the relationships of FIHOA score with other outcome measures including pain, grip and pinch hand strength, and EQ-5D in hand OA. In addition, correlation between functional impairment and radiographic damage was also explored. We found that FIHOA score was associated with patient-reported pain, hand strength, and quality of life based on the EQ-5D in hand OA. In addition, higher FIHOA score was associated with higher VAS pain score and lower EQ-5D index and EQ-VAS. However, there was no relationship between FIHOA score and radiographic outcome.

The outcome measures of hand OA include pain, hand physical function, and quality of life [3, 4]. Among the several hand OA-specific measures for physical disability that have been developed, such as the AUSCAN Index [5], the Cochin hand functional disability scale [6], and the FIHOA [7], FIHOA score is a unidimensional measure for functional impairment of hand OA and is considered a feasible and valid questionnaire commonly used in clinical study. Efforts have been made to verify the association between FIHOA score and other measures in OA. The Health Assessment Questionnaire (HAQ) [17], which is a rheumatoid arthritis-specific questionnaire for health status, was significantly associated with FIHOA score in hand OA ($r = 0.73$) and physical function scale of AUSCAN ($r = 0.80$) [18]. Similarly, EQ-5D, which is a generic measure for health-related quality of life [16], was also validated in patients with knee OA, showing a negative relationship of the Korean version of Western Ontario and McMaster Scale (KWOMAC) with the EQ-5D index [19]. There is a lack of data on the association between FIHOA score and EQ-5D in hand OA. As far as we know, this study is the first to find FIHOA score to be negatively related with EQ-5D index and EQ-VAS, and patients with high FIHOA score showed a trend toward a lower EQ-5D index but not EQ-VAS in hand OA. Based on these observations, functional impairment might be linked to health-related quality of life in hand OA.

Table 2 Comparison of variables according to FIHOA

	FIHOA ≤4 (*n* = 49)	FIHOA > 4 (*n* = 46)	*p* values
Age (year)	61.0 (54.6–67.5)	59.0 (54.0–63.3)	0.367
Sex, female (n, %)	46 (93.9)	44 (95.7)	0.530
Symptom duration (month)	24.0 (1.0–96.0)	4.0 (1.0–30.0)	0.120
BMI (kg/m^2)	23.4 (21.3–24.0)	23.8 (21.5–25.9)	0.295
SBP (mmHg)	126.0 (114.0–135.0)	127.5 (119.5–135.5)	0.690
DBP (mmHg)	74.0 (69.0–80.0)	75.5 (69.5–80.3)	0.463
ESR (mm/hr)	14.0 (9.0–27.3)	14.0 (8.0–20.5)	0.376
CRP (mg/L)	0.6 (0.6–0.8)	0.6 (0.6–1.3)	0.295
Grip strength			
Mean[a]	23.0 (19.3–25.0)	18.0 (13.9–22.3)	< 0.001
Right	22.0 (18.0–27.5)	18.0 (14.0–22.5)	0.004
Left	23.0 (10.0–26.0)	17.5 (12.8–23.0)	< 0.001
Pinch strength			
Mean[a]	6.3 (5.3–7.1)	5.4 (4.0–6.4)	< 0.001
Right	6.3 (5.1–7.3)	5.5 (3.5–6.5)	0.001
Left	6.0 (5.0–7.0)	5.5 (3.9–6.0)	0.002
VAS pain	22.0 (10.0–36.5)	48.5 (34.0–71.0)	< 0.001
EQ-5D index	0.87 (0.82–0.91)	0.82 (0.7–0.86)	< 0.001
EQ-VAS	70.0 (57.5–80.0)	50.0 (49.5–70.0)	< 0.001
Total radiographic severity scores[b]	6.0 (2.5–21.0)	8.5 (2.0–17.3)	1.000
Number of affected joints[b]	5.0 (2.0–12.0)	5.5 (2.0–9.0)	0.917

Data were described as median (Interquartile range) or number (%)
Abbreviation: *BMI* body mass index; *SBP* systolic blood pressure; *DBP* diastolic blood pressure; *ESR* erythrocyte sedimentation rate; *CRP* C-reactive protein; *VAS* visual analogue scale; *FIHOA* Functional Index for Hand Osteoarthritis; *EQ-5D* EuroQol-5 dimensio
[a]Average value of the sum of right and left hand scores
[b]Based on Kellgren-Lawrence grade

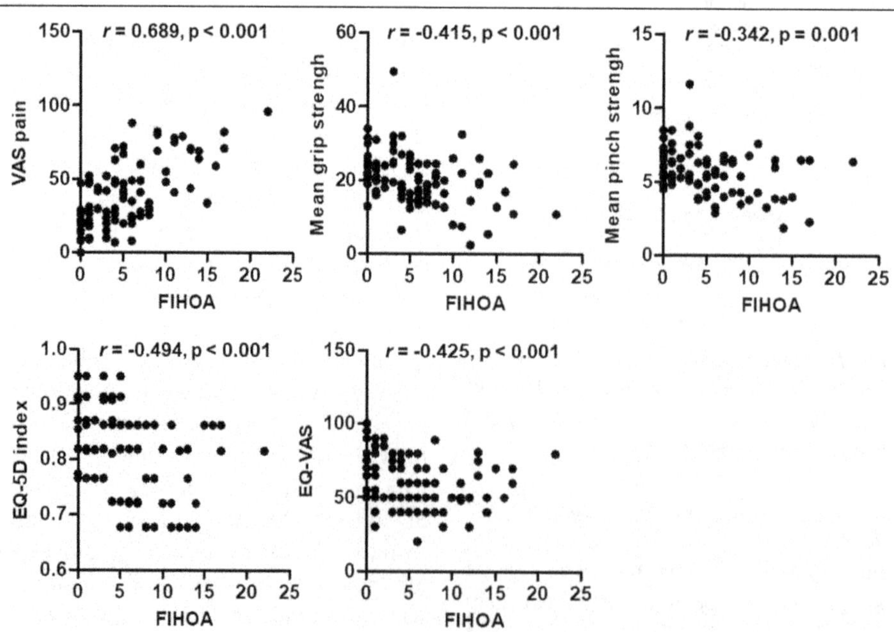

Fig. 1 Correlation of FIHOA with VAS pain, hand strength, and EQ-5D. Abbreviation: VAS, visual analogue scale; FIHOA, Functional Index for Hand Osteoarthritis; EQ-5D, EuroQol-5 dimension

Table 3 Determination of variables related with high FIHOA score

	Univariate regression			Multivariate regression		
Variables	OR	95% CI	*p* values	OR	95% CI	*p* values
Age (year)	0.978	0.934–1.025	0.362	0.940	0.864–1.022	0.149
Sex, female (n, %)	0.697	0.111–4.372	0.700	1.919	0.128–28.793	0.637
Symptom duration (month)	0.995	0.988–1.001	0.111	0.988	0.976–1.001	0.078
BMI (kg/m^2)	1.060	0.900–1.226	0.535			
ESR (mm/hr)	0.974	0.939–1.009	0.146			
CRP (mg/L)	1.137	0.856–1.512	0.375			
Mean grip strength	0.871	0.803–0.945	0.001	0.907	0.794–1.037	0.152
Mean pinch strength	0.525	0.368–0.748	< 0.001	0.803	0.445–1.448	0.466
Patient VAS	1.066	1.038–1.096	< 0.001	1.044	1.011–1.079	0.008
EQ-5D index	0.000	0.000–0.001	< 0.001	0.000	0.000–0.069	0.013
EQ-VAS	0.947	0.921–0.974	< 0.001	0.970	0.931–1.011	0.149
Total radiographic severity scores	0.996	0.963–1.030	0.815			
Number of affected joints	0.988	0.913–1.070	0.773			

Abbreviation: *BMI* body mass index; *ESR* erythrocyte sedimentation rate; *CRP* C-reactive protein; *VAS* visual analogue scale; *EQ-5D* EuroQol-5 dimension

It has been previously demonstrated that FIHOA score was relatively well associated with radiographic damages in hand OA [9, 10, 20, 21]. In assessment of correlation between hand functional limitation by AUSCAN function and FIHOA score and radiographic damage, FIHOA score was better correlated with radiographic structural changes than was the AUSCAN index [21]. FIHOA scores revealed larger physical disability in patients with erosive OA compared to those with non-erosive hand OA [20]. In addition, number of radiographic remodeled joints was markedly associated with FIHOA score in erosive OA. Number of joints with radiographic damage was shown to be a predictor of functional impairment ($\beta = 0.54$, 95% CI 0.24–0.84, $p < 0.01$). Compatible with these studies, radiographic severity determined by the Kellgren-Lawrence scale was significantly associated with FIHOA score [9, 10]. However, this study observed lack of association between radiographic outcomes such as total radiographic severity score and number of affected joints and FIHOA score. Similarly, Roux et al. showed that FIHOA score was not associated with number of OA joints with K-L grade ≥ 2, Verbruggen score, or osteophytes in Kallman score [10]. Ultrasound is a musculoskeletal imaging tool with many advantages over radiography in reliable and reproducible detection of intra- and extra-articular structural abnormalities, such as joint effusion, synovitis, bone erosions, and therapeutic monitoring in arthritis [22]. There is a close relationship between radiographic features and ultrasound findings [23]. However, FIHOA and AUSCAN scores were not associated with ultrasound findings [11, 24]. Important clinical questions about the relationship between functional impairment and diverse imaging tests, including conventional radiography, should be confirmed in large studies.

The VAS pain scale is frequently used to assess patient-reported pain in OA. Some studies have investigated whether physical function measures such as FIHOA and AUSCAN indexes are associated with VAS pain [11, 18]. A cross-sectional study revealed that FIHOA score was significantly associated with VAS pain and AUSCAN pain subscale ($r = 0.51$ and $r = 0.79$, respectively) [18]. It has been reported that tenderness on palpation was significantly related to FIHOA score [11]. Consistently, our study confirmed a close correlation between FIHOA score and VAS pain. In addition, high FIHOA score was positively dependent on VAS pain. This suggests that FIHOA score reflects to some extent the pain in hand OA patients, although this relationship should be validated in a larger study population.

Performance-based physical function tools such as pinch and grip strength for measurement of physical function of hands have been used in clinical studies of hand OA [25]. Substantial evidence of a negative association of grip or pinch strength with AUSCAN function subscale has been noted [5, 18, 26]. Interestingly, Moe et al. demonstrated a negative relationship between mean grip strength and FIHOA score ($r = -0.58$) [18]. Compatible with earlier data, the present study also found significant negative association between FIHOA score and two hand strength measures. This provides adequate evidence that there is comparable equivalence between questionnaire- and performance-based instruments in evaluating physical function of hand OA patients.

There are some limitations in this study. First, the results of this study originated from cross-sectional observation. Analysis of the causal relationships between FIHOA scores and clinical features, hand strength, and radiologic findings is needed in prospective studies. Second, the patient reported FIHOA index does not evaluate the relevance of AUSCAN function subscale and Cochin hand function scale. The clinical, physical, and radiographic measures related to FIHOA score in hand OA need to be verified using other hand function tools such as AUSCAN and Cochin hand function scale. In addition, most of the patients in this study consisted of women. Women have higher incidence and prevalence of knee, hand, feet OA than men [27]. Especially, decreased sex hormone contributes to an increased hand OA in female [28]. Musculoskeletal function and pain in knee OA was known to be dependent on gender [29]. This suggests that pain, functional impairment and quality of life in hand OA might be different between men and women. It is necessary to evaluate whether there is gender difference of functional outcome measures such as FIHOA.

Conclusion

This is the first observation that FIHOA score, an index for questionnaire-based physical function, is associated with EQ-5D, VAS pain, and grip and pinch strength in hand OA but not with radiographic changes. Longitudinal prospective analyses are needed to evaluate whether changes in FIHOA score are linked to those in other measures in hand OA.

Acknowledgements
None.

Disclosure statement

The authors do not have an actual or potential conflict of interest or not get interest of any kind to declare with regard to this work.

Authors' contributions

SK, UHJ, and JC contributed the conception and design of the study. SK and UHJ participated in data collection. SK and JC provided substantial supervision and interpretation of the statistical analysis. SK drafted and revised the manuscript. All authors have critically read this manuscript and approved the final version.

References

1. Marshall M, Watt FE, Vincent TL, Dziedzic K. Hand osteoarthritis: clinical phenotypes, molecular mechanisms and disease management. Nat Rev Rheumatol. 2018;14(11):641–56. https://doi.org/10.1038/s41584-018-0095-4.
2. Zhang W, Doherty M, Leeb BF, Alekseeva L, Arden NK, Bijlsma JW, Dincer F, Dziedzic K, Hauselmann HJ, Kaklamanis P, Kloppenburg M, Lohmander LS, Maheu E, Martin-Mola E, Pavelka K, Punzi L, Reiter S, Smolen J, Verbruggen G, Watt I, Zimmermann-Gorska I, ESCISIT. EULAR evidence-based recommendations for the diagnosis of hand osteoarthritis: report of a task force of ESCISIT. Ann Rheum Dis. 2009;68(1):8–17. https://doi.org/10.1136/ard.2007.084772.
3. Bellamy N, Kirwan J, Boers M, Brooks P, Strand V, Tugwell P, et al. Recommendations for a core set of outcome measures for future phrase III clinical trials in knee, hip and hand osteoarthritis. Consensus development at OMERACT III. J Rheumatol. 1997;24:799–802.
4. Maheu E, Altman RD, Bloch DA, Doherty M, Hochberg M, Mannoni A, Punzi L, Spector T, Verbruggen G, Osteoarthritis Research Society International Hand OA Task Force, Carr A, Cicuttini F, Dreiser RL, Haraoui BP, Hart D, Pelletier J, Ramonda R, Rovati L. Design and conduct of clinical trials in patients with osteoarthritis of the hand: recommendations from a task force of the osteoarthritis research society international. Osteoarthr Cartil. 2006; 14(4):303–22. https://doi.org/10.1016/j.joca.2006.02.010.
5. Bellamy N, Campbell J, Haraoui B, Gerecz-Simon E, Buchbinder R, Hobby K, MacDermid JC. Clinimetric properties of the AUSCAN osteoarthritis hand index: an evaluation of reliability, validity and responsiveness. Osteoarthr Cartil. 2002;10(11):863–9. https://doi.org/10.1053/joca.2002.0838.
6. Duruöz MT, Poiraudeau S, Fermanian J, Menkes CJ, Amor B, Dougados M, et al. Development and validation of a rheumatoid hand functional disability scale that assesses functional handicap. J Rheumatol. 1996;23: 1167–72.
7. Dreiser RL, Maheu E, Guillou GB, Caspard H, Grouin JM. Validation of an algofunctional index for osteoarthritis of the hand. Rev Rhum Engl Ed. 1995; 62(Suppl 1):43S–53S.
8. Dreiser RL, Maheu E, Guillou GB. Sensitivity to change of the functional index for hand osteoarthritis. Osteoarthritis Cartilage. 2000;8(Suppl A):S25–8.
9. Bagis S, Sahin G, Yapici Y, Bolgen Cimen O, Erdogan C. The effect of hand osteoarthritis on grip and pinch strength and hand function in post-menopausal women. Clin Rheumatol. 2003;22(6):420–4. https://doi.org/10.1007/s10067-003-0792-4.
10. Roux CH, Foltz V, Maheu E, Baron G, Gandjbakhch F, Lukas C, Wendling D, Loeuille D, Lafforgue P, Euler-Ziegler L, Richette P, Chevalier X, French Section on Osteoarthritis. MRI and serum biomarkers correlate with radiographic features in painful hand osteoarthritis. Clin Exp Rheumatol. 2016;34(6):991–8.
11. Koutroumpas AC, Alexiou IS, Vlychou M, Sakkas LI. Comparison between clinical and ultrasonographic assessment in patients with erosive osteoarthritis of the hands. Clin Rheumatol. 2010;29(5):511–6. https://doi.org/10.1007/s10067-009-1348-z.
12. Haugen IK, Bøyesen P, Slatkowsky-Christensen B, Sesseng S, van der Heijde D, Kvien TK. Associations between MRI-defined synovitis, bone marrow lesions and structural features and measures of pain and physical function in hand osteoarthritis. Ann Rheum Dis. 2012;71(6):899–904. https://doi.org/10.1136/annrheumdis-2011-200341.
13. Altman R, Alarcón G, Appelrouth D, Bloch D, Borenstein D, Brandt K, et al. The American College of Rheumatology criteria for the classification and reporting of osteoarthritis of the hand. Arthritis Rheum. 1990;33(11):1601–10. https://doi.org/10.1002/art.1780331101.
14. Kellgren JH, Lawrence JS. Radiological assessment of osteoarthrosis. Ann Rheum Dis. 1957;16(4):494–502. https://doi.org/10.1136/ard.16.4.494.
15. Ahn GY, Cho SK, Cha SJ, Nam E, Lee JE, Dreiser RL, Maheu E, Sung YK. Cross-cultural adaptation and validation of the Korean version of the functional index for hand osteoarthritis (FIHOA). Int J Rheum Dis. 2018; 21(12):2095–103. https://doi.org/10.1111/1756-185X.13412.
16. Kim MH, Cho YS, Uhm WS, Kim S, Bae SC. Cross-cultural adaptation and validation of the Korean version of the EQ-5D in patients with rheumatic diseases. Qual Life Res. 2005;14(5):1401–6. https://doi.org/10.1007/s11136-004-5681-z.
17. Fries JF, Spitz P, Kraines RG, Holman HR. Measurement of patient outcome in arthritis. Arthritis Rheum. 1980;23(2):137–45. https://doi.org/10.1002/art.1780230202.
18. Moe R, Garratt A, Slatkowsky-Christensen B, Maheu E, Mowinckel P, Kvien T, et al. Concurrent evaluation of data quality, reliability and validity of the Australian/Canadian osteoarthritis hand index and the functional index for hand osteoarthritis. Rheumatology (Oxford). 2010;49(12):2327–36. https://doi.org/10.1093/rheumatology/keq219.
19. Lim NY, Lee I, Lee EN, Lee KS, Cho KS, Rhee S, et al. A validation study of EQ-5D in the patients with osteoarthritis. J Muscle Joint Health. 2010;17(2): 203–11. https://doi.org/10.5953/JMJH.2010.17.2.203.
20. Wittoek R, Cruyssen BV, Verbruggen G. Predictors of functional impairment and pain in erosive osteoarthritis of the interphalangeal joints: comparison with controlled inflammatory arthritis. Arthritis Rheum. 2012;64(5):1430–6. https://doi.org/10.1002/art.33502.
21. Wittoek R, Verbruggen G. Correlation between FIHOA and AUSCAN and radiographic damage in patients with osteoarthritis of the hands. Osteoarthritis Cartilage. 2008;16(Suppl 4):S114.
22. McNally EG. Ultrasound of the small joints of the hands and feet: current status. Skelet Radiol. 2008;37(2):99–113. https://doi.org/10.1007/s00256-007-0356-9

23. Oo WM, Deveza LA, Duong V, Fu K, Linklater JM, Riordan EA, Robbins SR, Hunter DJ. Musculoskeletal ultrasound in symptomatic thumb-base osteoarthritis: clinical, functional, radiological and muscle strength associations. BMC Musculoskelet Disord. 2019;20(1):220. https://doi.org/10.1186/s12891-019-2610-4.
24. Keen HI, Wakefield RJ, Grainger AJ, Hensor EM, Emery P, Conaghan PG. An ultrasonographic study of osteoarthritis of the hand: synovitis and its relationship to structural pathology and symptoms. Arthritis Rheum. 2008; 59(12):1756–63. https://doi.org/10.1002/art.24312.
25. Visser AW, Bøyesen P, Haugen IK, Schoones JW, van der Heijde DM, Rosendaal FR, Kloppenburg M. Instruments measuring pain, physical function, or Patient's global assessment in hand osteoarthritis: a systematic literature search. J Rheumatol. 2015;42(11):2118–34. https://doi.org/10.3899/jrheum.141228.
26. Allen KD, Jordan JM, Renner JB, Kraus VB. Validity, factor structure, and clinical relevance of the AUSCAN osteoarthritis hand index. Arthritis Rheum. 2006;54(2):551–6. https://doi.org/10.1002/art.21615.
27. Srikanth VK, Fryer JL, Zhai G, Winzenberg TM, Hosmer D, Jones G. A meta-analysis of sex differences prevalence, incidence and severity of osteoarthritis. Osteoarthr Cartil. 2005;13(9):769–81. https://doi.org/10.1016/j.joca.2005.04.014.
28. Sowers MF, Hochberg M, Crabbe JP, Muhich A, Crutchfield M, Updike S. Association of bone mineral density and sex hormone levels with osteoarthritis of the hand and knee in premenopausal women. Am J Epidemiol. 1996;143(1):38–47. https://doi.org/10.1093/oxfordjournals.aje.a008655.
29. Phinyomark A, Osis ST, Hettinga BA, Kobsar D, Ferber R. Gender differences in gait kinematics for patients with knee osteoarthritis. BMC Musculoskelet Disord. 2016;17(1):157. https://doi.org/10.1186/s12891-016-1013-z.

9

Cardiovascular risk comorbidities in rheumatoid arthritis patients and the use of anti-rheumatic drugs

Gustavo Nogueira Schincariol Vicente[1*], Ivânio Alves Pereira[1], Gláucio Ricardo Werner de Castro[1], Licia Maria Henrique da Mota[2], Ana Paula Carnieletto[1], Dhara Giovanna Santin de Souza[1], Fabiana Oenning da Gama[1], Ana Beatriz Vargas Santos[3], Cleandro Pires de Albuquerque[2], Manoel Barros Bértolo[4], Paulo Louzada Júnior[5], Rina Dalva Neubarth Giorgi[6], Sebastião Cezar Radominski[7], Maria Fernanda Brandão Resende Guimarães[8], Karina Rossi Bonfiglioli[9], Maria de Fátima Lobato da Cunha Sauma[10], Claiton Viegas Brenol[11] and Geraldo da Rocha Castelar Pinheiro[3]

Abstract

Background: Rheumatoid arthritis (RA) is a common autoimmune systemic inflammatory disease. In addition to joint involvement, RA patients frequently have other comorbidities, such as cardiovascular diseases. Drugs used for RA treatment may increase or decrease the risk of a cardiovascular event. This study aims to analyze cardiovascular risk comorbidities in patients with RA and the correlation with the use of anti-rheumatic drugs.

Methods: Cross-sectional study conducted based on the real-life rheumatoid arthritis study database – REAL, a prospective observational cohort study. Associations between the use of anti-rheumatic drugs and the presence of comorbidities were represented by their prevalence ratio and evaluated using the Chi-square or Fisher's Exact tests.

Results: We assessed 1116 patients, 89.4% women, mean age of 55.15 years and predominance of seropositive disease. 63.3% had some cardiovascular comorbidity, predominantly hypertension (49.9%). The use of glucocorticoids was observed in 47.4% of patients and there was a significant tendency of lower use of these drugs in the presence of dyslipidemia (PR: 0.790; $p = 0.007$). We observed that the presence of cardiovascular comorbidities was associated with higher use of bDMARDs (PR:1.147; $p = 0.003$).

Conclusions: The presence of cardiovascular risk comorbidities was confirmed to be higher in RA patients. Different treatment strategies using less glucocorticoids in the presence of dyslipidemia and more common use of bDMARDs in patients with cardiovascular comorbidities suggest that rheumatologists are aware of the potential influence of the DMARDs in the risk of cardiovascular event. Reinforcing these results, we highlight the need for a better baseline assessment to guide the choice of anti-rheumatic drugs in RA patients who have comorbidities.

Keywords: Rheumatoid arthritis, Cardiovascular diseases, Treatment

* Correspondence: gustavo_schincariol@hotmail.com
[1]Universidade do Sul de Santa Catarina– UNISUL, Florianópolis, SC, Brazil

Background

Rheumatoid arthritis (RA) is a chronic, systemic and immune-mediated inflammatory disease that affects joints, connective and fibrous tissue, muscles, and tendons with preferential involvement in the third to fifth decade of life [1, 2]. Additionally, it causes lower life expectancy in 3 to 10 years and higher mortality rate in affected population compared to the general population [1, 3].

RA also involves the occurrence of extra-articular manifestations and comorbidities, with a higher prevalence of cardiovascular and pulmonary diseases, neoplasms, osteoporosis, changes in body composition and neuropsychiatric diseases [1, 4]. The most common and serious comorbidities are cardiovascular diseases (CVD) [5–7], being the main cause of increased premature mortality in this group [1, 8]. This fact is attributed to: the higher prevalence of traditional cardiovascular risk factors in these individuals, such as systemic arterial hypertension (SAH), diabetes mellitus (DM), dyslipidemia and obesity; the side effects of drugs used for treatment; and, mainly, the systemic inflammatory activity of RA, which determines endothelial injury and accelerated atherogenesis [5, 6, 8, 9]. Thus, it is possible to infer that the RA behaves as an independent risk factor for CVD [10].

The objective of RA treatment is its complete clinical remission, or, at least, to lower its activity [1, 11–13], thereby controlling systemic inflammation and reducing the risk of cardiovascular mortality [7, 14]. Drugs may positively or negatively influence cardiovascular risk comorbidities [15–18].

This study aims to analyze cardiovascular risk comorbidities in patients with RA and the correlation with the use of anti-rheumatic drugs.

Methods

The Rheumatoid Arthritis in Real Life (REAL) [19] is a prospective multi-center observational cohort study with 12 months of follow-up. The objectives were to describe the demographic, clinical, and therapeutic characteristics of Brazilian patients with RA and evaluate their treatment adherence, safety of pharmacological treatment and impact on the quality of life, physical function, and work ability.

Eleven tertiary care public health centers specialized in caring for RA patients were selected to represent the five geographic regions in Brazil. The recruitment period began on August 12, 2015 and ended on April 15, 2016. Patients were followed-up for approximately 12 months with systematic data collection at the initial visit (baseline), intermediate visit (6 months ±1 month), and final visit (12 months ±1 month) with an additional descriptive report of any other unscheduled visit. The present study is a cross-sectional evaluation of the data collected during the initial visit.

Patients included in the database were of both sexes, with RA according to the ACR 1987 [20] or ACR/EULAR 2010 [21] classification criteria, over 18 years of age, and with records of at least 6 months of medical clinical monitoring before the study. Patients with associated diseases that compromised the evaluation of the variables used in the study were excluded, namely: major depression, malignant neoplasia, use of dialysis and equivalent.

A sample of 1116 patients was calculated as statistically significant to detect the Prevalence Ratio of the outcomes of interest (use of non-steroidal anti-inflammatory drugs (NSAIDs), corticoids and disease modifying drugs (DMARDs) of at least double (PR: 2.0) when comparing patients with (exposed) and without (unexposed) comorbidities, with expected prevalence of 5% within significance level ($p < 0.05$) and statistical power of 80%.

The dependent variables included the drugs used for RA treatment: NSAIDs, glucocorticoids, synthetic and biological DMARDs. The sDMARDs included were methotrexate, leflunomide, antimalarials–chloroquine/hydroxychloroquine-, sulfasalazine and the JAK-kinase inhibitors (tofacitinib), a specific target synthetic DMAR D. All grouped biologicals were analyzed and subsequently separated into anti-TNFs (adalimumab, infliximab, etanercept, certolizumab, golimumab), anti-IL6r (tocilizumab), abatacept and rituximab. For glucocorticoids (prednisone), associations with use and dose were analyzed, with cut-off point at 10 mg (< 10 mg and ≥ 10 mg).

The independent variables analyzed were sociodemographic profile, laboratory parameters and comorbidities of cardiovascular risk. Sociodemographic factors used were gender, age, and education. The clinical laboratory parameters studied were the duration of the disease, presence or absence of erosive disease, the autoantibodies Rheumatoid Factor (RF) and anti–citrullinated protein antibody (ACPA), and disease activity, the latter by means of the Disease Activity Score using 28 Joint Counts (DAS28). Cardiovascular comorbidities were initially grouped in a single variable and later discriminated in the traditional risk factors - SAH, DM and dyslipidemia - and in the specific cardiovascular events - cerebrovascular disease, peripheral vascular disease, acute myocardial infarction (AMI) and congestive heart failure (CHF). Finally, Charlson comorbidity index (CCI) and age-adjusted Charlson comorbidity index (ACCI) were analyzed.

The Kolmogorov-Smirnov test was used to assess the normality of the Charlson Comorbidity Index variable. Due to the non-normal distribution, the data were presented in median (interquartile range).

The transversal data collected were tabulated on an electronic medium (Excel) and analyzed on SPSS 24.0 software (Statistical Package for the Social Sciences SPSS Version 24.0). Chicago: SPSS Inc.; 2016. The categorical variables were expressed as their absolute (n) and relative (%) frequencies. The means and standard deviations were calculated for the quantitative variables. The measure of association, represented by the Prevalence Ratio (PR), was evaluated by means of Chi-square Test or Fisher's Exact Test, at 5% significance level and 95% confidence interval (CI).

The present study was approved by the research ethics committee of the University of Southern Santa Catarina, under CAAE 45781015.8.2005.5369.

Results

A cohort of 1116 patients, 89.4% female and mean age of 55.15 years, participated in the study. As for the other sociodemographic characteristics of the participants, a more detailed analysis has already been published [19], reproduced in Table 1. When evaluating clinical and laboratory data, we found that 39.5% of them were smokers or former smokers; the mean disease duration was 14.5 years. There were predominance of erosive (54.9%) and seropositive diseases, with positive RF in 78.6% and anti-CCP in 76.8%.

Table 2 describes the comorbidities of cardiovascular risk in the study population. We observed that 63.6% of the patients had at least one of these comorbidities, more frequently SAH (49.9%), dyslipidemia (32.5%) and DM (14.9%).

Regarding the drugs used for RA treatment, we found that 47.4% of patients used glucocorticoids, of this percentage, 15.6% took doses higher than or equal to 10 mg. NSAIDs were used on demand by 66.6% of the participants. Methotrexate was the most used sDMARD (66.5%), followed by leflunomide (33.9%). Regarding bDMARDs, 35.7% of patients used some of them, most frequently anti-TNFs (19.9%). Other drugs and their frequencies of use can be found in Table 3.

Table 4 shows the association between the use of glucocorticoids and cardiovascular comorbidities. There was a significant association (PR:0.790; $p = 0.007$) between the presence of dyslipidemia and non-use of glucocorticoids.

We found no significant association between the use of NSAIDs and the presence of cardiovascular comorbidities.

The use of tofacitinib and sDMARDs (methotrexate, leflunomide, anti-malarial drugs and sulfasalazine) had no significant association with the presence of cardiovascular comorbidities. Table 5 shows the results obtained for methotrexate and leflunomide, the two main sDMARDs used by the population under study.

Table 1 Sociodemographic, clinical and laboratory characteristics of Rheumatoid Arthritis patients of the REAL study [19]

Variables	n (%)
Gender ($n = 1116$)	
Female	998 (89.4)
Age – Mean (standard deviation) ($n = 1116$)	55.15 (21–88)
Education time (years) ($n = 1076$)	
0–4 years	301 (28)
5–11 years	629 (58.4)
≥ 12 years	146 (13.6)
Disease duration (years) – mean (standard deviation) ($n = 1116$)	14.58 (1–57)
Erosive disease ($n = 1096$)	
Yes	602 (54.9)
DAS 28 VSH Score[a] **–** mean (standard deviation)	3.62 (0–8)
Smoking ($n = 1116$)	
Smoker	121 (10.8)
Former Smoker	320 (28.7)
Never Smoked	675 (60.5)
Rheumatoid Factor ($n = 1098$)	
Positive	863 (78.6)
ACPA[b] ($n = 479$)	
Positive	368 (768)

[a]*Disease Activity Score Index-28 Joints (DAS28);* [b] *Anti-citrullinated peptide antibody*

Table 2 Cardiovascular comorbidities of rheumatoid arthritis patients of the REAL study [19]

Variables ($n = 1116$)	n (%)
Cardiovascular Comorbidities	710 (63.6)
Systemic Arterial Hypertension -SAH	557 (49.9)
Dyslipidemia	363 (32.5)
Diabetes Mellitus	166 (14.9)
Congestive Heart Failure	24 (2.2)
Cerebrovascular Disease	24 (2.2)
Acute Myocardial Infarction - AMI	17 (1.5)
Peripheral Vascular Disease	8 (0.7)
Charlson Comorbidity Index- CCI – median (interquartile range)	0 (1.0)
Age-adjusted Charlson comorbidity index - CCI - median (interquartile range)	2 (2.0)

Table 3 Drugs used for rheumatoid arthritis treatment in the population of the REAL study [19]

Variables (n = 1116)	n (%)
Glucocorticoids	529 (47.4)
Dose ≥10 mg (n = 527)	82/527 (15.6)
Non-steroidal anti-inflammatory	743 (66.6)
Methotrexate	742 (66.5)
Leflunomide	378 (33.9)
Antimalarials (chloroquine/hydroxychloroquine)	146 (13.1)
Sulfasalazine	55 (4.9)
Tofacitinib	9 (0.8)
Biologicals	398 (35.7)
Anti-TNF (adalimumab, infliximab, etanercept, certolizumab, golimumab)	222 (19.9)
Anti-IL6r (tocilizumab)	55 (4.9)
Abatacept	72 (6.5)
Rituximab	49 (4.4)

Table 6 shows the association between the presence of comorbidities and the use of bDMARDs. The use of these drugs was higher in patients with some cardiovascular comorbidity (PR:1.147; p = 0.003) when compared to those without comorbidities. We found a similar association for SAH (PR:1.169; p = 0.011) and AMI (PR: 4.330; p = 0.002). The presence of dyslipidemia also followed an equivalent pattern (PR:1.186; p = 0.052). The main bDMARDs used by the population were anti-TNFs (19.9%), but no significant association was found between their use and the presence of comorbidities.

Regarding tocilizumab, no significant association was found between its use and the presence of cardiovascular comorbidities.

We observed that patients with cardiovascular comorbidities showed a significantly higher use of abatacept comparing to those without comorbidities (PR:1.194; p = 0.038). The use of rituximab was more frequent in patients with SAH (PR:1.327; p = 0.028), DM (PR:2.006; p = 0.006) and AMI (PR:9.073; p < 0.001) than in patients without these diseases.

Discussion

The present study analyzed whether the presence of cardiovascular comorbidities was associated with the use of different anti-rheumatic drugs in this large Brazilian cohort of RA patients.

RA patients show a higher prevalence of cardiovascular risk comorbidities compared to the general population [6, 16], which was confirmed in our study [22] by high rates of SAH (49.9%) and DM (14.9%), higher than those described in other cohorts [6, 23–25] . There was found in this cohort a higher prevalence of SAH when comparing to the prevalence of this commorbity in the Brazilian population, this fact may be explained by the fact that RA patients experience a higher cardiovascular risk explained by the systemic inflammation experienced by these patients, that contributes for a higher prevalence of cardiovascular commorbities. However, we found lower rates of dyslipidemia than those reported by other authors [7, 26]. There was a high prevalence of AMI, peripheral vascular disease, cerebrovascular disease and CHF, the most common causes of premature death in RA patients [1, 9].

Excessive cardiovascular risk in this population is multifactorial [8, 9]. It can be partially explained by the higher prevalence of traditional cardiovascular risk factors, such as SAH, type 2 DM, dyslipidemia, sedentary lifestyle and obesity [5, 6, 16], which was confirmed in our study [22]. However, the main factor associated with this increased risk is systemic inflammation due to RA [1, 8, 9]. A recent study demonstrated that these combined elements explain 69.6% of the increase in cardiovascular risk [27].

Pro-inflammatory state caused by RA [1, 9, 10], with elevated C-reactive protein (CRP) and pro-inflammatory cytokines, such as tumor necrosis factor-alpha (TNF-a), IL-6 and IL-1, are associated with accelerated atherosclerosis, changes in lipid patterns (quantitative and qualitative), insulin resistance and endothelial dysfunction [9, 10]. Other factors of the disease, such as presence of autoantibodies, extra-joint manifestations, disease activity and X-ray erosions, contribute to increasing cardiovascular risk [1, 10, 28, 29]. Therefore, we conclude that RA itself can be considered an independent risk factor for the development of CVD [9, 10].

A factor that can be associated with cardiovascular risk in RA patients is the drugs used for the management of the disease, which can influence cardiovascular risk positively or negatively [10, 15, 17]. Current recommendations state that the most important aspect in reducing the risk of cardiovascular events in RA patients is the reduction of disease activity using DMARDs, whether synthetic or biological, thus reducing chronic inflammation and its deleterious effects [11–13, 18, 30]. They are also proven to reduce atherosclerosis progression and, consequently, cardiovascular risk [18, 30, 31].

In addition, the use of different DMARDs should be individualized and take into account the presence of comorbidities that can be positively or negatively affected by these drugs [11, 18]. Indeed, there are specific agreements that guide the choice of drugs for RA treatment based on the presence of these comorbidities [13, 15].

The use of glucocorticoids is related to a large spectrum of adverse events, such as uncontrolled SAH, dyslipidemia and especially DM [24], and their use is associated with a 47% increase in relative risk of all

Table 4 Association of cardiovascular comorbidities with the use of glucocorticoids

		Glucocorticoids			
		Yes n*(%)	No n*(%)	PR^ (IC95%)	p‡
Cardiovascular Comorbidities	Yes	322 (66.9)	388 (66.1)	0.921 (0.842–1.007)	0.070
	No	207 (39.1)	199 (33.9)	1.154 (0.988–1.348)	
Systemic Arterial Hypertension	Yes	257 (48.6)	300 (51.1)	0.951 (0.845–1.070)	0.400
	No	272 (51.4)	287 (48.9)	1.052 (0.935–1.182)	
Dyslipidemia	Yes	151 (28.5)	212 (36.1)	0.790 (0.665–0.939)	0.007
	No	378 (71.5)	375 (63.9)	1.119 (1.031–1.213)	
Diabetes Mellitus	Yes	74 (14)	92 (15.7)	0.893 (0.673–1.184)	0.430
	No	455 (86)	495 (84.3)	1.020 (0.971–1.071)	
Congestive Heart Failure	Yes	11 (2.1)	13 (2.2)	0.939 (0.424–2.078)	0.876
	No	518 (97.9)	574 (97.8)	1.001 (0.984–1.019)	
Cerebrovascular Disease	Yes	12 (2.3)	12 (2)	1.110 (0.503–2.449)	0.797
	No	517 (97.7)	575 (98)	0.998 (0.980–1.015)	
Acute Myocardial Infarction	Yes	8 (1.5)	9 (1.5)	0.986 (0.383–2.538)	0.977
	No	521 (98.5)	578 (98.5)	1.000 (0.986–1.015)	
Peripheral Vascular Disease	Yes	4 (0.8)	4 (0.7)	1.110 (0.279–4.415)	1.000
	No	525 (99.2)	583 (99.3)	0.999 (0.989–1.009)	

*Absolute frequencies; ^ Prevalence Ratio ‡ Significance level

cardiovascular events and general mortality in RA patients, and this increase in risk is dependent on dose and time of use [17, 24, 32]. In the study population, the use of corticoids (47.2%) was lower than that reported by another Latin American study [33], but similar to that found in the cohort of Wilson et al [24].

Like corticosteroids, all NSAIDs [34], selective COX-2 in particular, are associated with a 20% increase in the relative risk of all cardiovascular events and lead to uncontrolled SAH [17, 35]. Therefore, it is recommended that NSAIDs be used as symptomatic medication for as little time as possible, and their use should be avoided in

Table 5 Association between cardiovascular comorbidities and the use of Methotrexate and Leflunomide

		Methotrexate			Leflunomide		
		Yes n*(%)	PR^ (IC95%)	p‡	Yes n*(%)	PR^ (IC95%)	p‡
Cardiovascular Comorbidities	Yes	463 (62.4)	0.945 (0.862–1.036)	0.232	251 (66.4)	1.068 (0.975–1.170)	0.167
	No	279 (37.6)	1.107 (0.935–1.311)		127 (33.6)	0.889 (0.750–1.053)	
Systemic Arterial Hypertension	Yes	365 (49.2)	0.958 (0.847–1.083)	0.499	195 (51.6)	1.052 (0.931–1.188)	0.423
	No	377 (50.8)	1.044 (0.921–1.184)		183 (48.4)	0.950 (0.838–1.078)	
Dyslipidemia	Yes	236 (31.8)	0.937 (0.785–1.117)	0.469	129 (34.1)	1.076 (0.903–1.283)	0.414
	No	506 (68.2)	1.033 (0.946–1.127)		249 (65.9)	0.965 (0.884–1.053)	
Diabetes Mellitus	Yes	111 (15)	1.017 (0.755–1.371)	0.910	52 (13.8)	0.891 (0.657–1.207)	0.453
	No	631 (85)	0.997 (0.947–1.050)		326 (86.2)	1.020 (0.970–1.073)	
Congestive Heart Failure	Yes	18 (2.4)	1.512 (0.605–3.777)	0.372	7 (1.9)	0.804 (0.336–1.922)	0.623
	No	724 (97.6)	0.992 (0.975–1.009)		371 (98.1)	1.005 (0.987–1.023)	
Cerebrovascular Disease	Yes	14 (1.9)	0.706 (0.316–1.574)	0.392	9 (2.4)	1.171 (0.517–2.652)	0.704
	No	728 (98.1)	1.008 (0.989–1.028)		369 (97.6)	0.996 (0.978–1.015)	
Acute Myocardial Infarction	Yes	12 (1.6)	1.210 (0.429–3.408)	0.718	3 (0.8)	0.418 (0.121–1.447)	0.200
	No	730 (98.4)	0.997 (0.982–1.012)		375 (99.2)	1.011 (0.998–1.025)	
Peripheral Vascular Disease	Yes	5 (0.7)	0.840 (0.202–3.496)	1.000	5 (1.3)	3.254 (0.782–13.543)	0.129
	No	737 (99.3)	1.001 (0.990–1.012)		373 (98.7)	0.991 (0.970–1.003)	

*Absolute frequencies; ^ Prevalence Ratio ‡ Significance level

Table 6 Association between cardiovascular comorbidities and use of biologicals, in particular those of the anti-TNF class

		Biologicals			Anti-TNF		
		Yes n*(%)	PR^ (IC95%)	p‡	Yes n*(%)	PR^ (IC95%)	p‡
Cardiovascular Comorbidities	Yes	276 (69.3)	1.147 (1.050–1.253)	0.003	148 (66.7)	1.060 (0.954–1.179)	0.292
	No	122 (30.7)	0.775 (0.652–0.922)		74 (33.3)	0.898 (0.731–1.101)	
Systemic Arterial Hypertension	Yes	219 (55)	1.169 (1.039–1.315)	0.011	116 (52.3)	1.059 (0.919–1.221)	0.436
	No	179 (45)	0.850 (0.747–0.967)		106 (47.7)	0.942 (0.808–1.097)	
Dyslipidemia	Yes	144 (36.2)	1.186 (1.000–1.407)	0.052	80 (36)	1.138 (0.932–1.390)	0.212
	No	254 (63.8)	0.918 (0.841–1.003)		142 (64)	0.936 (0.840–1.043)	
Diabetes Mellitus	Yes	65 (16.3)	1.161 (0.872–1.546)	0.308	31 (14)	0.925 (0.644–1.328)	0.670
	No	333 (83.7)	0.974 (0.924–1.020)		191 (86)	1.013 (0.955–1.076)	
Congestive Heart Failure	Yes	10 (2.5)	1.289 (0.578–2.874)	0.535	3 (1.4)	0.575 (0.173–1.911)	0.448
	No	388 (97.5)	0.994 (0.976–1.013)		219 (98.6)	1.010 (0.992–1.029)	
Cerebrovascular Disease	Yes	4 (1)	0.361 (0.124–1.048)	0.054	1 (0.5)	0.175 (0.024–1.289)	0.066
	No	394 (99)	1.018 (1.002–1.035)		222 (99.5)	1.022 (1.008–1.036)	
Acute Myocardial Infarction	Yes	12 (3)	4.330 (1.536–12.201)	0.002	3 (1.4)	0.863 (0.250–2.977)	1.000
	No	386 (97)	0.977 (0.959–0.995)		219 (98.6)	1.002 (0.985–1.020)	
Peripheral Vascular Disease	Yes	3 (0.8)	1.082 (0.260–4.505)	1.000	1 (0.5)	0.575 (0.071–4.652)	1.000
	No	395 (99.2)	0.999 (0.989–1.010)		221 (99.5)	1.003 (0.993–1.014)	

*Absolute frequencies; ^ Prevalence Ratio ‡ Significance level

those with some previous cardiovascular event (AMI, CCI) or with high risk based on traditional risk factors [11, 12, 15, 36]. In the present study, the use of NSAIDs was lower when compared to another cohort [7].

Since systemic inflammation caused by RA is the main determinant of increased cardiovascular risk, algorithms of RA treatment recommend the use of sDMARDs as the first line of treatment, methotrexate being the drug of choice [11–13, 18]. This finding was reproduced in our study, given that this was the most used DMARD by the population (66.5%). As it is the most used drug, evidence of cardiovascular risk is more robust for methotrexate. Recent meta-analysis in RA patients has shown that the risk of all cardiovascular events is reduced by 28% with the use of methotrexate, with a special reduction in risk and recurrence of AMI [17]. In our study, the presence of some comorbidity or cardiovascular event was not associated with the higher or lower use of this drug, which can be explained by the fact that, being the drug of choice, its use should be preferable in all patients, regardless of the presence of comorbidities or previous events.

In our population, frequent use of leflunomide was evidenced to the detriment of other sDMARDs in RA treatment. The available data regarding this drug are scarce. It is known that leflunomide is associated with the occurrence and bad control of SAH [13, 18]. Therefore, although it is not contraindicated, it should be avoided in hypertensive patients [13, 15, 18, 37]. In our population, we observed that this recommendation was not adopted, since the presence of hypertension was not associated with a lower use of this drug.

Biologicals are associated with reduced cardiovascular risk compared to patients who do not use them or those using sDMARDs [17, 25, 30]. Lee et al and Radner *et al* verified in their populations that the use of biological agents is less frequent in patients with comorbidities, especially cardiovascular ones [25, 38], which, according to recent protocols and recommendations, should in fact happen in the opposite way because of the cardiovascular benefit of these drugs [11–13, 18]. In the present study, we found that bDMARDs tended to be more frequently used ($p = 0.003$) in patients with some comorbidity or cardiovascular event, whereas individually this tendency was similar only for SAH ($p = 0.011$) and AMI ($p = 0.002$). This is an important finding, considering that the use of bDMARDs is associated to lower chance of future cardiocascular event. Besides that, bDMARDs use allows more easily the reduction or suspension of corticosteroids, which is well stabished associated with a pro-inflamatory state. However, this finding could be related to a selection bias, in which more severe patients and those with more inflammatory activity tend to receive bDMARDs.

The risk of all cardiovascular events, especially AMI (RR 0.85), is reduced with the use of anti-TNF drugs, more than that observed with the use of sDMARDs, specially in patients who respond well to the medication [17, 18, 30, 39]. Such protective effect was not identified for heart failure [17]. We found that the presence of comorbidities and cardiovascular events was not associated with use of anti-TNFs, contrasting with the guidelines [11–13, 18]. This absence of association is particularly important when evaluating heart failure, given the recommendations to avoid the use of anti TNFs in patients with CHF, especially in more advanced stages [14, 18, 30].

Abatacept and rituximab were the least frequently used drugs in our sample. The literature states that the risk reduction of cardiovascular events, such as AMI and stroke, with the use of abatacept is modestly higher comparing to anti-TNFs [40, 41], especially in patients with DM. For rituximab, data on cardiovascular outcomes are scarce, but their benefits seem to be comparable to those obtained with the use of anti-TNF [42]. In our study we observed that abatacept and rituximab tended to be used in patients with some cardiovascular risk factor like SAH, DM and AMI.

One limitations of this work is the impossibility to determine a causal relationship between the variables analyzed. Special care should also be taken in extrapolating these findings to the general population. Moreover, for some of the medications and comorbidities, the number of patients analyzed was small, which may have affected some of the associations found. One other limitation that should be mentioned is that the cardiovascular risk in these patients were not established by known formulas, which can influence at the analyses. In spite of the above, we underline that this work was a first attempt at evaluating the association between the presence of cardiovascular risk comorbidities and the use of anti-rheumatic drugs in the first large Brazilian RA cohort and may serve as a basis for further studies.

Conclusion

The findings of this study confirmed that the presence of comorbidities of cardiovascular risk is high in the RA population. Additionally, we observed that, for the patients of the REAL study, some of the recommendations by different algorithms, which advise taking into account the presence of cardiovascular comorbidities in the choice of some anti-rheumatic drugs, were adopted but could have been better implemented.

Given that RA is an independent risk factor for cardiovascular events itself, we highlight the need to better assess the cardiovascular risk of patients in order to guide the choice of different DMARDs, aiming at better cardiovascular outcomes.

Abbreviations

RA: Rheumatoid arthritis (RA); CVD: Cardiovascular diseases; SAH: Systemic arterial hypertension; DM: Diabetes mellitus; NSAIDs: Non-steroidal anti-inflammatory drugs; DMARDs: Disease-modifying antirheumatic drugs; sDMARDs: Synthetic disease-modifying antirheumatic drugs; JAK-quinase: Tirosina quinase; bDMARDs: Biological disease-modifying antirheumatic drugs; anti-TNF : Tumor necrosis factor inhibitor; anti-IL6r: Interleukin 6 nhibitor; BSR: Brazilian Society of Rheumatology; ACR: American College of Radiology; EULAR: European League Against Rheumatism; PR: Prevalence Ratio; P: Significance level; RF: Rheumatoid Factor; ACPA: Anti-citrullinated protein antibody; DAS 28 SCORE: Disease Activity Score Index 28 Joints; AMI: Acute myocardial infarction; CHF: Congestive heart failure; CCI: Charlson comorbidity index; ACCI: Age-adjusted Charlson comorbidity index; SPSS: Statistical Package for the Social Sciences; CI: Confidence interval; CRP: C-reactive protein; TNFa: Tumor necrosis factor-alpha; IL1: Interleukin 1; IL6: Interleukin 6; COX-2: Cyclooxygenase-2; RR: Relative risk; LDL: Low density lipoprotein; TC: Total cholesterol; TG: Triglycerides; HDL: High density lipoprotein

Acknowledgments

We thank the Brazilian Society of Rheumatology and the team of the University of Southern Santa Catarina for the statistical analysis of the data.

Authors' contributions

GNSV: medical student responsible for the study, participated in all planning, execution and preparation of the manuscript. IAP: advisor and supervisor, responsible for outlining the study, participated in the analysis, data interpretation and critical review of the content. APC, DGSS: participated in the process of execution and content review. FOG: participated in the content execution and review process. GRCP, ABVS, CPA, MBB, PLJR, DNG, SCR, MFBRG, JRB, MFLCS, CVB, LMHM, GRWC: responsible for the 'Rheumatoid Arthritis in Real Life' database. The author(s) read and approved the final manuscript.

Competing interests

GNSV: No financial disclosures; APC: No financial disclosures; DGSS: No financial disclosures; FOG: No financial disclosures; IAP: Has received consulting fees, speaking fees and supporting for internationals congresses from Roche, Pfizer, UCB Pharma, Eli-Lilly, Abbvie and Janssen; GRWC: No financial disclosures; GRCP: Has received consulting fees from AbbVie, Bristol-Myers Squibb, Eli Lilly, Glaxosmithkline, Janssen, Pfizer, Sanofi Genzyme and Roche; ABVS: Has received supporting for international medical events from AbbVie and Janssen; CPA: Has received personal fees and/or non-financial support from Pfizer, AbbVie, AstraZeneca, Janssen, Bristol-Myers Squibb, Roche, Novartis and UCB, outside the submitted work; MBB: Has participated in clinical and/or experimental studies related to this work and sponsored by Roche; has delivered speeches at events related to this work and sponsored by AbbVie and Pfizer; PLJ: Has received supporting for internationals congresses from Bristol-Myers Squibb, UCB and consulting fees from Pfizer; RDNG: Has received consulting fees, speaking fees and supporting for internationals congresses from Roche, Pfizer, Bristol-Myers Squibb, UCB, Eli-Lilly, AbbVie, Abbott and EMS; SCR: Has received consulting and speaking fees from Abbvie, Janssen, Pfizer, Roche and UCB; MFBRG: Has received speaking fees and supporting for congresses from AbbVie, Bristol-Myers Squibb, Janssen, Novartis, Pfizer, Roche and UCB; KRB: Has received speaking fees and supporting for international congresses from Roche, Pfizer, Bristol-Myers Squibb, Abbvie and Janssen; MFLCS: No financial disclosures; CVB: Has participated in clinical and/or experimental studies re- lated to this work and sponsored by AbbVie, BMS, Janssen, Pfizer and Roche; has received personal or institutional support from AbbVie, BMS, Janssen, Pfizer and Roche; has delivered speeches at events related to this work and sponsored by AbbVie, Janssen, Pfizer and Roche; CVB: Has participated in clinical and/or experimental studies related to this work and sponsored by AbbVie, BMS, Janssen, Pfizer and Roche; has received personal or institutional support from AbbVie, BMS, Janssen, Pfizer and Roche; has delivered speeches at events related to this work and sponsored by AbbVie, Janssen, Pfizer and Roche Ricardo Machado Xavier: Consultancies for Abbvie, BMS, GSK, Janssen, Lilly, Novartis, Pfizer, Roche, UCB. Clinical trials: Abbvie, UCB, Pfizer, GSK, Lilly; ESFC: No financial disclosures; LMHM: Has received personal or institutional support from AbbVie, Janssen, Pfizer and Roche; has delivered speeches at events related to this work and sponsored by AbbVie, Janssen, Pfizer, Roche and UCB.

Author details

[1]Universidade do Sul de Santa Catarina– UNISUL, Florianópolis, SC, Brazil.
[2]Hospital Universitário de Brasília, Universidade de Brasília, Brasília, DF, Brazil.

[3]Universidade do Estado do Rio de Janeiro, Rio de Janeiro, RJ, Brazil. [4]Faculdade de Ciências Médicas, Universidade Estadual de Campinas, Campinas, SP, Brazil. [5]Universidade de São Paulo, Ribeirão Preto, SP, Brazil. [6]Instituto de Assistência Médica ao Servidor Público Estadual, Hospital do Servidor Público Estadual de São Paulo, São Paulo, SP, Brazil. [7]Universidade Federal do Paraná, Curitiba, PR, Brazil. [8]Hospital das Clínicas, Universidade Federal de Minas Gerais, Belo Horizonte, MG, Brazil. [9]Faculdade de Medicina, Universidade de São Paulo, São Paulo, SP, Brazil. [10]Faculdade de Medicina, Universidade Federal do Pará, Belém, PA, Brazil. [11]Universidade Federal do Rio Grande do Sul, Porto Alegre, RS, Brazil.

References

1. Smolen JS, Aletaha D, Barton A, Burmester GR, Emery P, Firestein GS, et al. Rheumatoid arthritis. Nat Rev Dis Prim [Internet]. 2018;4:1800 [acesso em 2020 ago 14]. Disponível em: https://doi.org/10.1038/nrdp.2018.1.
2. World Health Organization (WHO). Chronic rheumatic conditions. 2019 [acesso em 2020 ago 18]; Disponível em: https://www.who.int/chp/topics/rheumatic/en/.
3. Myasoedova E, Davis JM, Crowson CS, Gabriel SE. Epidemiology of rheumatoid arthritis: rheumatoid arthritis and mortality. Curr Rheumatol Rep. 2010;12(5):379–85. https://doi.org/10.1007/s11926-010-0117-y.
4. Aletaha D, Smolen JS. Diagnosis and Management of Rheumatoid Arthritis: a review. JAMA. 2018;320(13):1360–72. https://doi.org/10.1001/jama.2018.13103.
5. Baghdadi LR, Woodman RJ, Shanahan EM. The impact of traditional cardiovascular risk factors on cardiovascular outcomes in patients with rheumatoid arthritis: a systematic review and meta-analysis. PLoS One. 2015; 10(2):e0117952. https://doi.org/10.1371/journal.pone.0117952.
6. Radner H, Lesperance T, Accortt NA, Solomon DH. Incidence and prevalence of cardiovascular risk factors among patients with rheumatoid arthritis, psoriasis, or psoriatic arthritis. Arthritis Care Res. 2017;69(10):1510–8. https://doi.org/10.1002/acr.23171.
7. Myasoedova E, Gabriel SE, Matteson EL, Davis JM 3rd, Therneau TM, Crowson CS. Decreased cardiovascular mortality in patients with incident rheumatoid arthritis (RA) in recent years: dawn of a new era in cardiovascular disease in RA? J Rheumatol. 2017;44(6):732–9. https://doi.org/10.3899/jrheum.161154.
8. Blum A, Adawi M. Rheumatoid arthritis (RA) and cardiovascular disease. Autoimmun Rev. 2019;18(7):679–90. https://doi.org/10.1016/j.autrev.2019.05.005.
9. England BR, Thiele GM, Anderson DR, Mikuls TR. Increased cardiovascular risk in rheumatoid arthritis: mechanisms and implications. BMJ. 2018;361:1–17.
10. Semb AG, Ikdahl E, Wibetoe G, Crowson C, Rollefstad S. Atherosclerotic cardiovascular disease prevention in rheumatoid arthritis. Nat Rev Rheumatol [Internet]. 2020;16(7):361–79 [acesso em 2020 out 18]. Disponível em: http://dx.doi.org/10.1038/s41584-020-0428-y.
11. da Mota LMH, Kakehasi AM, Gomides APM, Duarte ALBP, Cruz BA, Brenol CV, et al. 2017 recommendations of the Brazilian Society of Rheumatology for the pharmacological treatment of rheumatoid arthritis. Adv Rheumatol. 2018;58(1):1–17.
12. Singh JA, Saag KG, Bridges SL Jr, Akl EA, Bannuru RR, Sullivan MC, et al. 2015 American College of Rheumatology guideline for the treatment of rheumatoid arthritis. Arthritis Care Res. 2016;68(1):1–25. https://doi.org/10.1002/acr.22783.
13. Agca R, Heslinga SC, Rollefstad S, Heslinga M, McInnes IB, Peters MJL, et al. EULAR recommendations for cardiovascular disease risk management in patients with rheumatoid arthritis and other forms of inflammatory joint disorders: 2015/2016 update. Ann Rheum Dis. 2016;76(1):17–28. https://doi.org/10.1136/annrheumdis-2016-209775.
14. Gualtierotti R, Ughi N, Marfia G, Ingegnoli F. Practical management of cardiovascular comorbidities in rheumatoid arthritis. Rheumatol Ther. 2017; 4(2):293–308. https://doi.org/10.1007/s40744-017-0068-0.
15. Pereira IA, Mota LM, Cruz BA, Brenol CV, Fronza LS, Bertolo MB, et al. 2012 Brazilian Society of Rheumatology Consensus on the management of comorbidities in patients with rheumatoid arthritis. Rev Bras Reumatol. 2012; 52(4):474–95.
16. Nurmohamed MT, Heslinga M, Kitas GD. Cardiovascular comorbidity in rheumatic diseases. Nat Rev Rheumatol. 2015;11(12):693–704. https://doi.org/10.1038/nrrheum.2015.112.
17. Roubille C, Richer V, Starnino T, McCourt C, McFarlane A, Fleming P, et al. The effects of tumour necrosis factor inhibitors, methotrexate, non-steroidal anti-inflammatory drugs and corticosteroids on cardiovascular events in rheumatoid arthritis, psoriasis and psoriatic arthritis: a systematic review and meta-analysis. Ann Rheum Dis. 2015;74(3):480–9. https://doi.org/10.1136/annrheumdis-2014-206624.
18. Smolen JS, Landewé RBM, Bijlsma JWJ, Burmester GR, Dougados M, Kerschbaumer A, et al. EULAR recommendations for the management of rheumatoid arthritis with synthetic and biological disease-modifying antirheumatic drugs: 2019 update. Ann Rheum Dis. 2020;79(6):S685–99.
19. da Rocha C-PG, Vargas-Santos AB, de Albuquerque CP, Bértolo MB, Júnior PL, Giorgi RDN, et al. The REAL study: a nationwide prospective study of rheumatoid arthritis in Brazil. Adv Rheumatol. 2018;58(1):9.
20. Hutchinson D. Classification criteria: the 1987 American rheumatism association revised criteria for the classification of rheumatoid arthritis. CPD Rheumatol. 1999;1(1):13–4.
21. Aletaha D, Neogi T, Silman AJ, Funovits J, Felson DT, Bingham CO, et al. 2010 rheumatoid arthritis classification criteria: an American College of Rheumatology/European league against rheumatism collaborative initiative. Arthritis Rheum. 2010;62(9):2569–81. https://doi.org/10.1002/art.27584.
22. Ministério da Saúde. Secretaria de Vigilância em Saúde. Departamento de Vigilância de Doenças e Agravos não Transmissíveis e Promoção da Saúde. Vigitel Brasil 2017: Vigilância de fatores de risco e proteção para doenças crônicas por inquérito telefônico: estimativas sobre frequência e distribuição sociodemográfica de fatores de risco e de proteção para doenças crônicas nas capitais dos 26 estados brasileiros e no Distrito Federal em 2017 [recurso eletrônico]. Brasília: Ministério da Saúde, 2017. [acesso em 2020 fev 25]. Disponível em: https://bvsms.saude.gov.br/bvs/publicacoes/vigitel_brasil_2017_vigilancia_fatores_riscos.pdf.
23. Acosta-Mérida Á, Naranjo A, Rodríguez-Lozano C. Prognostic Factors for Sustained Remission in a "Real Life" Cohort of Rheumatoid Arthritis Patients. Reumatol Clin [Internet]. 2020;16(5Pt2):405–9 [acesso em 2020 set 07]. Disponível em: https://doi.org/10.1016/j.reuma.2018.10.002.
24. Wilson JC, Sarsour K, Gale S, Pethö-Schramm A, Jick SS, Meier CR. Incidence and risk of glucocorticoid-associated adverse effects in patients with rheumatoid arthritis. Arthritis Care Res. 2019;71(4):498–511. https://doi.org/10.1002/acr.23611.
25. Lee JL, Sinnathurai P, Buchbinder R, Hill C, Lassere M, March L. Biologics and cardiovascular events in inflammatory arthritis: a prospective national cohort study. Arthritis Res Ther. 2018;20(1):1–9.
26. Balsa A, Lojo-Oliveira L, Alperi-López M, García-Manrique M, Ordóñez-Cañizares C, Pérez L, et al. Prevalence of comorbidities in rheumatoid arthritis and evaluation of their monitoring in clinical practice: the spanish cohort of the COMORA study. Reumatol Clin. 2019;15(2):102–8. https://doi.org/10.1016/j.reuma.2017.06.002.
27. Crowson CS, Rollefstad S, Ikdahl E, Kitas GD, Van Riel PLCM, Gabriel SE, et al. Impact of risk factors associated with cardiovascular outcomes in patients with rheumatoid arthritis. Ann Rheum Dis. 2018;77(1):48–54. https://doi.org/10.1136/annrheumdis-2017-211735.
28. Myasoedova E, Chandran A, Ilhan B, Major BT, Michet CJ, Matteson EL, et al. The role of rheumatoid arthritis (RA) flare and cumulative burden of RA severity in the risk of cardiovascular disease. Ann Rheum Dis. 2016;75(3): 560–5. https://doi.org/10.1136/annrheumdis-2014-206411.
29. Humphreys JH, Warner A, Chipping J, Marshall T, Lunt M, Symmons DP, et al. Mortality trends in patients with early rheumatoid arthritis over 20 years: results from the Norfolk arthritis register. Arthritis Care Res. 2014;66(9): 1296–301. https://doi.org/10.1002/acr.22296.
30. Singh S, Fumery M, Singh AG, Singh N, Prokop LJ, Dulai PS, et al. Comparative risk of cardiovascular events with biologic and synthetic disease-modifying anti-rheumatic drugs in patients with rheumatoid arthritis: a systematic review and meta-analysis. Arthritis Care Res. 2020;72: 561–76.
31. Burggraaf B, Van Breukelen-Van Der Stoep DF, De Vries MA, Klop B, Liem AH, Van De Geijn GJM, et al. Effect of a treat-to-target intervention of cardiovascular risk factors on subclinical and clinical atherosclerosis in rheumatoid arthritis: a randomised clinical trial. Ann Rheum Dis. 2018:335–41.
32. del Rincon I, Battafarano DF, Restrepo JF, et al. Glucocorticoid dose thresholds associated with all-cause and cardiovascular mortality in rheumatoid arthritis. Arthritis Rheum. 2014;66(2):264–72. https://doi.org/10.1002/art.38210.

33. Cardiel MH, Pons-Estel BA, Sacnun MP, Wojdyla D, Saurit V, Marcos JC, et al. Treatment of early rheumatoid arthritis in a multinational inception cohort of Latin American patients: the GLADAR experience. J Clin Rheumatol. 2012; 18(7):327–35. https://doi.org/10.1097/RHU.0b013e31826d6610.
34. Nissen SE, Yeomans ND, Solomon DH, Lüscher TF, Libby P, Husni ME, et al. PRECISION trial investigators. Cardiovascular safety of Celecoxib, naproxen, or ibuprofen for arthritis. N Engl J Med. 2016;375(26):2519–29. https://doi.org/10.1056/NEJMoa1611593.
35. Lindhardsen J, Gislason GH, Jacobsen S, Ahlehoff O, Olsen AMS, Ole Rintek Madsen, et al. Non-steroidal anti-inflammatory drugs and risk of cardiovascular disease in patients with rheumatoid arthritis: a nationwide cohort study. Ann Rheum Dis. 2014;73(8):1515–21. https://doi.org/10.1136/annrheumdis-2012-203137.
36. Johnson TM, Mikuls TR, England BR. Assessment of cardiovascular disease risk in rheumatoid arthritis. J Clin Outcomes Manag. 2019;26(1):41–7.
37. Giollo A, Bissell LA, Buch MH. Cardiovascular outcomes of patients with rheumatoid arthritis prescribed disease modifying anti-rheumatic drugs: a review. Expert Opin Drug Saf [Internet]. 2018;17(7):697–708 [acesso em 2020 set 07]. Disponível em: https://doi.org/10.1080/14740338.2018.1483331.
38. Radner H, Yoshida K, Hmamouchi I, Dougados M, Smolen JS, Solomon DH. Treatment patterns of multimorbid patients with rheumatoid arthritis: results from an international cross-sectional study. J Rheumatol. 2015;42(7): 1099–104. https://doi.org/10.3899/jrheum.141534.
39. Low ASL, Symmons DPM, Lunt M, Mercer LK, Gale CP, Watson KD, et al. Relationship between exposure to tumour necrosis factor inhibitor therapy and incidence and severity of myocardial infarction in patients with rheumatoid arthritis. Ann Rheum Dis. 2017;76(4):654–60. https://doi.org/10.1136/annrheumdis-2016-209784.
40. Kang EH, Jin Y, Brill G, Lewey J, Patorno E, Desai RJ, et al. Comparative cardiovascular risk of Abatacept and tumor necrosis factor inhibitors in patients with rheumatoid arthritis with and without diabetes mellitus: a multidatabase cohort study. J Am Heart Assoc. 2018;7:e007393.
41. Jin Y, Kang EH, Brill G, Desai RJ, Kim SC. Cardiovascular (CV) risk after initiation of Abatacept versus TNF inhibitors in rheumatoid arthritis patients with and without baseline CV disease. J Rheumatol. 2018;45(9):1240–8. https://doi.org/10.3899/jrheum.170926 Epub 2018 May 15. PMID: 29764964.
42. Nurmohamed M, Choy E, Lula S, Kola B, DeMasi R, Accossato P. The impact of biologics and tofacitinib on cardiovascular risk factors and outcomes in patients with rheumatic disease: a systematic literature review. Drug Saf. 2018;41(5):473–88. https://doi.org/10.1007/s40264-017-0628-9.

10

Gout of feet and ankles in different disease durations: Diagnostic value of single-source DECT and evaluation of urate deposition with a novel semi-quantitative DECT scoring system

Jin Shang[1†], Xiao-Hu Li[1†], Shu-Qin Lu[1], Yi Shang[2], Lu-Lu Li[1] and Bin Liu[1*]

Abstract

Objectives: To investigate the diagnostic performance of single-source dual-energy computed tomography (DECT) based on gemstone spectral imaging technology (including Discovery CT750HD and Revolution CT) in patients with suspected feet/ankles gouty arthritis, and evaluate the urate deposition with a novel semi-quantitative DECT scoring system.

Methods: A total of 196 patients were consecutively included. Feet and ankles were evaluated in all patients by single-source DECT scan. The 2015 EULAR/ACR criteria were used as the reference for the diagnosis of gout. The sensitivity, specificity, and area under the receiver operating characteristic curve (AUC) of DECT for the diagnosis of gout in the early (≤1 year), middle (1–3 years), and late (> 3 years) disease durations were calculated. Besides, a novel semi-quantitative DECT scoring system was assessed for the measurement of urate deposition, and the correlation between the scores and the clinical and serological data were also evaluated. Moreover, the influences of artifacts on the diagnostic performance of DECT were also determined.

Results: The sensitivity, specificity, and AUC of DECT in 196 patients were 38.10, 96.43%, and 0.673 in the early-stage group; 62.96, 100.00%, and 0.815 in the middle-stage group; and 77.55, 87.50%, and 0.825 in the late-stage group, respectively. The overall diagnostic accuracies in the AUC of DECT (Discovery CT750HD and Revolution CT) in the middle and late stages of gout were higher than that in the early stage of gout. Besides, the monosodium urate crystals were deposited on the first metatarsophalangeal joints and ankles/midfeet. Age, the presence of tophus, bone erosion, and disease duration considerably affected the total urate score. No statistical difference in the positive detection of nail artifact, skin artifact, vascular calcification, and noise artifact was found between the case and control groups.

* Correspondence: lbhyz32@163.com
[†]Jin Shang and Xiao-Hu Li contributed equally to this work.
[1]Department of Radiology, The First Affiliated Hospital of Anhui Medical University, 210 Jixi Road, Hefei 230022, Anhui, China

Conclusion: DECT (Discovery CT750HD and Revolution CT) showed promising diagnostic accuracy for the detection of urate crystal deposition in gout but had limited diagnostic sensitivity for short-stage gout. Longer disease duration, the presence of tophus, and bone erosion were associated with the urate crystal score system. The artifacts do not remarkably affect the diagnostic performance of DECT in gout.

Keywords: Gout, Dual-energy spectral CT, Scoring method, Disease duration, Artifact, Clinical trial

Introduction

Gout is the most common form of inflammatory arthropathy resulting from monosodium urate (MSU) crystals deposition [1]. The long-term deposition of MSU crystals in the joints and periarticular soft tissues can contribute to progressive joint destruction, renal failure, and mortality given its association with coronary heart disease, metabolic syndrome, and diabetes [2, 3]. Early diagnosis and the timely initiation of therapy are imperative to improve the disease outcome of patients with gout. Gout diagnosis is based on the identification of negative birefringent MSU crystals in the joint fluid or tophi by polarized microscopy. However, this method is seldom used in clinical practice owing to many limitations, such as invasiveness, lack of training, and microscopy unavailability [4]. Thus, the clinical utilization of dual-energy computer tomography (DECT) for gout diagnosis has dramatically increased over the past decade. Image acquisition is based on two different spectra (often 80 and 140 kV) in DECT scanning that can operate at the source or detector level. Dual source–dual detector (DECT scanners with two X-ray tubes), single-source rapid kilovoltage switching, twin-beam single-source CT with gold filter, and dual-scan single-source are the most commonly used DECT technologies [5]. The validity of DECT as a measure for gout diagnosis has been confirmed in many previously published literatures [6–9]. Currently, DECT has been incorporated into the 2015 American College of Rheumatology/European League Against Rheumatism gout classification criteria (ACR /EULAR 2015) based on reliable previously published data and its diagnostic accuracy [10].

Most studies have shown that DECT is a highly accurate tool for gout diagnosis, but it has limited diagnostic accuracy for gout in short-term duration with widely varied results. Gamala et al. [11] conducted a meta-analysis of 10 studies on the diagnostic accuracy of DECT and revealed that the pooled sensitivity and specificity of DECT are 81 and 91%, respectively, whereas the pooled sensitivity is 55% in patients with recent onset disease (≤6 weeks). In a recent study of 15 patients with aspiration-proven gout with a disease duration of within 1 year, the sensitivity of DECT in identifying MSU deposition was only 26.6% [12]. Conversely, in a study of 40 patients in the early course of gout, the sensitivity and specificity of DECT for the diagnosis of gout are 90 and 83%, respectively [8]. However, currently most studies on gout were performed using dual-source DECT [8, 12–14]. and the performances of other types of DECT, such as single-source rapid kilovoltage switching DECT, and dual-scan single-source CT, were less studied. Thus, the present study was conducted using single-source rapid kilovoltage switching DECT based on gemstone spectral imaging (GSI) technology (including Discovery CT750HD and Revolution CT, GE Healthcare, Milwaukee, WI, USA), in which the single tube was switched between 80 and 140 kVp in less than 0.05 μs.

Moreover, DECT has a potential role in evaluating MSU crystals deposition in patients with gout receiving urate-lowering treatments. At present, urate deposition is assessed by automated volume assessment software, but this time-consuming method could not easily measure the volume of specific deposition sites. Therefore, Bayat et al. [15] developed a semi-quantitative DECT scoring system in a large sample set that allowed the evaluation of urate deposition at specific sites of feet/ankles. In this scoring system, each scan is divided into four areas, and each area is graded in accordance with the maximum amount of urate deposition measured during visual examination. They found that the DECT urate scores are highly correlated with urate volumes and can differentiate between responders and non-responders to intensive urate-lowering treatment. In the current study, we applied this semi-quantitative DECT scoring system for the evaluation of urate deposition in gout and assessed the correlation between the urate deposition scores evaluated by the DECT GSI at feet/ankles and the clinical data.

Furthermore, the artifacts produced during DECT scanning and post-processing may lead to false-positive results. However, the differentiation and clinical importance of artifacts in DECT for MSU deposition identification are still controversial. Chou et al. [3] summarized the common artifacts in DECT imaging for gout, such as nail bed artifact, skin artifact, clumpy artifacts along the tendon, beam hardening, patient motion during the scan, and urate-like pixelations in vascular calcification. Some scholars proposed that these artifacts are true artifacts [6, 16]. Roddy et al. [17] and other scholars [6, 18] suggested that nail bed and tendon artifacts have important influence on gout diagnosis. However, whether this influence is due to true gouty deposition or an artifact is unknown.

Thus, the aims of our study were:

- to evaluate the sensitivity, specificity, and accuracy of single-source DECT GSI (Discovery CT750HD and Revolution CT, GE Healthcare, Milwaukee, WI, USA) for the detection of MSU crystal deposition at feet/ankles in patients with suspected gout in early (≤1 year), middle (1–3 years), and late (> 3 years) stages;
- to determine the correlation between urate deposition evaluated by single-source DECT GSI at feet/ankles and clinical data;
- to investigate whether artifacts affect the diagnostic performance of single-source DECT in gout.

Methods

Study patients

Patients with suspected gout of the feet or ankles were consecutively included in the retrospective study from December 2016 to December 2020 in the hospital. The final gout diagnosis was determined by experienced rheumatologists using the 2015 EULAR/ACR classification criteria as the reference [10]. Characteristic data, including age, sex, disease duration, body mass index (BMI), serum uric acid (SUA) level at time of DECT (the interval between the test of SUA and performance of DECT within 3 days), urate-lowering treatments (ULT) at time of DECT (medication treatment on the day of DECT examination), Diuretic use at time of DECT, the presence of subcutaneous tophi, erosive disease, renal function described as eGFR, time from last gouty attack to DECT examination, and patient-reported concomitant disease (such as hypertension, ischemic heart disease, dyslipidemia, and type II diabetes), were obtained from the medical records.

Patients were selected using the following inclusion criteria: patients aged between 20 and 90 years old; patients undergoing two single-source DECT systems with same technique (Discovery CT750HD and Revolution CT, GE Healthcare, Milwaukee, WI, USA) of their feet and ankles; patients in the gout group receiving the final diagnosis using 2015 EULAR/ACR criteria after comprehensive musculoskeletal examinations; patients in the control with the final diagnosis of rheumatoid arthritis, inflammatory polyarthropathy, achilles tendinitis, and psoriatic arthritis. Exclusion criteria for patients were: relevant foot or ankle trauma, or surgery procedures. Moreover, there was no comparison with other imaging methods (ultrasonography, MRI, etc.).

Ethical approval was provided by the hospital ethics committee. The study was conducted according to the Helsinki Declaration.

DECT examination

All scans were performed using single-source DECT systems (Discovery CT750HD and Revolution CT). The tube voltage of the two systems was switched between 80 and 140 kVp in less than 0.05 µs. In the Discovery CT750HD DECT system (GE Healthcare, Milwaukee, WI, USA), the pitch was 0.984, the beam collimation was 40 mm, the gantry rotation time was 0.6 s, the slice thickness was 5 mm, and the reconstruction increment was 1.25 mm. In the Revolution CT system (GE Healthcare, Milwaukee, WI, USA), the pitch was 0.992, the beam collimation was 80 mm, the gantry rotation time was 0.8 s, the slice thickness was 5 mm, and the reconstruction increment was 1.25 mm. Both feet were scanned simultaneously in supine position without an intravenous contrast agent.

DECT GSI translated two sets of absorption projection data to material density projection data and provided different base material mapping (such as uric acid/calcium pairing, water/iodine pairing, water/calcium pairing, etc.). Base material concentration imaging can better reflect the content of the corresponding components of the tissue, and the uric acid crystal can be visualized more accurately in the uric acid-based map than that in the calcium-based map [19].

Image analysis

Two musculoskeletal radiologists blinded to the patients' information independently reviewed the images for the detection and localization of MSU deposits. Each site was deemed positive or negative for the presence of MSU crystals. One positive presence in a single joint was enough to count the patient as having gout. Four regions were involved in the scoring system: the first metatarsophalangeal (MTP1st) joints, other joints of the toes (2nd–5th MTP and interphalangeal joints), ankles/midfeet, and tendons. Each joint was scored as follows: 0 = no deposit, 1 = dots, 2 = single deposit, 3 = more than one deposit. The presence of artifacts at the feet/ankles was also recorded. If discordant results arose after the consultation of the two readers, the two reviewer and a third co-author with more than 30 years of experience in musculoskeletal radiology jointly re-examined the controversial images to achieve a consensus that would be used for final analyses described in this current study.

Statistical analyses

The SPSS software version 26.0 (SPSS Inc., Chicago, IL, USA) and MedCalc statistical software version 19.2.6 (MedCalc Software bvba, Ostend, Belgium) were used for statistical analyses. Sensitivity, specificity, and area under receiver operating characteristic curve (AUC) were calculated. Continuous data were described as means and standard deviation (SD), while categorical data were expressed as frequencies and percentages. The statistical significance for the differences between quantitative variables without normal distribution were calculated by Mann-Whitney test, whereas for those with normal distribution we used the Student's t-test. The inter-reader reliability analyses for the diagnostic performance of DECT were assessed using Cohen's kappa statistic that was interpreted as follows: the values of 0.00–0.20 representing as "slight" reliability; 0.21–0.40 as "fair" reliability; 0.41–0.60 as "moderate" reliability; 0.61–0.80 as "substantial" reliability; and > 0.80 as "almost perfect" reliability. Cramer's V was utilized to correlate the DECT findings that indicate the presence of MSU crystal deposits at feet/ankles with the clinical and serological variables. Statistical significance was evaluated by Chi-square and Fisher's exact test. $P < 0.05$ was regarded as the statistical significance.

Results

Clinical characteristic

An overall number of 196 patients were recruited in the study. The demographic characteristics of the patients are shown in Table 1. Among the included patients, 125 (mean age, 56.16 ± 16.93 years) were examined using the Discovery CT750HD, whereas 71 (mean age, 51.68 ± 17.59 years) were examined using the Revolution CT. Mean disease duration was 7.52 ± 7.94 years. A history of tophus was found in 16.8% (33/196) of patients, and the mean uric acid level at recruitment was 456.11 ± 123.16 mmol/L. Thirty-seven patients were receiving urate-lowering treatment during evaluation. There were significant differences in disease duration, presence of tophus, and diuretic use between the gout and control groups (P<0.05), and the related outcomes should be interpreted cautiously. Meanwhile, subgroup analysis on disease duration was performed regarding the early-, middle-, and late- stages to reduce the bias. Moreover, we recorded positive DECT results (Fig. 1) and scored the urate deposition in four locations (MTP1st joints, other joints of the toes, ankles/midfeet, and tendons).

Diagnostic performance of single-source DECT GSI in different stages of gout

The sensitivity, specificity, and AUC of single-source DECT GSI in 196 patients for the diagnosis of gout were 38.10, 96.43%, and 0.673 in the early-stage group; 62.96, 100.00%, and 0.815 in the middle-stage group; 77.55, 87.50%, and 0.825 in the late-stage group, and 69.18, 94.00%, and 0.816 in the total-stages group, respectively (Table 2 and Fig. 2). The sensitivity, specificity, and AUC of gout diagnosis using Discovery CT750HD (n = 125) were 55.56, 100.00%, and 0.778 in the early-stage group; 59.09, 100.00%, and 0.795 in the middle-stage group; 75.71, 85.71%, and 0.807 in the late-stage group, and 70.30, 95.83%, and 0.831 in the total-stages group, respectively (Table 2 and Additional files 1). The sensitivity, specificity, and AUC in gout diagnosis using Revolution CT (n = 71) were 25.00, 93.33%, and 0.592 in the early-stage group; 80.00, 100.00%, and 0.900 in the middle-stage group; 82.14, 88.89%, and 0.855 in the late-stage group, and 66.67, 92.31%, and 0.795 in the total-stages group, respectively (Table 2 and Additional files 2). The overall diagnostic accuracies of AUC in DECT GSI (Discovery CT750HD and Revolution CT) in the late and middle stages of gout were higher than that in the early stage of gout. Moreover, the cross-tabulations of diagnostic performance of DECT based on different disease durations are shown in Additional files 3, 4, 5, and 6.

The inter-reader reliability analyses for the diagnostic performance

The values for inter-reader agreements of Discovery CT, Revolution CT, and both CT scanners were 0.879, 0.867, and 0.874 in the early stage; 0.923, 0.720, and 0.879 in the middle stage; and 0.853, 0.885, and 0.864 in the late stage. The strength of agreements was considered good or very good.

Measurement of urate deposition using the semi-quantitative DECT scoring system

The MSU crystals were deposited on MTP1st joints (1.43 ± 2.06 scores) and ankles/midfeet (1.44 ± 2.32 scores), followed by tendons (0.71 ± 1.68 scores) and other joints of the toes (0.54 ± 1.46 scores). The scores were significantly higher in patients with a disease duration of more than 3 years than those with a duration of less than 3 years (Table 3).

Associations between total urate deposit score and gout characteristics

Age, presence of tophus, bone erosion, and disease duration significantly affected the total urate score (P < 0.050), whereas gender, SUA level at time DECT, urate-lowering treatments, BMI, time from last gouty attack to DECT exam, and renal function did not significantly affect the total urate score (P > 0.050, Table 4).

Artifacts in gout and non-gout groups

Four types of artifacts, namely, nail artifact, skin artifact, noise artifact, and vascular calcification, were found in the current study (Fig. 3). No statistical difference in the detection of these four types of artifacts including nail artifact (P = 0.143), skin artifact (P = 0.307), vascular calcification (P = 0.341), and noise artifact (P = 1.000) was found between the case and control groups (Table 5). Therefore, artifacts do not remarkably affect the diagnostic performance of DECT in gout.

Discussion

Gout is caused by the deposition of MSU crystals in the joints or surrounding tissues, among which, the MTP1st joint is the most common joint involved in gout [20].

Table 1 Demographic, clinical and serological data for both patients with gout and controls

Variables	Overall single source DECT (Discovery 750HD and Revolution CT)				Discovery 750HD				Revolution CT			
	Total	Gout patients	Controls	*P*	Total	Gout patients	Controls	*P*	Total	Gout patients	Controls	*P*
Male/Female	175/21	133/13	42/8	0.161	115/10	94/7	21/3	0.627	60/11	39/6	21/5	0.508
Age (years)	54.54 ± 17.27	56.02 ± 16.98	50.20 ± 17.52	0.163	56.16 ± 16.93	56.65 ± 16.65	54.08 ± 18.28	0.441	51.68 ± 17.59	54.60 ± 17.81	46.62 ± 16.31	0.065
Disease duration (yrs)	6.36 ± 7.07	7.60 ± 7.56	2.75 ± 3.48	0.031	7.52 ± 7.94	8.69 ± 8.27	2.63 ± 3.42	<0.001	4.32 ± 4.59	5.07 ± 4.92	2.95 ± 3.64	0.049
Tophus (n, %)	33 (16.8)	33 (22.6)	0	<0.001*	20 (16.0)	20 (19.8)	0	0.013*	13 (18.3)	13 (28.9)	0	0.001*
Erosive disease (n, %)	79 (40.3)	73 (50.0)	6 (12.0)	<0.001	60 (48.0)	57 (56.4)	3 (12.5)	<0.001	19 (26.8)	16 (35.6)	3 (11.5)	0.054
IHD (n, %)	74 (37.8)	61 (41.8)	13 (26.0)	0.047	47 (37.6)	41 (40.6)	1 (25.0)	0.156	27 (38.0)	20 (44.4)	7 (26.9)	0.143
Hypertension (n, %)	113 (57.7)	93 (63.7)	20 (40.0)	0.003	75 (60)	65 (64.4)	10 (41.7)	0.041	38 (53.5)	28 (62.2)	10 (38.5)	0.053
Type II diabetes (n, %)	84 (42.9)	68 (46.6)	16 (32.0)	0.072	56 (44.8)	49 (48.5)	7 (29.2)	0.087	28 (39.4)	19 (42.2)	9 (34.6)	0.527
Dyslipidemia (n, %)	10 (5.1)	9 (6.2)	1 (2.0)	0.434	47 (37.6)	41 (40.6)	6 (25.0)	0.841	1 (1.4)	1 (2.2)	0 (0)	1.000*
Diuretic use (n, %)	39 (19.9)	38 (26.0)	1 (2.0)	0.001	23 (18.4)	23 (22.8)	0	0.007*	16 (22.5)	15 (33.3)	1 (3.8)	0.010
ULT at time of DECT (n, %)	37 (18.9)	35 (24.0)	2 (4.0)	0.004	22 (17.6)	21 (20.8)	1 (4.2)	0.104	15 (21.1)	14 (31.1)	1 (3.8)	0.016
BMI ≥ 28 (n, %)	32 (16.3)	22 (15.1)	10 (20.0)	0.415	21 (16.8)	18 (17.8)	3 (12.5)	0.747	11 (15.5)	4 (8.9)	7 (26.9)	0.092
serum uric acid at time of DECT, (μmol/L)	456.11 ± 123.16	471.69 ± 119.96	410.64 ± 122.29	0.003	451.54 ± 117.82	466.61 ± 114.98	388.08 ± 110.24	0.005	466.42 ± 126.56	486.62 ± 120.73	431.46 ± 131.11	0.096
serum uric acid at time of DECT with ULT, (μmol/L)	435.81 ± 146.94	443.37 ± 145.37	303.50 ± 147.79	0.243	399.73 ± 143.50	409.29 ± 139.69	199.00	0.091	475.40 ± 133.0	480.21 ± 136.71	408.00	0.933
serum uric acid at time of DECT without ULT, (μmol/L)	459.21 ± 118.43	480.62 ± 110.00	415.10 ± 120.90	0.001	462.60 ± 109.24	481.66 ± 103.41	396.30 ± 104.93	0.004	464.02 ± 125.91	489.52 ± 115.11	432.40 ± 133.73	0.081
eGFR				0.012				0.058				0.014
eGFR>90 (n, %)	96 (49.0)	64 (43.8)	32 (64.0)		63 (50.4)	49 (48.5)	14 (58.3)		33 (46.5)	15 (33.3)	18 (69.2)	
eGFR60–90 (n, %)	64 (32.7)	49 (33.6)	15 (30.0)		42 (33.6)	32 (31.7)	10 (41.7)		22 (31.0)	17 (37.8)	5 (19.2)	
eGFR<60 (n, %)	36 (18.4)	33 (22.6)	3 (6.0)		20 (16.0)	20 (19.8)	0		16 (22.5)	13 (28.9)	3 (11.5)	

Abbreviations: *IHD* ischemic heart disease, *ULT* urate lowering treatment, *BMI* body mass index, *yrs*. years
**P* value was calculated by Fisher Exact Test

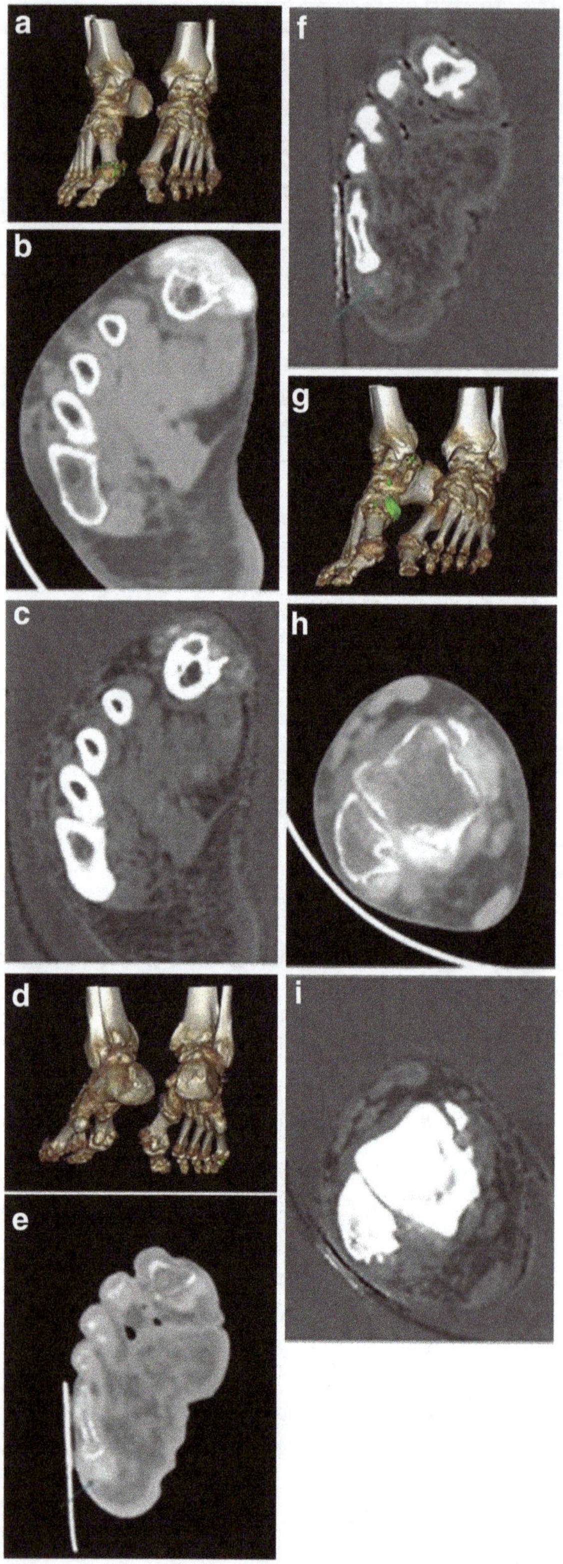

Fig. 1 3D reconstruction (**a**), uric acid base image (**b**), calcium base image (**c**) of the same patient showed the identification of score 3 for MTP1st in the foot. (**d**), uric acid base image (**e**), calcium base image (**f**) of the same patient showed the identification of score 2 for other joints of the toes in the foot. (**g**), uric acid base image (**h**), calcium base image (**i**) of the same patient showed the identification of score 3 for MTP1st in the foot for ankle/midfoot in the foot

The incidence of gout has been increasing annually with the improvement of living standards and changes in diet [6]. Long-term urate deposition is closely related to diabetes mellitus, coronary heart disease, metabolic disorder, and other diseases, which result in serious complications, including joint destruction [21]. Therefore, the early diagnosis and timely treatment of gout are important for the prognosis of patients with gout. Most of the experimental studies on urate deposition were conducted using dual-source devices [12–14, 22]. The current study used single-source systems (DECT GSI: Discovery CT750HD and Revolution CT) to explore the diagnostic performance of DECT in patients with different disease durations and correlate urate deposition score with clinical characteristics. Furthermore, whether artifacts have impacts on gout diagnosis was also investigated.

Dual-source DECT has been reported as a highly accurate tool for gout diagnosis [6, 7, 9]. However, the studies regarding the diagnostic performance of single-source DECT were rare. Glazebrook et al. [6] conducted a retrospective study on 12 patients with aspiration-proven gout, and reported that the sensitivity and specificity of dual-source DECT are 100 and 89%, respectively. Jia et al. [14] concluded that the sensitivity of dual-source DECT is lower by 35.7% in patients with onset gout. Zhang et al. [12] compared the diagnostic accuracies of dual-source DECT and ultrasonography in patients with different gouty disease durations and reported that the sensitivities of DECT for gout within 1 year, 1–3 years, and more than 3 years are 26.6, 66.6, and 90%, respectively. They also revealed that the sensitivity of ultrasonography is remarkably higher than that of dual-source DECT in early gout and suggested ultrasonography as the first choice for the diagnosis of early-stage gout. By contrast, Bongartz et al. [8] reported a higher sensitivity of 80% using dual-source DECT in 20 gout patients with symptom duration of < 6 weeks. In the present study, the sensitivities of single-source DECT in middle- and late-stage gout were remarkably higher than that in early-stage gout. The outcomes demonstrated that disease duration strongly affects the diagnostic accuracy of single-source DECT, and DECT has limited diagnostic value in early-stage gout.

The results could be explained as follows. First, DECT could only detect the smallest size of 2 mm in diameter

Table 2 Sensitivity and specificity of DECT GSI in different stages of gout

Group	Overall single source DECT of Discovery and Revolution					Discovery CT					Revolution CT				
	No.	Sensitivity (95% CI)	Specificity (95% CI)	AUC (95% CI)	*P**	No.	Sensitivity (95% CI)	Specificity (95% CI)	AUC (95% CI)	*P**	No.	Sensitivity (95% CI)	Specificity (95% CI)	AUC (95% CI)	*P**
Early stage (≤1 yr)	49	38.10 (18.1–61.6)	96.43 (81.7–99.9)	0.673 (0.524–0.800)	0.003	22	55.56 (21.2–86.3)	100.00 (75.3–100.0)	0.778 (0.552–0.925)	0.002	27	25.00 (5.5–57.2)	93.33 (68.1–99.8)	0.592 (0.387–0.775)	0.211
Middle stage (≤3 yrs)	33	62.96 (42.4–80.6)	100.00 (54.1–100.0)	0.815 (0.642–0.928)	<0.001	26	59.09 (36.4–79.3)	100.00 (39.8–100.0)	0.795 (0.593–0.927)	<0.001	7	80.00 (28.4–99.5)	100.00 (15.8–100.0)	0.900 (0.467–0.999)	<0.001
Late stage (>3 yrs)	114	77.55 (68.0–85.4)	87.50 (61.7–98.4)	0.825 (0.743–0.890)	<0.001	77	75.71 (64.0–85.2)	85.71 (42.1–99.6)	0.807 (0.701–0.888)	<0.001	37	82.14 (63.1–93.9)	88.89 (51.8–99.7)	0.855 (0.700–0.949)	<0.001
Total	196	69.18 (61.0–76.5)	94.00 (83.5–98.7)	0.816 (0.754–0.868)	<0.001	125	70.30 (60.4–79.0)	95.83 (78.9–99.9)	0.831 (0.753–0.892)	<0.001	71	66.67 (51.0–80.0)	92.31 (74.9–99.1)	0.795 (0.682–0.882)	<0.001

Abbreviations: No. number, *CI* confidence intervals, *AUC* area under receiver operating characteristic curve, *yrs.* years
* the *P* values refer to the AUC

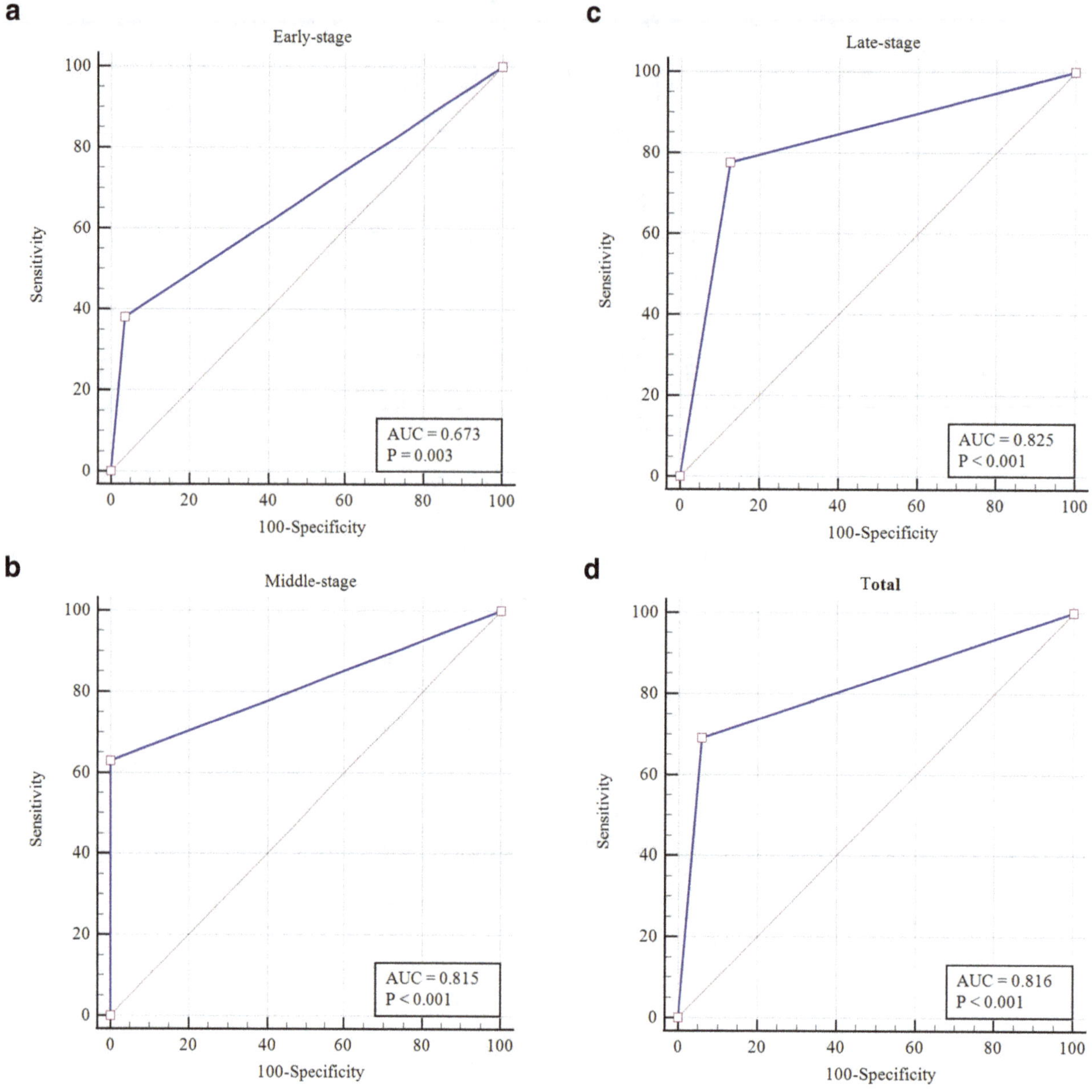

Fig. 2 a ROC curve for sensitivity, 1-specificity, and AUC regarding the early-stage of gout with overall single source DECT Discovery and Revolution. **b** ROC curve for sensitivity, 1-specificity, and AUC regarding the middle-stage of gout with overall single source DECT Discovery and Revolution. **c** ROC curve for sensitivity, 1-specificity, and AUC regarding the late-stage of gout with overall single source Discovery CT750 HD and Revolution CT. **d** ROC curve for sensitivity, 1-specificity, and AUC regarding the total-stages of gout with overall single source Discovery CT750 HD and Revolution CT

and a minimum volume concentration of 15–20% [16, 23]. However, the volume of MSU crystals in patients with short disease course was small and undetected. Thus, the sensitivity of single-source DECT is decreased in the early stages of gout. Wu et al. [9] and Jia et al. [14] found a strong relationship between disease duration and MSU crystal volume, which can partly explain the higher diagnostic effect of DECT in patients with late-stage gout. Most studies on gout presented a relatively long disease duration, and the overall high diagnostic accuracy is largely attributed to the high MSU crystal volume in the late stage of gout [12, 14, 24]. Moreover, the deposition of MSU crystals in the early stage of gout is also affected by the active chemotaxis and phagocytosis of leukocytes. The detection of single-source DECT for MSU crystals might be adversely affected by these chemical compositions [22]. Future researches should test the reliability of single-source DECT in early gout and find an optimal imaging approach for the identification of MSU deposits in early-stage disease.

Table 3 Measurement of urate deposition using the semi-quantitative DECT scoring system and the stratification by disease duration

Value	No. of patients (n, %)							Total urate scores (x ± s)			Z of duration ≤ 3 yrs versus duration>3 yrs	*P* value of duration ≤ 3 yrs versus duration>3 yrs
	Score of 0	Score of 1	Score of 2	Score of 3	Score of 4	Score of 5	Score of 6	Overall disease duration	Disease ≤3 yrs. duration	Disease>3 yrs. duration		
MTP 1st joint	65 (44.5)	16 (11.0)	13 (8.9)	15 (10.3)	11 (7.5)	8 (5.5)	18 (12.3)	1.43 ± 2.06	1.13 ± 1.81	2.30 ± 2.26	− 3.085	0.002
Other joints of the toes	116 (79.5)	4 (2.7)	8 (5.5)	6 (4.1)	1 (0.7)	3 (2.1)	8 (5.5)	0.54 ± 1.46	0.10 ± 0.37	1.02 ± 1.93	−2.798	0.005
Ankles/ Midfeet	83 (56.8)	3 (2.1)	13 (8.9)	4 (2.7)	6 (4.1)	6 (4.1)	31 (21.2)	1.44 ± 2.32	1.06 ± 2.10	2.35 ± 2.59	−3.306	0.001
Tendons	111 (76.0)	1 (0.7)	8 (5.5)	8 (5.5)	3 (2.1)	4 (2.7)	11 (7.5)	0.71 ± 1.68	0.48 ± 1.26	1.18 ± 2.10	− 1.996	0.046
All joints and tendons	_							4.12 ± 6.27	2.77 ± 4.16	6.85 ± 7.32	−3.723	<0.001

Abbreviations: *MTP 1st joint* the first metatarsophalangeal joint, *No.* number, *yrs.* years

Table 4 Associations between total urate deposit score and gout characteristics

Factors	n	Total urate deposit score	t/Z/F[a]	*P*-value
Age (years)			−2.040	0.041
<56	63	4.27 ± 5.78		
≥ 56	83	6.45 ± 7.25		
Gender			−0.91	0.928
Men	133	5.62 ± 6.87		
Women	13	4.38 ± 5.06		
Tophus			−6.157	<0.001
Yes	33	12.45 ± 7.65		
No	113	3.48 ± 4.84		
Erosive disease			−6.188	<0.001
Yes	73	8.55 ± 7.52		
No	73	2.47 ± 3.96		
Disease duration (yrs)			−3.723	<0.001
≤ 3	48	2.77 ± 4.16		
>3	98	6.85 ± 7.32		
Urate at DECT (μmol/L)			−1.752	0.080
≤ 585	26	8.12 ± 7.90		
> 585	120	4.94 ± 6.33		
ULT use at DECT			−1.528	0.127
Yes	35	7.20 ± 7.88		
No	111	4.97 ± 6.26		
BMI (kg/m^2)			−0.756	0.450
<28	124	5.53 ± 6.56		
≥ 28	22	5.36 ± 7.73		
Time from last gouty attack to DECT examination (day)			−0.883	0.405
≤ 10	66	4.94 ± 6.90		
> 10	66	5.45 ± 6.84		
Renal function by eGFR			0.981	0.378
≥ 90	64	4.62 ± 6.06		
60–90	49	6.18 ± 6.77		
< 60	33	6.21 ± 7.81		

[a]The t value, Z value, and F value were obtained by Student's t-test, Mann-Whitney test, and Analysis of variance, respectively, according to the result of the test for normal distribution

Besides, growing evidence shows that DECT can determine disease activity and therapy efficacy in gout [25]. Bayat et al. [15] developed a semi-quantitative DECT scoring method for the evaluation of MSU crystal deposits at specific sites in the feet/ankles during therapy, and the scores were highly correlated with urate volumes. Dalbeth et al. [26] measured the MSU crystal deposition in patients with gout who received stable-dose allopurinol and demonstrated that the higher crystal deposition on DECT was associated with higher SUA and lower allopurinol dose. However, the results of our study showed that SUA level at time of DECT. are not correlated with the total urate deposit score, which might be attributed to the fact that for some patients with gout, the SUA levels are in the normal range, or even lower [27]. Urano et al. [27] concluded that the decrease in SUA during acute gouty arthritis was associated with increased urinary excretion of uric acid. In addition, we also found that there was no correlation of use of urate-lowering treatment with the total urate deposit score. Dehlin et al. [28] showed the suboptimal treatment using urate-lowering treatment in gout and suggested that the efficiencies of urate-lowering treatment with long-term periods were limited for patients

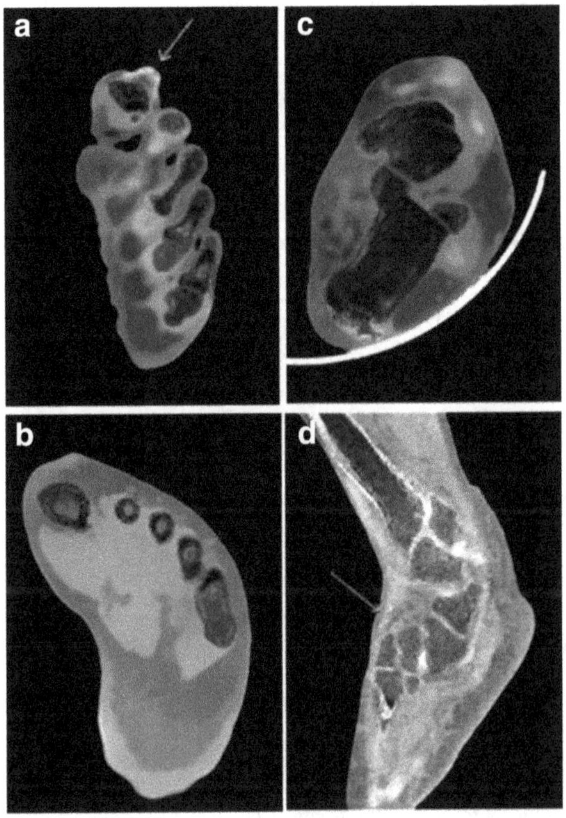

Fig. 3 a Uric acid base image (a) depicted typical artifact from the nail bed. **b** Uric acid base image (b) depicted typical artifact from the skin. **c** Uric acid base image (c) depicted typical artifact from the noise. **d** Uric acid base image (d) depicted typical artifact from the vascular calcification

who had difficulties in compliance to the advice of doctor, thereby contributing to a health care problem of urate-lowering treatment management. Moreover, well-treated patients are slow "MSU deposit depletors" and still have substantial urate volumes even after 2 years. Patients unevenly reduce their MSU burden after urate-lowering treatment. Thus, adding a density measurement of MSU crystal deposition to the apparent volume assessment may help understand the varying kinetics of MSU burden depletion [29, 30]. In addition, some of the patients enrolled in our study used urate-lowering treatment for a short time after gout diagnosis. These factors above could explain the unrelatedness of urate-lowering treatment use and the total urate deposit scores. Furthermore, the results of our study also showed that the total urate deposit score was higher in patients with longer disease duration and correlated strongly to the presence of tophus, bone erosion, and disease duration. Similarly, Svensson et al. [31] applied this urate scoring method and found that the amount of MSU deposits is associated with the presence of tophus and disease duration. Dalbeth et al. [26] found that higher urate deposits are correlated with tophi and bone erosion. The reason why the presence of tophus, bone erosion, and longer disease duration caused higher amount of urate deposition could be explained by the following reasons. First, disease duration is the major contributor to urate deposition; urate deposition increases with disease duration [9, 14]. Second, the presence of tophus is a dominant factor for bone erosion in gout [32]. Moreover, the presence of tophus and bone erosion result in a longer disease duration in patients with gout.

There are differences between single- and dual-source DECT. As for the dual-source DECT, two tube-detector pairs are employed and the tube voltages can be adjustable with the advantage of fast single energy combinations. However, the two separate tubes are offset by approximately 90° to each other, thereby contributing to the material decomposition that is required to be performed only on the image domain because of the spatial offset between acquisitions [33]. In terms of the single-source rapid kilovoltage switching scanners (Discovery CT750 HD and Revolution CT), there are almost no-temporal mismatch and full feilds of view with the X-ray tube switching between 80 and 140 kVp in less than 0.2 ms. [34] Thus, multiple spectral images are generated by projection-space decomposition. As opposed to dual-source DECT systems, projection-space decomposition has the advantages of greater flexibility in the types of materials that can be used of data to minimize beam hardening artifacts [33].

DECT has limitations in gout diagnosis. First, the artifacts are commonly observed in the feet and ankles and

Table 5 Presence of artifacts in both patients with gout and controls

Group		Nailartifact		Skinartifact		Noise		Vascular calcification	
		+	-	+	-	+	-	+	-
Gout patients	146	67	79	30	116	6	140	1	145
Controls	50	17	31	7	43	0	50	0	50
Cramer's V		0.105		0.073		0.104		0.042	
χ^2		2.150		1.043		–		–	
P-value		0.143		0.307		0.341*		1.000*	

**P* value was calculated by Fisher Exact Test

might interfere with radiologists' performance and experience. Some scholars believed that tiny scattered green pixelation within tendons may be the result of the subclinical deposition of MSU crystals [6, 18]. Besides, Chen et al. [35] demonstrated that nail urate could be a proxy for the burden of MSU deposition. We found no statistical difference in the positive detection of nail artifact, skin artifact, vascular calcification, and noise artifact between the case and control groups. Furthermore, the artifacts caused by noise and motion were not seen in the present study, which is probably attributed to the ultrafast reconstruction algorithms by the scintillator of the DECT GSI equipment with fast sampling capabilities (~ 50 μs) [36]. Moreover, the ionizing radiation of DECT is harmful to patients, although the radiation doses of DECT are comparable to or even lower than the dose reference level of body CT [37]. In addition, DECT has been described as a highly accurate tool for the detection and measurement of disease burden and is thus well-suited to evaluate the treatment response of gout. However, the presence of MSU deposits is not necessarily associated with gout, although they increase the risk of its occurrence. Meanwhile, DECT cannot be utilized for the establishment of inflammation. Thus, DECT can diagnose these deposits that contribute to the diagnosis of gout instead of directly diagnosing gout. In the criteria of ACR /EULAR 2015, DECT is one of the criteria, not the only and sufficient one. Moreover, DECT is not widely available and only restricted to certain radiology centers. Nevertheless, DECT provides material characterization via two or more X-ray photon energy-dependent attenuation, which allows the qualitative and quantitative determination of MSU deposition in joints and tissues. Furthermore, DECT performs an excellent visualization of deeper or complex structures and display the anatomic extent of gouty deposits.

This study has several limitations. First, this study was a cross-sectional study and therefore cannot determine the relationship between changes in urate deposition and urate-lowering treatment. Second, no reliable information on the characteristics of gout attack, such as the severity and frequency of attacks, was obtained in the medical records. Third, we did not compare our method with other types of DECT techniques to determine any difference in gout diagnosis. Finally, a few cases were confirmed by arthrocentesis, which is the gold standard for gout diagnosis. Alternatively, we utilized the 2015 EULAR/ACR classification criteria as reference instead of the invasive method.

Conclusion

DECT GSI (Discovery CT750HD and Revolution CT) showed promising diagnostic accuracy for the detection of MSU crystal deposition in gout but had limited diagnostic sensitivity for short-stage gout. Longer disease duration, the presence of tophus, and bone erosion were associated with the novel semi-quantitative DECT scoring system. Artifacts do not remarkably affect the diagnostic performance of DECT in gout.

Supplementary Information

Additional file 1. a. ROC curve for sensitivity, 1-specificity, and AUC regarding the early-stage of gout with Discovery CT750 HD. **b**. ROC curve for sensitivity, 1-specificity, and AUC regarding the middle-stage of gout with Discovery CT750 HD. **c**. ROC curve for sensitivity, 1-specificity, and AUC regarding the late-stage of gout with Discovery CT750 HD. **d**. ROC curve for sensitivity, 1-specificity, and AUC regarding the total-stages of gout with Discovery CT750 HD.

Additional file 2. a. ROC curve for sensitivity, 1-specificity, and AUC regarding the early-stage of gout with Revolution CT. **b**. ROC curve for sensitivity, 1-specificity, and AUC regarding the middle-stage of gout with Revolution CT. **c**. ROC curve for sensitivity, 1-specificity, and AUC regarding the late-stage of gout with Revolution CT. **d**. ROC curve for sensitivity, 1-specificity, and AUC regarding the total-stages of gout with Revolution CT.

Additional file 3. The cross-tabulation of diagnostic performance of DECT in the early stage (≤1 yrs).

Additional file 4. The cross-tabulation of diagnostic performance of DECT in the middle stage (≤3 yrs).

Additional file 5. The cross-tabulation of diagnostic performance of DECT in the late stage (>3 yrs).

Additional file 6. The cross-tabulation of diagnostic performance of DECT in all the disease durations.

Acknowledgements

The authors thank Lu-Ping Zhou for his invaluable assistance in the editing of this manuscript.

Authors' contributions

Jin Shang: Conceptualization, Data curation, Formal analysis, Investigation, Methodology, Software, Validation, Visualization, Writing - original draft, Writing - editing. Xiao-hu Li: Conceptualization, Project administration, Data curation, Formal analysis, Methodology, Writing - review. Shu-qin Lu: Conceptualization, Data curation, Formal analysis, Methodology, Supervision, Validation, Visualization, Writing - review. Yi Shang: Conceptualization, Data curation, Formal analysis, Methodology, Validation, Visualization, Writing - review. Lu-lu Li: Data curation, Formal analysis, Methodology, Validation, Visualization, Writing - review. Bin Liu: Conceptualization, Project administration, Supervision, Validation, Writing - review. The author(s) read and approved the final manuscript.

Authors' information

Jin Shang: MD, Department of Radiology, the First Affiliated Hospital of Anhui Medical University, 210 Jixi Road, Hefei, Anhui 230022, China.
Xiao-Hu Li: PhD, Department of Radiology, the First Affiliated Hospital of Anhui Medical University, 210 Jixi Road, Hefei, Anhui 230022, China.
Shu-Qin Lu: MD, Department of Radiology, the First Affiliated Hospital of Anhui Medical University, 210 Jixi Road, Hefei, Anhui 230022, China.
Yi Shang: MD, Outpatient Department of The Second Central Division, The General Hospital of PLA, 28 Fuxing Road, Beijing 100853, China.
Lu-Lu Li: MD, Department of Radiology, the First Affiliated Hospital of Anhui Medical University, 210 Jixi Road, Hefei, Anhui 230022, China.
Bin Liu: MD, Department of Radiology, the First Affiliated Hospital of Anhui Medical University, 210 Jixi Road, Hefei, Anhui 230022, China.

References

1. Kuo CF, Grainge MJ, Zhang W, Doherty M. Global epidemiology of gout: prevalence, incidence and risk factors. Nat Rev Rheumatol. 2015;11(11):649–62. https://doi.org/10.1038/nrrheum.2015.91.
2. Perez-Ruiz F, Dalbeth N, Bardin T. A review of uric acid, crystal deposition disease, and gout. Adv Ther. 2015;32(1):31–41. https://doi.org/10.1007/s12325-014-0175-z.
3. Chou H, Chin TY, Peh WC. Dual-energy CT in gout - a review of current concepts and applications. J Med Radiat Sci. 2017;64(1):41–51. https://doi.org/10.1002/jmrs.223.
4. Pascual E, Sivera F, Andrés M. Synovial fluid analysis for crystals. Curr Opin Rheumatol. 2011;23(2):161–9. https://doi.org/10.1097/BOR.0b013e328343e458.
5. Coupal TM, Mallinson PI, Gershony SL, McLaughlin PD, Munk PL, Nicolaou S, et al. Getting the Most from your dual-energy scanner: recognizing, reducing, and eliminating artifacts. Am J Roentgenol. 2016;206(1):119–28. https://doi.org/10.2214/AJR.14.13901.
6. Glazebrook KN, Guimarães LS, Murthy NS, Black DF, Bongartz T, Manek NJ, et al. Identification of intraarticular and periarticular uric acid crystals with dual-energy CT: initial evaluation. Radiology. 2011;261(2):516–24. https://doi.org/10.1148/radiol.11102485.
7. Hu MG, Li SL, Lyu GR, Wang CF. Diagnostic value of high frequency ultrasound and dual-energy CT for gouty arthritis. Chin J Med Imaging Technol. 2014;30(6):909–12.
8. Bongartz T, Glazebrook KN, Kavros SJ, Murthy NS, Merry SP, Franz WB, et al. Dual-energy CT for the diagnosis of gout: an accuracy and diagnostic yield study. Ann Rheum Dis. 2015;74(6):1072–7. https://doi.org/10.1136/annrheumdis-2013-205095.
9. Wu HX, Xue J, Ye L, Zhou QJ, Shi D, Xu RZ. The application of dual-energy computed tomography in the diagnosis of acute gouty arthritis. Clin Rheumatol. 2014;33(7):975–9. https://doi.org/10.1007/s10067-014-2606-2.
10. Neogi T, Jansen TLTA, Dalbeth N, Fransen J, Schumacher HR, Berendsen D, et al. 2015 gout classification criteria: an American College of Rheumatology/European league against rheumatism collaborative initiative. Ann Rheum Dis. 2015;74(10):1789–98. https://doi.org/10.1136/annrheumdis-2015-208237.
11. Gamala M, Jacobs JWG, Laar JM. The diagnostic performance of dual energy CT for diagnosing gout: a systematic literature review and meta-analysis. Rheumatology (Oxford). 2019;58(12):2117–21. https://doi.org/10.1093/rheumatology/kez180.
12. Zhang B, Yang M, Wang H. Diagnostic value of ultrasound versus dual-energy computed tomography in patients with different stages of acute gouty arthritis. Clin Rheumatol. 2020;39(5):1649–53. https://doi.org/10.1007/s10067-020-05014-6.
13. Wang Y, Deng X, Xu Y, Ji L, Zhang Z. Detection of uric acid crystal deposition by ultrasonography and dual-energy computed tomography a cross-sectional study in patients with clinically diagnosed gout. Medicine (Baltimore). 2018;97(42):e12834. https://doi.org/10.1097/MD.0000000000012834.
14. Jia E, Zhu J, Huang W, Chen X, Li J. Dual-energy computed tomography has limited diagnostic sensitivity for short-term gout. Clin Rheumatol. 2018;37(3):773–7. https://doi.org/10.1007/s10067-017-3753-z.
15. Bayat S, Aati O, Rech J, Sapsford M, Cavallaro A, Lell M, et al. Development of a dual-energy computed tomography scoring system for measurement of Urate deposition in gout. Arthritis Care Res (Hoboken). 2016;68(6):769–75. https://doi.org/10.1002/acr.22754.
16. Melzer R, Pauli C, Treumann T, Krauss B. Gout tophus detection-a comparison of dual-energy CT (DECT) and histology. Semin Arthritis Rheum. 2014;43(5):662–5. https://doi.org/10.1016/j.semarthrit.2013.11.002.
17. Roddy E, Doherty M. Epidemiology of gout. Arthritis Res Ther. 2010;12(6):223. https://doi.org/10.1186/ar3199.
18. Dalbeth N, Kalluru R, Aati O, Horne A, Doyle AJ, McQueen FM. Tendon involvement in the feet of patients with gout: a dual-energy CT study. Ann Rheum Dis. 2013;72(9):1545–8. https://doi.org/10.1136/annrheumdis-2012-202786.
19. Li X, Wang X, Yu Y, Liu B, Cai J, Xia L, et al. Detection of uric acid depositing in tophaceous gout using a new dual energy spectral CT technology. J Xray Sci Technol. 2014;22(4):541–9. https://doi.org/10.3233/XST-140444.
20. Monu JUV, Pope TL. Gout: a clinical and radiologic review. Radiol Clin N Am. 2004;42(1):169–84. https://doi.org/10.1016/S0033-8389(03)00158-1
21. Choi HK, Curhan G. Independent impact of gout on mortality and risk for coronary heart disease. Circulation. 2007;116(8):894–900. https://doi.org/10.1161/CIRCULATIONAHA.107.703389.
22. Lee SK, Jung J-Y, Jee W-H, Lee JJ, Park S-H. Combining non-contrast and dual-energy CT improves diagnosis of early gout. Eur Radiol. 2019;29(3):1267–75. https://doi.org/10.1007/s00330-018-5716-4.
23. Diekhoff T, Kiefer T, Stroux A, Pilhofer I, Juran R, Mews J, et al. Detection and characterization of crystal suspensions using single-source dual-energy computed tomography: a phantom model of crystal arthropathies. Investig Radiol. 2015;50(4):255–60. https://doi.org/10.1097/RLI.0000000000000099.
24. Ogdie A, Taylor WJ, Weatherall M, Fransen J, Jansen TL, Neogi T, et al. Imaging modalities for the classification of gout: systematic literature review and meta-analysis. Ann Rheum Dis. 2015;74(10):1868–74. https://doi.org/10.1136/annrheumdis-2014-205431.
25. Filippou G, Pascart T, Iagnocco A. Utility of ultrasound and dual energy CT in crystal disease diagnosis and management. Curr Rheumatol Rep. 2020;22(5):15. https://doi.org/10.1007/s11926-020-0890-1.
26. Dalbeth N, Nicolaou S, Baumgartner S, Hu J, Fung M, Choi HK. Presence of monosodium urate crystal deposition by dual-energy CT in patients with gout treated with allopurinol. Ann Rheum Dis. 2018;77(3):364–70. https://doi.org/10.1136/annrheumdis-2017-212046.
27. Urano W, Yamanaka H, Tsutani H, Nakajima H, Matsuda Y, Taniguchi A, et al. The inflammatory process in the mechanism of decreased serum uric acid concentrations during acute gouty arthritis. J Rheumatol. 2002;29(9):1950–3.
28. Dehlin M, Ekstrom EH, Petzold M, Stromberg U, Telg G, Jacobsson LT. Factors associated with initiation and persistence of urate-lowering therapy. Arthritis Res Ther. 2017;19(1):6. https://doi.org/10.1186/s13075-016-1211-y.
29. Dalbeth N, Billington K, Doyle A, Frampton C, Tan P, Aati O, et al. Effects of allopurinol dose escalation on bone Erosion and Urate volume in gout: a dual-energy computed tomography imaging study within a randomized, controlled trial. Arthritis Rheumatol. 2019;71(10):1739–46. https://doi.org/10.1002/art.40929.
30. Ellmann H, Bayat S, Araujo E, Manger B, Kleyer A, Cavallaro A, et al. Effects of conventional uric acid-lowering therapy on monosodium Urate crystal deposits. Arthritis Rheumatol. 2020;72(1):150–6. https://doi.org/10.1002/art.41063.
31. Svensson E, Aurell Y, Jacobsson LTH, Landgren A, Sigurdardottir V, Dehlin M. Dual energy CT findings in gout with rapid kilovoltage-switching source with gemstone scintillator detector. BMC Rheumatol. 2020;4(1):7. https://doi.org/10.1186/s41927-019-0104-5.
32. Dalbeth N, Clark B, Gregory K, Gamble G, Sheehan T, Doyle A, et al. Mechanisms of bone erosion in gout: a quantitative analysis using plain radiography and computed tomography. Ann Rheum Dis. 2009;68(8):1290–5.
33. Megibow AJ, Kambadakone A, Ananthakrishnan L. Dual-energy computed tomography: image acquisition, processing, and workflow. Radiol Clin N Am. 2018;56(4):507–20. https://doi.org/10.1016/j.rcl.2018.03.001.
34. Agostini A, Borgheresi A, Mari A, Floridi C, Bruno F, Carotti M, et al. Dual-energy CT: theoretical principles and clinical applications. Radiol Med. 2019;124(12):1281–95. https://doi.org/10.1007/s11547-019-01107-8.
35. Chen H, Zhao L, Liu F, Chen S, Hu Z, Chen L, et al. Urate in fingernail represents the deposition of urate burden in gout patients. Sci Rep. 2020;10(1):15575. https://doi.org/10.1038/s41598-020-72505-6.
36. Rajiah P, Parakh A, Kay F, Baruah D, Kambadakone AR, Leng S. Update on multienergy CT: physics, principles, and applications. Radiographics. 2020;40(5):1284–308. https://doi.org/10.1148/rg.2020200038.
37. Foley WD, Shuman WP, Siegel MJ, Sahani DV, Boll DT, Bolus DN, et al. White paper of the Society of Computed Body Tomography and Magnetic Resonance on dual-energy CT, part 2: radiation dose and iodine sensitivity. J Comput Assist Tomogr. 2016;40(6):846–50. https://doi.org/10.1097/RCT.0000000000000539.

11

Pathogenic implications, incidence and outcomes of COVID-19 in autoimmune inflammatory joint diseases and autoinflammatory disorders

Piero Ruscitti[1*†], Alessandro Conforti[1†], Paola Cipriani[1], Roberto Giacomelli[2], Marco Tasso[3†], Luisa Costa[3†] and Francesco Caso[3†]

Abstract

As the coronavirus disease 2019 (COVID-19) pandemic caused by severe acute respiratory syndrome coronavirus 2 (SARS-CoV-2) continues to spread rapidly, there are still many unresolved questions of how this virus would impact on autoimmune inflammatory joint diseases and autoinflammatory disorders. The main aim of this paper is to describe the main studies focusing their attention on COVID-19 incidence and outcomes of rheumatoid arthritis (RA), spondylarthritis (SpA), and autoinflammatory disease cohorts. We also revised possible pathogenic mechanisms associated with. Available data suggest that, in patients with RA and SpA, the immunosuppressive therapy, older age, male sex, and the presence of comorbidities (hypertension, lung disease, diabetes, CVD, and chronic renal insufficiency/end-stage renal disease) could be associated with an increased risk of infections and high rate of hospitalization. Other studies have shown that lower odds of hospitalization were associated with bDMARD or tsDMARDs monotherapy, driven largely by anti-TNF therapies. For autoinflammatory diseases, considering the possibility that COVID-19 could be associated with a cytokine storm syndrome, the question of the susceptibility and severity of SARS-CoV-2 infection in patients displaying innate immunity disorders has been raised. In this context, data are very scarce and studies available did not clarify if having an autoinflammatory disorder could be or not a risk factor to develop a more severe COVID-19. Taking together these observations, further studies are likely to be needed to fully characterize these specific patient groups and associated SARS-CoV-2 infection.

Keywords: Rheumatoid arthritis, Spondiloarthritis, Psoriatic arthritis, COVID-19, SARS-COV-2

Introduction

As the coronavirus disease 2019 (COVID-19) pandemic caused by severe acute respiratory syndrome coronavirus 2 (SARS-CoV-2) continues to spread rapidly, there are still many unresolved questions of how this virus would impact on rheumatic musculoskeletal diseases (RMDs) [1–3]. Evidence have highlighted that mechanisms underlining autoimmune and autoinflammatory conditions are critically involved in the host defense and response versus SARS-COV-2, and in more severe cases, leading to a cytokine storm syndrome (CSS), with an acute respiratory distress syndrome (ARDS), multiorgan failure and death [4–6]. Not at last, several studies have been conducted and are ongoing to evaluate the efficacy of biologic disease modifying antirheumatic drugs (bDMARDs) and targeted synthetic DMARDs (tsDMARDs) to treat COVID-19 CSS [7, 8]. Of note, among those, there are agents targeting interleukin-6 (IL-6) and IL-1, and Janus Kinase Inhibitors (JAKis),

* Correspondence: piero.ruscitti@univaq.it
†Piero Ruscitti, Alessandro Conforti, Marco Tasso, Luisa Costa and Francesco Caso have contributed equally to this work
[1]Rheumatology Unit, Department of Biotechnological and Applied Clinical Sciences, University of L'Aquila, L'Aquila, Italy

currently used for the treatment of inflammatory arthropathies and autoinflammatory disorders. However, due to the heterogeneity of randomized controlled trials (RCTs) design and cohorts, and the presence of limitations, as for example concomitant steroidal treatment, studies have showed mixed results on the impact of these therapies on COVID-19 outcomes [7, 8]. Many questions remain still open and one of the most important is whether patients with autoimmune arthropathies and autoinflammatory disorders may have different responses to the SARS-CoV-2 infection, because of impaired immunological and genetic background and/or concomitant antirheumatic treatment [9–11].

Until today, scientific literature has described high incidence and severe outcomes of COVID-19 in middle-aged and elderly subjects and/or patients with underlining diseases, such as diabetes, cardiovascular disease, chronic obstructive pulmonary disease (COPD) [12, 13]. Whether patients with RMDs, especially those receiving Disease Modifying Antirheumatic drugs (DMARDs), are at an increased risk of SARS- CoV-2 infection or severe COVID-19 disease remains to be clarified. On the other hand, it is well known that viral infection susceptibility and clinical aspects may be influenced both by inflammatory diseases, as well as immunomodulant and immunosuppressive therapies [14–16]. For this last point, several studies highlighted that patients with immunoinflammatory diseases on biologic (bDMARDs) may be at higher risk to test positive for COVID-19 and hospitalized, but with a not increased risk of Intensive Care Units (ICU) admission or death in comparison with general population. Hence, the COVID-19 pandemic has represented a hard challenge for Rheumatologists [17, 18].

Today, most studies on incidence and clinical outcomes are available. Thus, the aims of this paper are to describe the main studies focusing their attention on COVID-19 incidence and outcomes of rheumatoid arthritis (RA), spondylarthritis (SpA), and autoinflammatory disease cohorts. We also revised possible pathogenic mechanisms associated with.

Methods

We designed a comprehensive research of literature on incidence and outcomes of COVID-19 during RMDs and autoinflammatory disorders by a review of reports published in international journals. We searched relevant English-language articles in MEDLINE (via Pubmed) until up February 2021, with the research terms: ("SARSCoV2" OR "COVID-19") AND ("RMDs OR "autoinflammatory disorders"). We also revised possible pathogenic mechanisms involved with. In preparing this work, we followed the proposed guidelines for narrative review [19]. Furthermore, we hand-searched reference lists of the relevant articles to find possible additional studies. Out of retrieved 417 articles, both observational studies and case series were assessed if reporting data about COVID-19 incidence and outcomes in patients with RA, SpA, or autoinflammatory diseases.

SARS-CoV-2 infection and immune response

The host immune response has a crucial role for the resolution of COVID-19, but, at the same time, it is implicated in the occurrence of major clinical manifestations of the disease, mostly in more severe patients, as shown in Fig. 1 [20]. Thus, SARS-CoV-2 infection is an example of environmental factor which could trigger an aberrant inflammatory reaction [20]. As for previous evidence, it is well known that an infective trigger may exacerbate an inflammatory disease [21]. In fact, a persistent infection may result in the uptake of microbial antigens by antigen presenting cells (APCs) and presentation of these antigens to microbe-specific T cells [21]. The consequent activation of the pro-inflammatory cascade in a persistently infected site may lead to a tissue damage and uptake of self-antigens by APCs [21]. The presentation of these self-antigens to self-reactive T cells may induce an immune reaction against self-tissues, spreading from a one against microbial antigen epitopes to some non-cross-reactive self-epitopes [21]. This mechanism leading to a reaction against self-antigens is recognized as epitope spreading. Simultaneously, a molecular mimicry may occur. This is a step related to a sufficient similarity between the amino acid sequences of the pathogen and some of the host antigens producing a reaction directed against the host [21]. Furthermore, the pro-inflammatory process during an infection may enhance the production of proteases and the processing of self-antigens by APCs. Additionally, subdominant cryptic antigens, which are unnoticed by the immune system under normal conditions, may be implicated in this process. Infections may also result in the development of pro-inflammatory disorders by driving the APCs to process and display such cryptic antigens [21].

SARS-CoV-2 infection may cause a significant reduction in circulating T cell subsets [22]. The specific depletion of CD4+T cells may lead to an enhanced immune-mediated interstitial pneumonitis and delayed clearance of SARS-CoV in the lungs [22]. In fact, in the pulmonary *interstitium* of SARS-CoV-infected patients, CD8+T cells are the most common infiltrative inflammatory cells, playing an important role in virus clearance as well as in immune-mediated injury [22]. In addition, SARS-CoV2 infection may activate lymphocytes and macrophage by the binding with angiotensin-converting enzyme 2 (ACE-2) receptor [23]. During COVID-19, it has been shown that ACE2-expressing macrophages contained SARS-CoV-2 nucleoprotein antigen. These cells

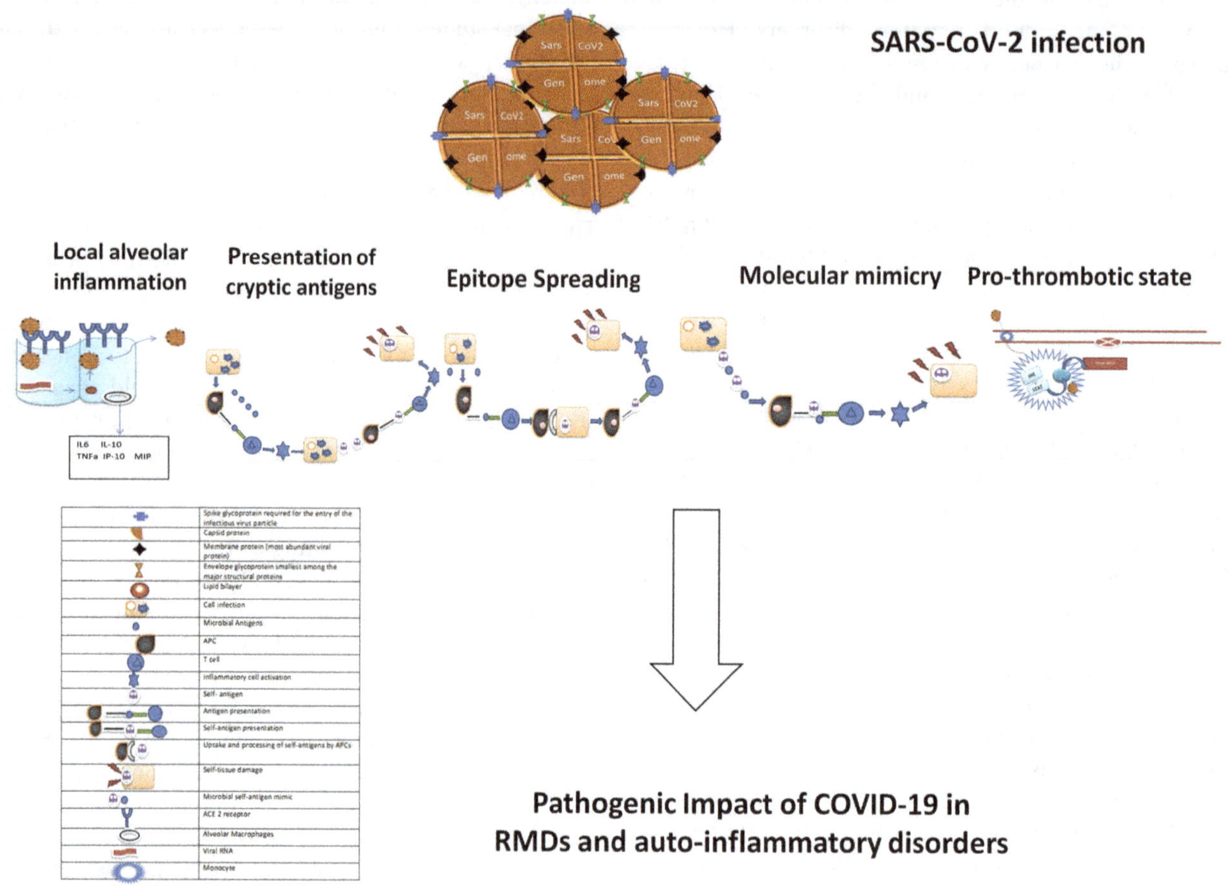

Fig. 1 The figure describes the structure of SARS-CoV2 and the possible infection associated mechanism of autoimmunity. SarsCov2 infects epitelial cells by receptors angiotensin converting enzyme 2 (ACE2) resulting in replication and release of the virus with consequent pyroptosis and the release of damage associated molecular patterns. This process leads to local inflammation and secretion by alveolar macrophages of pro-inflammatory cytokines such as IL-6, IL-10, macrophages inflammatory protein 1 alfa (MIPa), and TNF. Furthermore, this figure describes epitope spreading where persistent infection leads to the uptake of microbial antigens by antigen presenting cells (APCs) and antigen presentation of T-cells. This mechanism carries an inflammatory cascade resulting in a tissue damage, a possible uptake of self-antigens by APC and subsequent presentation of these self-antigens to Tc ells causing an anti-self-reaction. After microbial infection self-antigens could be recognised and processed by APC; subsequently cryptic epitopes could be exposed and presented to self-reactive T-cells leading to an autoimmune response. This figure also describes the mechanism of molecular mimicry where microbial antigens could share antigenic similarly with self-antigens. The presentation of these self-antigen mimics by APC to cross reactive cells leads to an inflammatory response because T cells recognize both the microbial mimic and its respective self-antigens. Finally, viral particles and proinflammatory cytokines induce the activation of blood monocytes which respond by inducing tissue factor membrane expression contributing to a pro-thrombotic state

also showed an upregulation of IL-6, which may contribute to the excessive inflammatory burden and correlate with the disease severity [23]. Moreover, other pro-inflammatory chemokines and pro-inflammatory cytokines may be secreted by SARS-CoV-2-infected alveolar macrophages, which may further enhance the inflammation [23]. Interestingly, during COVD-19, two chemokines (CCL2 and CCL7) resulted to be increased in the bronchoalveolar fluid [24]. Thus, the recruitment of CC-chemokine receptor 2-positive (CCR2+) pro-inflammatory monocytes is favored in COVID-19 with an associated depletion of tissue-resident alveolar macrophages [24]. These pro-inflammatory macrophages have been described to be enriched in genes associated with tissue repair and fibrosis, possibly leading to the fibrotic complications in these patients under mechanical ventilation [24]. In addition, a massive expansion of CD8+T cells with a tissue-resident memory T cell gene signature has been observed in bronchoalveolar fluid patients with mild COVID-19, associated with a minimal infiltration of pro-inflammatory monocytes [24]. This finding suggested that some pre-existing populations of tissue-resident memory T cells, with a possible cross-reactivity against SARS-CoV-2, may limit the activation of pathological macrophages, thus resulting in a protection against a more severe pro-inflammatory process. These observations paralleled with infections due to other highly pathogenic coronaviruses, such as SARS-

CoV and MERS-CoV [24, 25]. In fact, an extensive cellular infiltration dominated by macrophages was found in post-mortem lungs from these patients [24, 25]. Similarly, high levels of interferon-γ (IFN-γ), IL-6, IL-12, transforming growth factor-β (TGF-β), CCL2, CXCL10, CXCL9, and IL-8 were reported in patients with SARS-CoV [25, 26]. Probably, during these disease, high rates of viral replication may lead to host cell cytolysis and the production of pro-inflammatory cytokines and chemokines by infected epithelial cells [26]. In addition, a delayed induction of antiviral interferon responses, owing to specific virus escape mechanisms, could promote the accumulation of pro-inflammatory cells in the lungs. This finding could be probably related to viral structural and non-structural proteins antagonizing IFN responses [26]. The antagonism could occur at various stages of the IFN signaling pathway: (1) preventing the pattern-recognition receptors (PRRs) recognition of viral; (2) impairing the PRR signaling through TBK1/inhibitor of nuclear factor-κB kinase subunit-ε (IKKε), TRAF3 and IRF3; (3) inhibiting the downstream of IFN signaling through STAT1; (4) promoting the host mRNA degradation and inhibiting host protein translation [26]. Furthermore, SARS-COV 2 replication in airway epithelial cells could cause high levels of virus-linked pyroptosis with associated vascular leakage [26]. This could also be a trigger for the subsequent pro-inflammatory response [26]. By PRRs, alveolar epithelial cells and alveolar macrophages may detect the released pathogen-associated molecular patterns (PAMPs), such as viral RNAs, and damage-associated molecular patterns (DAMPs) [26]. This may lead to a local inflammation resulting in an increased secretion of the pro-inflammatory cytokines and chemokines IL-6, IFN-γ, MCP1, and IP-10 into the blood of COVID-19 patients [26]. In addition, the pulmonary recruitment of immune cells from the blood and the infiltration of lymphocytes into the airways may explain the lymphopenia and an increased neutrophil–lymphocyte ratio observed in patients with SARS-CoV-2 infection [26]. Finally, some studies reported the development of autoantibodies in patients with COVID-19, particularly anti-cardiolipin, anti-β2-glycoprotein, and antinuclear antibodies [27, 28]. An increase of ACPA was reported after SARS-CoV2 infection suggesting an epitope spreading before the clinical onset of arthritis [27, 28]. Additional studies reported that the onset of anti-cardiolipin, anti-β2-glycoprotein, and lupus anti-coagulant could be associated with the thromboembolic complications occurring in COVID-19 [29].

Risk of infections in RMDs and autoinflammatory disorders

Patients with RMDs are recognized to have an increased risk of infections related to disease activity, comorbidities, and immunomodulatory therapy [30]. This is due to a combination of underlying disease characteristics and treatment-related factors. In fact, it must be pointed out that inflammatory diseases may also be associated with some immunological dysfunctions increasing the risk of infections [30]. In addition, both csDMARDs and bDMARDs are associated with a higher risk for serious infections [30]. These drugs, targeting key molecules involved in the immune response against infectious antigens, may consequently increase the susceptibility to viruses and bacteria. At the same time, these therapies could provide substantial benefit for controlling RMDs and limiting long-term disability and improving the quality of life [30].

In this context, it is well-known that glucocorticoids (GCs) usage is associated with an enhanced risk of infections, which is correlated with dosages and time of treatment. In fact, a prolonged therapy, even if at low dosages, may enhance the risk of serious infections, which is further increased by the concomitant administration of csDMARDs [31, 32]. Among these drugs, methotrexate (MTX) is the most common administered in RMDs and it is also associated with an increased risk of infection [33, 34]. In fact, recently a meta-analysis showed that MTX is associated with a higher risk of all infections, mainly in RA [35].

In addition, TNFis are associated with an increased risk of serious infections, since the inhibition of this molecule may impair its regulation of immune cell proliferation, differentiation, and survival [36]. In fact, it has been shown that TNF knockout mice rapidly succumb to tuberculosis infection [36]. National registries, open-label extension studies, and retrospective cohorts showed that TNF inhibition may enhance the risk of tuberculosis in patients with RMD [36–39] TNFi could also influence the odds of clearance or reactivation of chronic hepatitis B virus infection [40]. Furthermore, TNFi may increase the risk of fungal infections, such as cryptococcosis, aspergillosis, and pneumocystis jirovecii pneumonia [36, 38].

IL-6-targeted agents are largely used in the treatment of patients with RMDs and autoinflammatory disorders [40–43]. The inhibition of this cytokine, whose signaling pathway uses the protein gp130 as a common signal transducer, could impair the host capacity for generating acute phase responses, including Th17 differentiation and long-lived plasma cell generation [36, 42, 43]. In fact, some clinical data derived from RCTs supports the notion that IL-6-targeting agents increase the risk of infection to a degree similar to TNFis [36, 40, 52, 53]. On the other hand, neutropenia induced by IL-6 inhibition would frequently occur, due to a margination of neutrophils rather than peripheral sequestration. This finding could increase the risk of infection following this therapeutic strategy [40, 41].

Different IL-17-targeted agents have been recently approved for patients with PsA and SpA. IL-17 stimulates neutrophil granulopoiesis and chemotaxis, expression of antimicrobial peptides (β-defensin-2) [41–44]. Thus, patients with RMDs treated with IL-17-targeted agents may be exposed to an increased risk of mucocutaneous candidiasis [42–44]. No cases of active tuberculosis have been reported in a review of clinical trial data [37, 42, 43, 45].

Abatacept is a fusion protein designed to interfere with the binding of CD80/86 molecules on antigen presenting cells/dendritic cells with their CD28 receptors on the surface of CD4 T cells, used in the treatment of RA. Although lower than TNFis, the risk of infection-related hospitalizations is further recognized in patients treated with abatacept [36, 43, 46].

Furthermore, rituximab (RTX), a chimeric monoclonal antibody against the B-cell specific CD20-antigen, is commonly administered in RMDs. Considering that RTX is related to the development of hypogammaglobulinemia, it could increase the risk of infections [47]. In this context, it has been suggested that patients with low levels of IgG post-RTX may be at increased risk of serious infections since IgG levels are relevant for protective immunity. Infections seem to be more frequent during the first 3 months post-treatment, but they may occur anytime [47]. In addition to the immunosuppression caused by the hypogammaglobulinemia and the collapse of B and T cell immunity, RTX may also induce neutropenia, which may furtherly contribute to the risk of infections in these patients [47]. Finally, JAKis are approved for the treatment of RA, and they may enhance the risk of pneumonia and skin and soft tissues infections [48]. JAK are transmembrane proteins that mediate and amplify extracellular signals from growth factors and cytokines [43, 48, 49]. In accordance, JAKis exert a deleterious impact on adaptive immunity by decreasing CD4+T-cell expansion and Th1 and Th17 differentiation, among other effects [48–51]. Particularly, it was reported than the incidence rate for Herpes Zooster was higher than those estimated for other infectious events [49–51].

Incidence and outcomes of COVID-19 in arthritis patients

RA and SpA are chronic inflammatory diseases, mainly affecting the joint, mediated by autoimmune and inflammatory process [52, 53].

More specifically, whereas RA is characterized by predominant peripheral synovial inflammation sustained by autoantibodies and B- and T-lymphocytes mechanisms, SpAs provide a main innate-immunity mediated pathogenesis leading to inflammation of synovial-entheseal structures and axial skeleton. SpA group includes ankylosing spondylitis (AS), psoriatic arthritis (PsA), reactive arthritis (ReA), enteropathic, and undifferentiated spondylarthritis (uSpA) [52, 53]. In patients with RA and SpA, it is recognized that the immunosuppressive therapy and the presence of comorbidities are associated with an increased risk of infections [54–57]. On these bases, a growing body of evidence described the characteristics of COVID-19 patients affected by RA [54–57]. In this context, it is unclear whether these patients may have an increased risk of infection or a higher risk of a severe course for COVID-19 [55–57]. On one hand, the host immunity could provide a strong immunological response adequate for virus clearance, whereas, on the other hand, an aberrant production of pro-inflammatory cytokines induced by the uncontrolled immune response may contribute to a development of cytokine storm syndrome worsening the prognosis of COVID-19 [58].

A recent nationwide Swedish study by Bower et al., comparing March-September 2020 inflammatory joint diseases cohort and 2015–2019 population referent, has evidenced that the risks of hospitalisation (0.5% vs 0.3% in their population referents), admission to intensive care (0.04% vs 0.03%) and death (0.10% vs 0.07%) due to COVID-19 were low in patients with RMDs and similar to general population [55]. This study has reported that overall absolute and excess risks for patients with inflammatory joint diseases are low and the level of risk increases are largely proportionate to those in the general population and explained by comorbidities [55]. Thus, this study showed a similar risk of severe COVID-19 in either RMDs or general population and suggested the negative prognostic impact of comorbidities in this context.

In a German registry, 468 patients with RMDs and a PCR-confirmed SARS-CoV-2 infection were studied [59]. Patients were stratified into three groups by using the hospitalization as indicator for a more severe course: (1) non-hospitalised patients, (2) hospitalised patients without the need for invasive ventilation, (3) hospitalised patients with the need for invasive ventilation. In this cohort, the most common disease was RA, affecting 225 patients (48%) and it was associated with a high rate of hospitalization. Out of those, 62 were hospitalised and 17 needed an invasive ventilation [59]. Out of 140 SpA patients with a PCR-confirmed SARS-CoV-2 infection showed that 20 were hospitalized and 5 needed an invasive ventilation [59]. In this cohort, when compared with RA, patients with SpA showed a lower risk of hospitalization (OR 0.46; 95% CI 0.23–0.91) [59]. In this cohort, only 38% did not have any other chronic condition, frequently concomitant comorbidities were registered in these patients. The most frequent one was high blood pressure, followed by obesity, cardiovascular disease (CVD), and diabetes. Regarding the administered therapy for the RMD, 193 patients were treated with csDMARD monotherapy, 167 patients with bDMARDs, and 145 patients with GCs, mostly low dose GCs of ≤ 5 mg/day. Older age, associated comorbidities, GCs at doses of > 5 mg/day, and moderate to high RMD disease activity were related to the rate of hospitalization [59].

In the COVID-19 Global Rheumatology Alliance physician-reported registry, a large collection of data about COVID-19 infection in RMD was reported, evaluating 600 patients from 40 countries, of whom 277 were hospitalized and 55 were deceased [60]. COVID-19 were predominately diagnosed through PCR testing. In this cohort, 230 patients were affected by RA which was the most represented RMD. A high percentage of these patients with RA (104 out of 230) were hospitalized. Results showed that 48 and 74 SpA and PsA patients, respectively, were diagnosed with COVID-19 predominately diagnosed through PCR testing [60]. A lower proportion of patients who were hospitalized had PsA and other SpA (8% and 6%, respectively) compared with those who were not (16% and 10%, respectively) [60]. Furthermore, a higher prevalence of comorbidities was also registered (hypertension 199 patients, lung disease 127 patients, diabetes 69 patients, CVD 63 patients and chronic renal insufficiency/end-stage renal disease 40 patients) [60]. The authors showed that older age and comorbidities were associated with the rate of hospitalization. On the contrary, the therapy with b/tsDMARD monotherapy, just before COVID-19 diagnosis, was significantly associated with a lower rate of admission to the hospital when compared with no DMAR D therapy [60].

In addition, an observational French cohort described the characteristics of 694 patients with RMDs affected by COVID-19 [61]. The severity of COVID-19 was stratified as follows: (1) mild/ambulatory, (2) moderate/hospitalized out of intensive care unit, (3) severe/intensive care unit or deceased. SARS-CoV2 infection was mostly confirmed by PCR and/or specific antibodies. A large percentage of patients (492 out of 694) had at least one comorbidity (182 hypertension, 146 obesity, 99 respiratory disease, 85 CVD). Fifty-eight patients in this cohort died, resulting in an overall death rate of 8.3%, and of 22.6% in the hospitalized subgroup. In this study, 213 patients were affected by RA [61]. In this study the Authors described the characteristics of 165 patients with SpA and 70 patients with PsA [61]. Of those, great part of SpA patients showed mild infection [n. SpA patients: 135 (30.8%); n. PsA patients: 52 (11.9%)] and moderate infection (n. SpA patients: 25 (14.8%); n. PsA patients: 12 (7.1%)). SpA and PsA patients showing severe infection were 5 (5.8%) and 6 (6.9%), respectively. One patient with SpA and three patients with PsA died during the follow-up [61]. In a Spanish retrospective observational study, the Authors assessed patients with RMDs attending their rheumatology department and who were infected by SARS-CoV2 [62]. They described 62 patients with COVID-19, 42 were hospitalized and 20 were followed-up at home [62]. The most common RMD was RA in 20 affected patients (32%), of whom 3 patients died. Male gender, preexisting lung disease and treatment with GCs (≥ 5 mg per day) were associated with a more severe infection requiring hospitalization [62]. The Authors also described 16 patients with SpA/PsA, representing the 26% of the entire enrolled cohort with RMD and COVID-19 [62]. Eleven of those were hospitalized and 5 were followed-up at home. One of those died [62].

When compared with non-rheumatic hospitalized patients with SARS-COV2 infections, greater odds of hospitalization for patients with inflammatory arthropathies and connective tissue diseases were described by a Spanish group [63]. In a retrospective observational matched cohort study [63], 456 RMDs and non-rheumatic hospitalized patients with SARS-COV2 infection were described. Amongst them, 65 patients were affected by RA and 35 patients were affected by SpA [63]. This study also showed that comorbidities are associated with severe COVID-19 [63]. In this cohort, independent factors associated with severe COVID-19 were increased age, male sex, and having a connective tissue disease, but nor inflammatory arthritis nor previous immunosuppressive therapies were associated with severe COVID-19 [63].

In addition, an observational multicenter study (ReumaCoV Brasil register) assessed adult RMD patients with COVID-19 [64]. In this study, 334 patients with SARS-COV2 infection were included; the most common RMD was RA (28.4%). Hydroxychloroquine (34.9%), GCs (34.2%), MTX (20.1%), and TNFi (75/338; 22.2%) were the most common therapies [64]. This study showed that older age, use of GCs and cyclophosphamide were associated with unfavorable outcomes of SARS-CoV-2 infection. Conversely, TNFi appeared to have a protective role being associated with a reduction of the development of a more severe COVID-19 [64]. Finally, other small case series were available furtherly confirming these findings, as described in Table 1 [65, 66].

Arthritis and potential risk factors for severe COVID-19

In describing the characteristics of RA and SpA with COVID-19, many potential risk factors for a more severe disease have been suggested [59–63]. Similarly, to general population, age is considered a poor prognostic factor of COVID-19 for RA patients [67]. The possible age-associated shift in both innate and adaptive immune systems could reduce the capacity to deal infections and could contribute to the development of a chronic inflammatory state [68]. Moreover, a chronic low-grade

Table 1 Main studies focusing on Incidence, outcomes, and prognostic factors of COVID-19 in rheumatoid arthritis and spondiloarthritis patients

First author	Study design	Sample size	RA patients	SpA patients	PsA patients	Outcome of COVID-19 patients with inflammatory arthropathies	Prognostic factors
FAI2R /SFR/SNFMI/SOFREMIP/CRI/ IMIDIATE consortium and contributors	Observational study	694	213	165	70	Severe COVID-19/hospitalization in RA: 29; SpA: 5; PsA: 6 Death in RA: 20; SpA: 1; PsA: 3	Older age Comorbidities Longer term of GCs
Gianfrancesco et al.	Observational study	600	225	48	74	Severe COVID-19/hospitalization in RA: 104; SpA: 16; PsA: 22 Death in the overall cohort including also CTD: 55	Older age Comorbidities Higher doses of GCs
Hasseli et al.	Retrospective observational study	468	146	125	*	Severe COVID-19/hospitalization in RA: 79; SpA: 20 severe COVID-19 Death in the overall cohort including also CTD: 19	Older age Comorbidities Treatment with GCs at doses > 5 mg/day Moderate to high RMD disease activity
Montero et al.	Retrospective observational study	62	20	16	*	Severe COVID-19/hospitalization in RA: 15; SpA: 11 Death in the overall cohort including also CTD: 10	Male Gender Preexisting lung disease Treatment with GC at dose > 5 mg/day
Pang et al.	Observational study	21	15	–	–	Severe COVID-19/hospitalization in RA: 15 0 death	Comorbidities
Cheng et al.	Observational study	5	4	–	–	5 hospitalised 0 death	Not reported
Marques et al.	Observational study	334	95	45	23	110 hospitalised 28 death	Age > 50 years Treatment with GCs and cyclophosphamide

GCs: Glucocorticoids; PsA: Psoriatic arthritis; RA: Rheumatoid arthritis; RMD: Rheumatic Diseases; SpA: Spondiloarthritis
*In these studies, PsA patients are included in the SpA group

inflammation called inflammaging is associated with immunosenescence, driven by a reduced ability to endure inflammatory triggers as well as an increased production of pro-inflammatory cytokines, acute phase proteins, and oxidative stressors, may lead to higher rates of infection and disease [68].

In addition, comorbidities, including chronic respiratory disease, CVD, diabetes, hypertension, obesity, and renal failure increased the risk for severe COVID-19, as reported in general population [55–62]. In fact, these comorbidities could modulate host-viral or host-immune system interactions favoring a more aggressive course of the disease [69]. Furthermore, the metabolic alterations produced by COVID-19 could decrease cardiorespiratory reserves following a possible stressor agent, enhancing the dysregulation of the immune system, and favoring a pro-thrombotic and pro-inflammatory state. The presence of diabetes would be considered one of the major risk factors for in-hospital mortality increasing the risk of thromboembolism in COVID-19 patients, disease severity, and mortality [69].

Antirheumatic drugs have been reported as not associated with increased risk of serious COVID-19 outcomes, although data accuracy was partial for certain drugs [55]. Moreover, some studies concerning the treatment of RA reported that the use of GCs was associated with a poorer outcome which may parallel with previous studies showing an increased risk of infection with higher doses of these drugs [31]. On the contrary, it has been suggested that no substantial risk was detected neither csDMARDS nor ts/bDMARD. mostly TNFis. Interestingly, the use of ts/bDMARD was also associated with a lower rate of complications during COVID-19 [61]. These findings are consistent with previous studies that found lower odds of hospitalization with ts/bDMARD monotherapy [60–63]. It could be possible that bDMARDs could reduce the high levels of cytokines, including IL-6 and TNF, associated with a more severe COVID-19, thus reducing the possibility to develop a CCS [61–63]. Of note, similar observations, about a beneficial effect of bDMARDs, were suggested on the risk of sepsis after serious infection or a fatal outcome [70].

Taking together these observations, to fully manage patients with RMDs and SARS-CoV-2 infection, it would be of crucial importance to understand how the characteristics of the underlying disease, associated comorbidities, and the use of immunotherapies could be associated with a more severe COVID-19 and a poorer outcome of affected patients [57, 60–63, 71]

Incidence and outcomes of COVID-19 in patients affected by autoinflammatory disorders

Autoinflammatory diseases are caused by self-directed inflammation due to an alteration of innate immunity leading to episodic systemic inflammation attacks [72, 73]. Familial Mediterranean Fever (FMF) is the most common monogenic autoinflammatory diseases. It is an autosomal recessive disease characterized by recurrent systemic inflammatory attacks with fever and serositis [74]. Considering the possibility that COVID-19 could be associated with a CCS [58], the question of the susceptibility and severity of SARS-CoV-2 infection in patients displaying innate immunity disorders, such as FMF, has been raised. In this context, a survey on SARS-CoV-2 infection in patients with FMF followed in Paris area was conducted, including patients fulfilling the international FMF criteria and a genetic confirmed FMF diagnosis [63]. The authors collected the data of 342 patients, of whom 27 FMF patients (7.8%) were infected by SARS-CoV-2. Specifically, 7 patients were hospitalized, 6 required oxygen therapy, 3 developed acute respiratory distress syndrome and required admission to the intensive care unit, and 2 patients died. Severe SARS-CoV-2 infection occurred in patients with risk factors including advanced age, chronic kidney disease, hypertension, vascular disease, obesity, and lung dysfunction [63]. Based on these results, a dysfunction of the innate immune system of FMF could not appear to be a risk factor to develop a more severe COVID-19 [63]. In addition, a French national cohort study described 27 patients out of 694 with autoinflammatory disease affected by SARS-Cov2 infections [61]. Fifteen patients were affected by periodic fever syndromes, 7 patients by other autoinflammatory diseases, and 5 patients were diagnosed with adult onset Still's disease (AOSD) [61]. Five patients experienced a severe COVID-19 and 4 died. Although of interest, these results should be cautiously interpreted due to the very low number of patients assessed by the authors [61]. Finally, a growing body of evidence points out that severe COVID-19 is characterized by an overlapping clinical picture with AOSD and macrophage activation syndrome (MAS), since these are characterized by fever, hyperferritinemia, and a hyper-inflammatory process with a massive release of pro-inflammatory cytokines [74, 75]. These findings would suggest that a hyperinflammatory lung injury, either in severe COVID-19 or MAS, would amplify the immune response leading to an overwhelming release of inflammatory mediators and the occurrence of a CCS [76].

Appraisal of literature

As catastrophic COVID-19 pandemic continues to spread rapidly, many unresolved questions of how this virus would impact on RMDs and autoinflammatory disorders needs to be fully clarified [1–3]. Whether patients with RMDs could be at an increased risk of SARS-CoV-2 infection or severe COVID-19 disease remains to be entirely evaluated [14–16]. Incidence and outcomes of COVID-19 among RMDs and autoinflammatory disorders patients would appear to be consistent with general population affected by SARS-CoV-2 infection. In fact, patients with such diseases who are older and/or have comorbidities may have a higher odd of a more severe COVID-19 [55–57, 60, 63]. For the autoinflammatory disorders, the question is about a possible increased susceptibility to develop CCS in the context of COVID-19 since the prominent pathogenic involvement of the innate immune system in these diseases. However, the available data did not fully clarify this issue due to the low prevalence of these patients suggesting the need of further studies on this topic.

In addition, some data suggested that the real risk of developing severe forms of COVID-19 in patients with RMDs treated with csDMARD or bDMARDs might not increase [60–63]. It could be possible that these medications could reduce the high levels of proinflammatory cytokines thus possibly reducing the risk of a more severe disease during COVID-19 [60–63]. However, the risk of infections is reported to be consistent with such drugs [36–43] and further studies with a longer follow-up are needed to fully understand the real risk of these patients to develop a more severe SARS- CoV-2 infection. In this context, a possible theory could be that patients with RMDs could avoid risky behavior for infections being more aware for the possible risks associated with their immunosuppressive therapies. Furthermore, patients with RMDs may be associated with an increase frailty, which is defined as a syndrome characterized by a decrease of strength, endurance, reduced physiological function, and increased the individual's vulnerability [77]. The chronic RMD inflammation may possibly contribute to the development of frailty associated with a characteristic pro-inflammatory T-lymphocyte phenotype as well as with an elevated concentration of IL-6 [78].

In addition, coagulation abnormalities are increasingly associated with a poor prognosis in COVID- [24]. Microthrombi of the lungs have been described in these patients [1, 24]. In fact, the activation of intravascular coagulation is a hallmark of organ injury in SARS-CoV-2 infection, which is mediated by pro-inflammatory cytokines [24, 73]. Furthermore, IL-1, IL-6, and TNF production and the endothelial cell dysfunction, associated with COVID-19, may play an important role in the thrombo-inflammatory processes ultimately impairing normal vascular haemostasis, fibrinolysis, and vessel wall permeability [79]. Thus, a high thrombotic risk of COVID-19 is clearly recognized which could be further increased by the concomitant RMDs [70, 79]. In fact, during these diseases, the pro-inflammatory milieu may induce a hyper-coagulation by an upregulation of procoagulant factors and a simultaneous downregulation of anticoagulant and fibrinolytic systems, thus leading to this clinical phenotype [79]. This risk is also associated with traditional CVD risk factors, such as an older age and diabetes, but also with the burden of the pro-inflammatory process over time and specific disease features [80, 81]. Taking together these observations, an accurate evaluation of the hyper-coagulation burden in the patients with RMDs affected by SARS-CoV2 infection is needed, since possibly associated with a worse prognosis.

Vaccination against SARS-CoV-2 is now available leading to a significant improvement in the management of COVID-19 [82, 83]. However, it could be matter of debate if the development of protective immunity could occur in patients with RMDs due to a possible impairment of the immune system by underlying inflammatory disease or therapies [82, 83]. Conflicting results are available in literature about this point [82, 83]. In a monocentric study enrolling 26 patients with immune-mediated inflammatory diseases (IMIDs), mainly RMDs, SARS-CoV-2 mRNA vaccines led to development of antibodies in immunosuppressed patients without considerable side effects [82]. Differently, another study on 84 patients with IMIDs, mostly RMDs, showed that immune responses against the SARS-CoV-2 were delayed and reduced [83]. In fact, the concomitant use of MTX appeared to adversely affect both humoral and cellular immune response to COVID-19 vaccines as shown in a more recent cohort study [84]. Taking together these observations, further studies are needed to entirely clarify this topic.

Conclusions

The challenging situation of the SARS-CoV-2 infection is associated with the need of rapid access to the evolving evidence to close the gaps of knowledge which could make difficult to manage patients with chronic conditions. Since the early stages of the COVID-19 pandemic, many concerns arose regarding the potential consequences of SARS-CoV-2 infection in patients with RMDs or autoinflammatory disorders, given the potential negative effects of immunosuppressive drugs on viral clearance, thus speculating a possible increased COVID-19 severity and excess mortality in these patients. However, based on the current literature, available data would suggest that the real risk of developing severe forms of COVID-19 in patients with RMDs or autoinflammatory disorders treated with csDMARD or bDMARDS might not increase. Disease severity in COVID-19 is either similar or slightly higher among those with RMD, and risk appears to be largely associated with risk factors similar to the general population. In this context, it must be pointed out that further studies are likely to be needed to fully characterize these specific patient groups and associated SARS-CoV-2 infection.

Acknowledgements

We thank Mrs. Federica Sensini for her technical assistance.

Authors' contributions

All authors made substantial contributions to the conception or design of the work, the acquisition and interpretation of data. All authors contributed to the critical review and revision of the manuscript and approved the final version. All the authors agreed to be accountable for all aspects of the work. PR, AC, MT, LC, and FC contributed the conception and design of the review. PC and RG provided substantial supervision and interpretation of the review. All authors drafted and revised the manuscript. All authors read and approved the final manuscript.

Author details

[1]Rheumatology Unit, Department of Biotechnological and Applied Clinical Sciences, University of L'Aquila, L'Aquila, Italy. [2]Rheumatology and Immunology Unit, Department of Medicine, University of Rome 'Campus Biomedico', Rome, Italy. [3]Rheumatology Unit, Department of Clinical Medicine and Surgery, School of Medicine, University of Naples Federico II, Naples, Italy.

References

1. van Eijk LE, Binkhorst M, Bourgonje AR, Offringa AK, Mulder DJ, Bos EM, et al. COVID-19: immunopathology, pathophysiological mechanisms, and treatment options. J Pathol. 2021;5642:307–31.
2. Caso F, Costa L, Ruscitti P, Navarini L, Del Puente A, Giacomelli R, et al. Could Sars-coronavirus-2 trigger autoimmune and/or autoinflammatory mechanisms in genetically predisposed subjects? Autoimmun Rev. 2020;19:24.
3. Mehta P, McAuley DF, Brown M, Sanchez E, Tattersall RS, Manson JJ. On behalf of the HLH Across Speciality Collaboration, UK. COVID-19: consider cytokine storm syndromes and immunosuppression. Lancet. 2020;28:395.
4. Qin C, Zhou L, Hu Z, Zhang S, Yang S, Tao Y, et al. Dysregulation of immune response in patients with COVID-19 in Wuhan. China Clin Infect Dis. 2020;28:71.
5. Opdenakker G, Van Damme J. Interferons and other cytokines, genetics and beyond in COVID-19 and autoimmunity. Cytokine Growth Factor Rev. 2021; 29:S1359-610100004–6.
6. Shah VK, Firmal P, Alam A, et al. Overview of immune response during SARS-CoV-2 infection: lessons from the past. Front Immunol. 2020;7(11):1949.
7. Fajgenbaum DC, June CH. Cytokine storm. N Engl J Med. 2020;383:2255–73.
8. Randy QC. COVID-19 cytokine storm: targeting the appropriate cytokine. Lancet Rheumatol. 2021.
9. Gasparotto M, Framba V, Piovella C, Doria A, Iaccarino L. Post-COVID-19 arthritis: a case report and literature review. Clin Rheumatol. 2021;15:1–6.
10. Pelechas E, Drossou V, Voulgari PV, Drosos AA. Anti-rheumatic drugs for the fight against the novel coronavirus infection (SARSCoV-2): what is the evidence? Mediterr J Rheumatol. 2020;31(Suppl 2):259–67.
11. Rosenbaum JT, Hamilton H, Weisman MH, Reveille JD, Winthrop KL, Choi D. The effect of HLA-B27 on susceptibility and severity of COVID-19. J Rheumatol. 2020;15:939.
12. Sanyaolu A, Okorie C, Marinkovic A, Patidar R, Younis K, Desai P, et al. Comorbidity and its impact on patients with COVID-19. SN Compr Clin Med. 2020;25:1–8.
13. Scarpa R, Costa L, Del Puente A, Caso F. Role of thymopoiesis and inflamm-aging in COVID-19 phenotype. Pediatr Neonatol. 2020;61:364–5.
14. Scarpa R, Caso F, Costa L, Passavanti S, Vitale MG, Trojaniello C, et al. May the analysis of 1918 influenza pandemic give hints to imagine the possible magnitude of Corona Virus Disease-2019 (COVID-19)? J Transl Med. 2020;18:489.
15. Rosenbaum JT, Hamilton H, Choi D, Weisman MH, Reveille JD, Winthrop KL. Biologics, spondylitis and COVID-19. Ann Rheum Dis. 2020;79:1663–5.

16. Hyder Pottoo F, Abu-Izneid T, Mohammad Ibrahim A, Noushad Javed M, AlHajri N, Hamrouni AM. Immune system response during viral Infections: Immunomodulators, cytokine storm (CS) and Immunotherapeutics in COVID-19. Saudi Pharm J. 2021;29:173–87.
17. Damiani G, Pacifico A, Bragazzi NL, Malagoli P. Biologics increase the risk of SARS-CoV-2 infection and hospitalization, but not ICU admission and death: Real-life data from a large cohort during red-zone declaration. Dermatol Ther. 2020;33:e13475.
18. Gisondi P, Piaserico S, Naldi L, Dapavo P, Conti A, Malagoli P, et al. Collaborators in the studies of COVID-19 pandemic. Incidence rates of hospitalization and death from COVID-19 in patients with psoriasis receiving biological treatment: a Northern Italy experience. J Allergy Clin Immunol. 2021;147:558–60.
19. Gasparyan AY, Ayvazyan L, Blackmore H, Kitas GD. Writing a narrative biomedical review: considerations for authors, peer reviewers, and editors. Rheumatol Int. 2011;31:1409–17.
20. Ungaro RC, Agrawal M, Park S, Hirten R, Colombel JF, Twyman K, et al. Autoimmune and chronic inflammatory disease patients with COVID-19. ACR Open Rheumatol. 2021;3:111–5.
21. Hussein HM, Rahal EA. The role of viral infections in the development of autoimmune diseases. Crit Rev Microbiol. 2019;45:394–412.
22. Zhao JM, Zhou GD, Sun YL, Wang SS, Yang JF, Meng EH, et al. Clinical pathology and pathogenesis of severe acute respiratory syndrome. Zhonghua Shi Yan He Lin Chuang Bing Du Xue Za Zhi. 2003;17:217.
23. Li J, Liu HH, Yin XD, Li CC, Wang J. COVID-19 illness and autoimmune diseases: recent insights. Inflamm Res. 2021;28:1–22.
24. Merad M, Martin JC. Pathological inflammation in patients with COVID-19: a key role for monocytes and macrophages. Nat Rev Immunol. 2020;20:355–62.
25. Berardicurti O, Conforti A, Ruscitti P, Cipriani P, Giacomelli R. The wide spectrum of Kawasaki-like disease associated with SARS-CoV-2 infection. Expert Rev Clin Immunol. 2020;16:1205–15.
26. Tay MZ, Poh CM, Rénia L, MacAry PA, Ng LFP. The trinity of COVID-19: immunity, inflammation and intervention. Nat Rev Immunol. 2020;20:363–74.
27. Vlachoyiannopoulos PG, Magira E, Alexopoulos H, Jahaj E, Theophilopoulou K, Kotanidou A. Autoantibodies related to systemic autoimmune rheumatic diseases in severely ill patients with COVID-19. Ann Rheum Dis. 2020;79: 1661–3.
28. Perrot L, Hemon M, Busnel JM, Muis-Pistor O, Picard C, Zandotti C, et al. First flare of ACPA-positive rheumatoid arthritis after SARS-CoV-2 infection. Lancet Rheumatol. 2021;3:e6–8.
29. Chen G, Wu D, Guo W, Cao Y, Huang D, Wang H, et al. Clinical and immunological features of severe and moderate coronavirus disease 2019. J Clin Investig. 2020;130:2620–9.
30. Curtis JR, Xi J, Patkar N, et al. Drug-specific and time-dependent risks of bacterial infection among patients with rheumatoid arthritis who were exposed to tumor necrosis factor alpha antagonists. Arthritis Rheum. 2007; 56:4226–7.
31. Berardicurti O, Ruscitti P, Pavlych V, Conforti A, Giacomelli R, Cipriani P. Glucocorticoids in rheumatoid arthritis: the silent companion in the therapeutic strategy. Expert Rev Clin Pharmacol. 2020;13:593–604.
32. Dixon WG, Abrahamowicz M, Beauchamp ME, Ray DW, Bernatsky S, Suissa S, Sylvestre MP. Immediate and delayed impact of oral glucocorticoid therapy on risk of serious infection in older patients with rheumatoid arthritis: a nested case-control analysis. Ann Rheum Dis. 2012;71:1128–33.
33. Cipriani P, Ruscitti P, Carubbi F, Liakouli V, Giacomelli R. Methotrexate: an old new drug in autoimmune disease. Expert Rev Clin Immunol. 2014;10: 1519–30.
34. Cipriani P, Ruscitti P, Carubbi F, Liakouli V, Giacomelli R. Methotrexate in rheumatoid arthritis: optimizing therapy among different formulations. Current Emerg Paradig Clin Ther. 2014;1(36):427–35.
35. Ibrahim A, Ahmed M, Conway R, Carey JJ. Risk of infection with methotrexate therapy in inflammatory diseases: a systematic review and meta-analysis. J Clin Med. 2018;21(8):15.
36. Godfrey MS, Friedman LN. Tuberculosis and biologic therapies: anti-tumor necrosis factor-α and beyond. Clin Chest Med. 2019;40:721–39.
37. Dobler CC. Biologic agents and tuberculosis. Microbiol Spectr. 2016;4(6):56.
38. Fabroni C, Gori A, Prignano F, Lotti T. A severe complication of anti-TNF alfa treatment. G Ital Dermatol Venereol. 2010;145:775–7.
39. Michel M, Duvoux C, Hezode C, Cherqui D. Fulminant hepatitis after infliximab in a patient with hepatitis B virus treated for an adult onset still's disease. J Rheumatol. 2003;30:1624–5.
40. Narazaki M, Tanaka T, Kishimoto T. The role and therapeutic targeting of IL-6 in rheumatoid arthritis. Expert Rev Clin Immunol. 2017;2017:535–51.
41. Ishihara K, Hirano T. IL-6 in autoimmune disease and chronic inflammatory proliferative disease. Cytokine Growth Factor Rev. 2002;13:357–68.
42. Shoor S. Risk of serious infection associated with agents that target T-cell activation and interleukin-17 and interleukin-23 cytokines. Infect Dis Clin North Am. 2020;34:179–89.
43. Siegel SAR, Winthrop KL. In the real world: infections associated with biologic and small molecule therapies in psoriatic arthritis and psoriasis. Curr Rheumatol Rep. 2019;6(21):36.
44. Wu KK, Lee MP, Lee EB, Wu JJ. Risk of herpes zoster with IL-17 inhibitor therapy for psoriasis and other inflammatory conditions. J Dermatolog Treat. 2020;31:359–65.
45. Nogueira M, Warren RB, Torres T. Risk of tuberculosis reactivation with interleukin (IL)-17 and IL-23 inhibitors in psoriasis—time for a paradigm change. J Eur Acad Dermatol Venereol. 2021;35:824–34.
46. Chen SK, Liao KP, Liu J, Kim SC. Risk of hospitalized infection and initiation of abatacept versus tumor necrosis factor inhibitors among patients with rheumatoid arthritis: a propensity score-matched cohort study. Arthritis Care Res (Hoboken). 2020;72:9–17.
47. Christou EA, Giardino G, Worth A, Ladomenou F. Risk factors predisposing to the development of hypogammaglobulinemia and infections post-Rituximab. Int Rev Immunol. 2012;36(6):352–9.
48. Ghoreschi K, Jesson MI, Li X, Lee JL, Ghosh S, Alsup JW. Modulation of innate and adaptive immune responses by tofacitinib (CP-690,550). J Immunol. 2011;186:4234–43.
49. Favoino E, Prete M, Catacchio G, Ruscitti P, Navarini L, Giacomelli R. Working and safety profiles of JAK/STAT signaling inhibitors. Are these small molecules also smart? Autoimmun Rev. 2021;20:102750.
50. Alves C, Penedones A, Mendes D, Batel-Marques F. Risk of infections and cardiovascular and venous thromboembolic events associated with JAK inhibitors in rheumatoid arthritis: protocols of two systematic reviews and network meta-analyses. BMJ Open. 2020;31(10):e041420.
51. Sunzini F, McInnes I, Siebert S. JAK inhibitors and infections risk: focus on herpes zoster. Ther Adv Musculoskelet Dis. 2020;29(12): 1759720X20936059.
52. Conforti A, Di Cola I, Pavlych V, Ruscitti P, Berardicurti O, Ursini F, et al. Beyond the joints, the extra-articular manifestations in rheumatoid arthritis. Autoimmun Rev. 2021;20:102735.
53. Chimenti MS, Perricone C, Conigliaro P, Triggianese P, D'Antonio A, de Martino E, et al. Tackling the autoimmune side in Spondyloarthritis: a systematic review. Autoimmun Rev. 2020;19:102648.
54. Cipriani P, Berardicurti O, Masedu F, D'Onofrio F, Navarini L, Ruscitti P, et al. Biologic therapies and infections in the daily practice of three Italian rheumatologic units: a prospective, observational study. Clin Rheumatol. 2017;36:251–60.
55. . Bower H, Frisell T, Di Giuseppe D, Delcoigne B, Ahlenius GM, Baecklund E, et al. ARTIS Study Group. Impact of the COVID-19 pandemic on morbidity and mortality in patients with inflammatory joint diseases and in the general population: a nationwide Swedish cohort study. Ann Rheum Dis. 2021:annrheumdis-2021-219845.
56. Emmi G, Bettiol A, Mattioli I, Silvestri E, Di Scala G, Urban ML, et al. SARS-CoV-2 infection among patients with systemic autoimmune diseases. Autoimmun Rev. 2020;19:102575.
57. Hyrich KL, Machado PM. Rheumatic disease and COVID-19: epidemiology and outcomes. Nat Rev Rheumatol. 2021;17:71–2.
58. Ruscitti P, Berardicurti O, Iagnocco A, Giacomelli R. Cytokine storm syndrome in severe COVID-19. Autoimmun Rev. 2020;19:102562.
59. Hasseli R, Mueller-Ladner U, Hoyer BF, Krause A, Lorenz HM, Pfeil A, et al. Older age, comorbidity, glucocorticoid use and disease activity are risk factors for COVID-19 hospitalisation in patients with inflammatory rheumatic and musculoskeletal diseases. RMD Open. 2021;7:e001464.
60. Gianfrancesco M, Hyrich KL, Al-Adely CL, Danila MI, Gossec L, et al. COVID-19 Global Rheumatology Alliance. Characteristics associated with hospitalisation for COVID-19 in people with rheumatic disease: data from the COVID-19 Global Rheumatology Alliance physician-reported registry. Ann Rheum Dis. 2020;79:859–66.
61. FAI2R /SFR/SNFMI/SOFREMIP/CRI/IMIDIATE consortium and contributors. Severity of COVID-19 and survival in patients with rheumatic and

inflammatory diseases: data from the French RMD COVID-19 cohort of 694 patients. Ann Rheum Dis.:annrheumdis-2020-218310.
62. Montero F, Martínez-Barrio J, Serrano-Benavente B, González T, Rivera J, Molina Collada J, et al. Coronavirus disease 2019 (COVID-19) in autoimmune and inflammatory conditions: clinical characteristics of poor outcomes. Rheumatol Int. 2020;40:1593–8.
63. Pablos JL, Galindo M, Carmona L, Lledó A, Retuerto M, Blanco R, et al. RIER Investigators Group; RIER investigators group. Clinical outcomes of hospitalised patients with COVID-19 and chronic inflammatory and autoimmune rheumatic diseases: a multicentric matched cohort study. Ann Rheum Dis. 2020;79:1544–9.
64. Marques CDL, Kakehasi AM, Pinheiro MM, Mota LMH, Albuquerque CP, Silva CR, et al. High levels of immunosuppression are related to unfavorable outcomes in hospitalized patients with rheumatic diseases and COVID-19: first results of ReumaCoV Brasil registry. RMD Open. 2021;7:e001461.
65. Pang R, Zhao J, Gan Z, Hu Z, Xue X, Wu Y, et al. Evolution of COVID-19 in patients with autoimmune rheumatic diseases. Aging (Albany NY). 2020; 3(12):23427–35.
66. Cheng C, Li C, Zhao T, Yue J, Yang F, Yan Y, et al. COVID-19 with rheumatic diseases: a report of 5 cases. Clin Rheumatol. 2020;39:2025–9.
67. Akiyama S, Hamdeh S, Micic D, Sakuraba A. Prevalence and clinical outcomes of COVID-19 in patients with autoimmune diseases: a systematic review and meta-analysis. Ann Rheum Dis. 2020:annrheumdis-2020-218946.
68. Bajaj V, Gadi N, Spihlman AP, Wu SC, Choi CH, Moulton VR. Aging, immunity, and COVID-19: how age influences the host immune response to coronavirus infections? Front Physiol. 2021;12(11):571416.
69. Safdarian AR, Momenzadeh K, Kahe F, Farhangnia P, Rezaei N. Death due to COVID-19 in a patient with diabetes, epilepsy, and gout comorbidities. Clin Case Rep. 2020;25(9):461–4.
70. Shakoory B, Carcillo JA, Chatham WW, Amdur RL, Zhao H, Dinarello CA, et al. Interleukin-1 receptor blockade is associated with reduced mortality in sepsis patients with features of macrophage activation syndrome: reanalysis of a prior phase III trial. Crit Care Med. 2016;44:275–81.
71. Singh S, Facciorusso A, Dulai PS, Jairath V, Sandborn WJ. Comparative risk of serious infections with biologic and/or immunosuppressive therapy in patients with inflammatory bowel diseases: a systematic review and meta-analysis. Clin Gastroenterol Hepatol. 2020;18:69-81.e3.
72. Caso F, Costa L, Nucera V, et al. From autoinflammation to autoimmunity: old and recent findings. Clin Rheumatol. 2018;37:2305–21.
73. Caso F, Costa L, Nucera V, Barilaro G, Masala IF, Talotta R, et al. Monogenic autoinflammatory syndromes: state of the art on genetic, clinical, and therapeutic issues. Int J Rheumatol. 2013;56:513782.
74. Ruscitti P, Berardicurti O, Di Benedetto P, et al. Severe COVID-19, another piece in the puzzle of the hyperferritinemic syndrome. An immunomodulatory perspective to alleviate the storm. Front Immunol. 2020;11:1130.
75. Peter AE, Sandeep BV, Rao BG, Kalpana VL. Calming the storm: natural immunosuppressants as adjuvants to target the cytokine storm in COVID-19. Front Pharmacol. 2021;11:583777.
76. Ruscitti P, Bruno F, Berardicurti O, Acanfora C, Pavlych V, Palumbo P, et al. Lung involvement in macrophage activation syndrome and severe COVID-19: results from a cross-sectional study to assess clinical, laboratory and artificial intelligence-radiological differences. Ann Rheum Dis. 2020;79:1152–5.
77. Bąk E, Młynarska A, Marcisz C, Bobiński R, Sternal D, Młynarski R. Factors that affect the assessment of the quality of life of rheumatoid arthritis patients depending on the prevalence of frailty syndrome. Health Qual Life Outcomes. 2020;6(18):216.
78. Motta F, Sica A, Selmi C. Frailty in rheumatic diseases. Front Immunol. 2020; 11:576134.
79. McGonagle D, O'Donnell JS, Sharif K, Emery P, Bridgewood C. Immune mechanisms of pulmonary intravascular coagulopathy in COVID-19 pneumonia. Lancet Rheumatol. 2020;2:e437–45.
80. Ketfi C, Boutigny A, Mohamedi N, Bouajil S, Magnan B, Amah G, et al. Risk of venous thromboembolism in rheumatoid arthritis. Jt Bone Spine. 2020;17: 105122.
81. Bezuidenhout JA, Venter C, Roberts TJ, Tarr G, Kell DB, Pretorius E. Detection of citrullinated fibrin in plasma clots of rheumatoid arthritis patients and its relation to altered structural clot properties, disease-related inflammation and prothrombotic tendency. Front Immunol. 2020;4(11):577523.
82. Geisen UM, Berner DK, Tran F, Sümbül M, Vullriede L, Ciripoi M, et al. Immunogenicity and safety of anti-SARS-CoV-2 mRNA vaccines in patients with chronic inflammatory conditions and immunosuppressive therapy in a monocentric cohort. Ann Rheum Dis. 2021:annrheumdis-2021-220272.
83. Simon D, Tascilar K, Fagni F, Krönke G, Kleyer A, Meder C, et al. SARS-CoV-2 vaccination responses in untreated, conventionally treated and anticytokine-treated patients with immune-mediated inflammatory diseases. Ann Rheum Dis. 2021; 6:annrheumdis-2021-220461.
84. Haberman RH, Herati R, Simon D, Samanovic M, Blank RB, Tuen M, et al. Methotrexate hampers immunogenicity to BNT162b2 mRNA COVID-19 vaccine in immune-mediated inflammatory disease. Ann Rheum Dis. 2021: annrheumdis-2021-220597.

12

Dentists' knowledge about osteoporosis and their ability to identify the disease

Renato Vicente Ferreira[1], Suely Roizenblatt[2*] and Vera Lucia Szejnfeld[2]

Abstract

Background: Osteoporosis is an underdiagnosed condition, and its seriousness is not considered until severe complications arise. This study aimed to evaluate general dentists' knowledge about osteoporosis and their ability to identify patients with this disease by assessing mandibular cortical width (MCW) and mandibular cortical index (MCI) on panoramic dental radiographs using a visual method.

Methods: In this cross-sectional study, an email questionnaire regarding the diagnosis and prevention of osteoporosis was sent to 20,773 dentists in 2016. Those who completed the questionnaire were invited to participate in radiomorphometric training and then to analyze the MCI and MCW of 114 panoramic radiographs of postmenopausal women who underwent both panoramic radiography and bone densitometry. Based on the radiomorphometric indices and while blinded to the densitometry results, the dentists determined whether they would indicate densitometry for these patients.

Results: The response rate was 2.3%: 485 dentists completed the questionnaire, and 50 evaluated panoramic radiographs using the MCW and MCI. All of them reported some knowledge about osteoporosis, but 41.6% demonstrated a misleading conceptualization of the disease. Approximately 90% reported minimal access to this information during graduation, and only 27.0% were exposed to the topic during their postgraduate studies. Interest in osteoporosis prevention was expressed by 70.7% of the respondents, and interest in learning the radiomorphometric indices was expressed by 99.0%. The sensitivity in the detection of low bone mineral density through the MCW and MCI was 52.9%, and the specificity was 64%.

Conclusions: Brazilian dentists demonstrated insufficient knowledge about osteoporosis and a low ability to detect osteopenia or osteoporosis by applying radiomorphometric indices.

Keywords: Osteoporosis, Radiography, Dental education, Educational methods

Background

Osteoporosis is characterized by microstructural deterioration and loss of bone mass, leading to decreased bone strength and quality and an increased risk of fragility fractures. Osteoporosis is typically an underdiagnosed condition, and the identification of affected individuals before the condition is established and a fracture occurs is a major challenge.

* Correspondence: suely.roizenblatt@unifesp.br
[2]Department of Internal Medicine, Universidade Federal de Sao Paulo (UNIFESP), Rua Angelina Maffei Vita 670, Sao Paulo, SP CEP:01455070, Brazil

Dual-energy X-ray absorptiometry (DXA) scans are currently considered the standard diagnostic approach for osteoporosis, and peripheral imaging techniques, such as peripheral quantitative tomography, peripheral DXA, quantitative ultrasound methods, and peripheral magnetic resonance imaging, have been used as screening tests to identify individuals who are most likely to benefit from further bone density testing. In this context, an increasing number of studies have proposed the use of quantitative/qualitative indices on dental panoramic radiographs to identify low bone mass [1, 2]. Assessment of the trabecular pattern of the mandible using panoramic radiographs has been considered a valid tool for identifying individuals with osteoporosis, as a substantial number of patients are subjected to dental radiographs each year for diagnostic and treatment purposes [3]. Therefore, it would be of great clinical benefit if dentists could identify patients at a high risk for osteoporosis using these radiographs. In the academic environment, radiomorphometric indices applied to panoramic radiographs have been used to estimate osteopenia and osteoporosis based on established cutoff values [4].

As shown in the large European multicenter study OSTEODENT [5, 6], much interest was expressed on the cortical bone layer at the lower border of the mandible. In this study involving five European centers between 2003 and 2005, mandibular cortical width (MCW) was considered an alternative method for assessing bone changes related to osteoporosis in panoramic X-rays of patients who had undergone radiographic evaluation for the usual dental reasons, not as a formal risk assessment tool [5, 6].

Strategies have been implemented to encourage dentists' involvement in general health promotion activities, particularly for diabetes and cardiovascular diseases [7, 8]. Regarding osteoporosis, few studies have addressed dentists' knowledge, and most of these studies are related to mandibular osteonecrosis and its association with bisphosphonates [9, 10].

In this study, we aimed to investigate dentists' knowledge about the prevention and diagnosis of osteoporosis and to verify their ability to detect this disease by applying a simple visual method for evaluating radiomorphometric cortical indices on panoramic dental radiographs.

Methods

Participants

This cross-sectional study included general dentists with ≥2 years of registration at the Regional Dentistry Council of the State of São Paulo (CROSP). After approval by its internal scientific council, CROSP released an e-mail message to 20,733 actively practicing dentists requesting information about their general profile (age, gender, years since graduation), excluding those specialized in dental radiography. The participants were then directed to a structured questionnaire regarding osteoporosis.

The dentists who answered the questionnaire were invited to evaluate the panoramic dental radiographs of 114 postmenopausal female patients, consecutively selected from the Osteoporosis Ambulatory of the Outpatient Clinic for Osteometabolic Diseases in the Rheumatology Division of Federal University of São Paulo (UNIFESP) between January 2016 and January 2017. These women (age range 50–78 years) were concomitantly imaged with panoramic radiographs and DXA of the spine and femur. There were 38 women in each of the following conditions: normal DXA, osteopenia and osteoporosis.

The study was approved by the Ethics Committee of UNIFESP - CEP # 2.193.407. After providing written informed consent, patients underwent mandibular panoramic radiography and DXA of the spine and femur. Electronic signed consent was obtained from the dentists who agreed to participate in this research.

Questionnaire

To evaluate the knowledge about osteoporosis, we used a structured questionnaire [11] previously applied to Brazilian physicians [12]. From a total of 27 questions, 14 items related to medical specialties, such as treatment, were removed, and five other items were added: three about previous osteoporosis knowledge selected from the BRAZOS questionnaire [13] and two regarding the methods used to evaluate osteoporosis on panoramic dental radiographs. Thus, the final questionnaire had a total of 18 questions.

Distribution and collection of the questionnaire

For the approach through e-mail, CROSP requested voluntary participation by dentists through a message that included a link to the online Survio™ survey platform (SurveyGizmo, Boulder, CO). The participant was then directed to an online interface displaying the research questionnaire. The e-mail message was sent only once to each CROSP member, and the platform remained open for 6 months. The interested members could access the platform only once during this period. No advantages or remuneration was offered to the participants.

Acquisition and evaluation of panoramic radiographs

The panoramic radiographs were obtained with an Eagle 2D panoramic OP 3000 2D (Dabi Atlante, Ribeirão Preto, Brazil) by the same experienced operator, with the patient in a standardized position predefined by the equipment.

The modified visual method for evaluating cortical indices, such as the MCW and the mandibular cortical index (MCI), was used in this research [14] by 50 dentists who agreed to be trained on both indices through e-learning classes using Klickmembers™ (Klickpages information technology and services, DF, Brazil). This platform includes video classes and secure-access exercises. For training purposes, restrictive access for each dentist was provided by means of an individual password for a period of 7 to 10 days. After completing all classes and clarifying any lingering doubts, those 50 dentists were invited to assess the panoramic radiographs in this study and to answer the following question: "Would you recommend DXA to this patient?" The possible answers were "yes", "no", and "I do not know".

In a small room provided with individual X-ray illuminators, there was a box containing the panoramic radiographs of the 114 postmenopausal women. The dentists were asked to randomly select 10 radiographs per turn for visual evaluation of the MCW and MCI while blinded to the DXA results, and then to return the radiographs to the box. Finally, we obtained 1170 views, with an average of 26 views per dentist.

Statistical analysis

The results are expressed as frequencies and percentages. Correlations between radiomorphometric indices and bone density were analyzed using the Spearman correlation coefficient test. The kappa coefficient was used to assess the agreement between the dentists' opinions based on the panoramic radiographs and the DXA results. We used SPSS software version 22.0 (Chicago, IL, USA), and the significance level was 5%.

Results

The response rate of the 20,733 contacted dentists was 2.3%: 485 of them answered the questionnaire, and 50 agreed to evaluate the 114 panoramic dental examinations of postmenopausal female patients. Figure 1 shows a flow chart detailing the response outcomes for the delivered questionnaires. Among the 20,733 dentists invited, 15,840 were nonresponders, 4893 (23.9%) opened their e-mails, 902 (4.3%) accessed the platform, and only 485 (2.3%) answered the full questionnaire.

The demographic characteristics of the dentists are shown in Table 1. The majority of the responders (82.1%) had > 15 years of dentistry practice experience. The frequencies of the responses to osteoporosis questions by the general dentists are presented in Table 2. Although 41.6% of the dentists had a misleading concept of osteoporosis, most of them knew that bone densitometry was used to diagnose osteoporosis and identified the commonly affected age groups. In addition, 58.6% were not aware of which dentistry methods were available for the diagnosis of osteoporosis. Nevertheless, 99% demonstrated interest in learning these techniques. The dentists' responses to information about osteoporosis obtained during graduation and postgraduate courses are presented in Table 3. Most dentists had little or no exposure to this topic, but 58.8% of them rated the access to information about osteoporosis as "easy".

The 50 previously trained dentists randomly and blindly analyzed these radiographs, completing 1170 views. The correlation of bone mineral density status and the radiomorphometric indices was 0.326 for MCI and 0.283 for MCW ($p < 0.01$). The agreement between the dentists' opinions and the densitometry results is presented in Table 4. The dentists' evaluations had a sensitivity of 52.9% and a specificity of 64.0%.

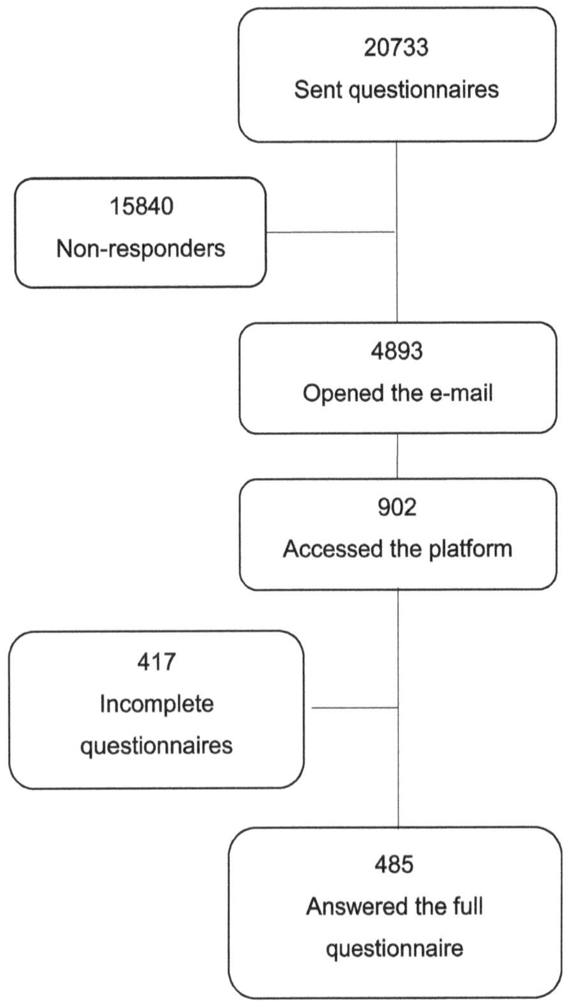

Fig. 1 Response outcomes to the mailed questionnaire

Discussion

This study showed a low return rate for the questionnaire and, among the responders, superficial knowledge about osteoporosis and a low ability to evaluate cortical indices on panoramic dental radiographs.

Only 4.0% of the 20,733 dentists accessed the platform, and 2.3% completed the questionnaire. This low return

Table 1 Demographic characteristics of the dentists

	Number	%
Gender		
Male	201	41.1%
Female	284	58.6%
Years since graduation		
0–5	17	3.5%
5–10	24	4.9%
10–15	46	9.5%
> 15	398	82.1%

Table 2 frequencies of response to osteoporosis questions by general dentists

Question	Answer	Frequency
Have you heard about osteoporosis?	Yes	485 (100%)
	No	0 (0.0%)
Which of these phrases best define osteoporosis?	Stronger bones, rich in calcium	0 (0%)
	Fragile bones that break easily	283 (58.4%)
	Lack of calcium in the bones	202 (41.6%)
From the tests below, which is the main one to diagnose osteoporosis?	Outpatient visit	3 (0.6%)
	X-ray	3 (0.6%)
	Computed tomography	3 (0.6%)
	Urine analysis	0 (0.0%)
	Blood test	8 (1.6%)
	Bone densitometry	466 (96.1%)
	Magnetic resonance imaging	2 (0.4%)
Which are the appropriate age group(s) to start screening for osteoporosis?	Childhood (0–8 years)	0 (0%)
	Preteen (8–12 years)	1 (0.2%)
	Teen (12–19 years)	0 (0.0%)
	Early adulthood (19–40 years)	1 (0.2%)
	Mid-life (40–66 years)	230 (47.4%)
	Elderly (> 66 years)	253 (52.2%)
Do you know any method in dentistry that can indicate the presence of osteoporosis in the patient?	Yes	201 (41.4%)
	No	284 (58.6%)
Would you like to know a method to identify osteoporosis using panoramic maxilla and mandible X-rays?	Yes	480 (99.0%)
	No	5 (1.0%)
Are you interested in advising your patients on this disease preventively?	Yes	480 (99.0%)
	No	5 (1.0%)

rate is in accordance with a previous *survey* carried out by our group [12], in which we administered a similar questionnaire to 11,000 Brazilian general practitioners (GPs) and achieved a response rate of 3%. International surveys have achieved higher return rates than these Brazilian surveys. In a study involving GPs from the United Kingdom, 1153 out of the 2515 sent questionnaires were answered, resulting in a response rate of 46% [11]. A Canadian survey achieved a response rate of 30% by using an online questionnaire focused on a dentistry theme of interest: osteonecrosis of the jaw [15].

A systematic review compared the performance on electronic questionnaires and face-to-face interviews among health professionals and demonstrated a variable response rate, with better results for the presential ones. The return rates of the questionnaires sent via e-mail were between 0.3 and 70% [16]. There was no difference in the quality of the results obtained by electronic survey with those obtained with other methods. In contrast, another systematic review reported that surveys with electronic questionnaires had a lower return rate than those conducted by other routes [17] and that there is great variation between the methods used for online and in-person surveys, impeding a clear idea about this topic. The authors suggested that monetary incentives did not influence the return rate of the questionnaires. Therefore, the low return rate of our questionnaire cannot be attributed to its straightforward design that lacked any incentives or rewards. We assume, unfortunately, that there is a lack of interest among our dentists in osteoporosis and its consequences, as we previously observed in the study with Brazilian GPs, who also demonstrated low interest in this subject [12].

Surveys on topics closer to dentistry clinical practice typically have a higher return rate than those regarding osteoporosis. Research involving dental trauma achieved a return rate of 9.6% [18], while that involving pins in endodontically treated teeth achieved a return rate of 68% [19], and that involving toward composite resins achieved a return rate of 68% [20].

The responses obtained in our study indicate that dentists, even with many years of dentistry practice experience (> 15 years), have superficial knowledge about osteoporosis, with 41.6% considering that the best phrase to define osteoporosis was a "lack of calcium in bones". This is a popular but incorrect concept since in

Table 3 Frequencies of responses to questions about exposure to information on osteoporosis

Question	Answer	Number (%)
How would you rate your knowledge about osteoporosis acquired in *dentistry* school?	None	238 (49.1%)
	Minimal	204 (42.1%)
	Excessive	0 (0.0%)
	Sufficient	43 (8.9%)
How would you rate your knowledge about osteoporosis acquired during postgraduate training?	None	167 (58.4%)
	Minimal	188 (38.8%)
	Excessive	12 (2.5%)
	Sufficient	118 (24.3%)
How would you rate the access to information about osteoporosis?	Very difficult	9 (1.9%)
	Difficult	144 (29.7%)
	Very easy	47 (9.7%)
	Easy	285 (58.8%)
What type of information regarding osteoporosis are you interested in?	Prevention	343 (70.7%)
	Treatment	64 (13.2%)
	Services	18 (3.7%)
	Research	60 (12.4%)

osteoporosis, there is microstructural deterioration and loss of bone mass. Exposure to the topic in the graduate coursework was practically nil. When asked about the possibility of using tools for diagnosing osteoporosis on panoramic radiographs, most (99.0%) were interested; however, 58.6% had no knowledge about these techniques. Although it is very important to target middle-aged and postmenopausal women for osteoporosis screening and prevention programs, 52.2% of dentists considered the elderly age group to be most appropriate to screen for osteoporosis.

There are few studies in the literature on the specific knowledge of dentists about osteoporosis. A recent qualitative study based on focus group discussions analyzed the knowledge and attitudes of 17 Swedish dentists toward patients with osteoporosis [21]. Dentists from both public and private practice expressed insufficient knowledge of what osteoporosis is, how it is diagnosed and treated, and its consequences. Knowledge on the topic was lacking and almost entirely limited to academia. Interestingly, dentists were more familiar with osteoporosis studies involving osteonecrosis of the jaw, periodontitis, and absence of teeth than with those involving osteoporosis itself [15].

Table 4 Agreement between the dentist's opinion and the DXA results regarding osteoporosis

DXA	Dentist's opinion			Total
	Yes	No	Do not know	
Yes	421	299	75	795
No	100	240	35	375
Total	521	539	110	1170

Kappa (S.E.) = 0.209 (0.023), $p < 0{,}001$
Agreement (%): for "Yes" = 52.9% (sensitivity) and for "No" = 64.0% (specificity)
DXA dual-energy X-ray absorptiometry

There is a tendency to encourage dentists to refer patients for DXA based on the changes noted in panoramic radiographs [22]. The OSTEODENT multicenter study aimed to identify the most valid and effective radiographic index or the combination of radiography and the Osteoporosis Index of Risk (OSIRIS) applicable for dentists to diagnose osteoporosis. Although the MCW demonstrated better efficacy than the MCI in the detection of osteoporosis, the OSIRIS showed higher diagnostic validity than radiographic measurements [6]. This indicates that measurement of the MCW should be viewed as an alternative possibility for risk assessment among patients who have undergone radiography for usual dental reasons [6]. The same group from Manchester reported a good correlation between the radiomorphometric indices MCW and MCI obtained manually on panoramic radiographs by well-trained observers and computerized measurements [5].

A systematic review and meta-analysis [23] noted that manual measurement of the MCW could introduce operator-related bias. Nevertheless, the costs and complexity of semi or totally computer-driven techniques of panoramic radiograph analysis are little applicable to general dental practice and to the reality of many dental care scenarios. In addition, computer software that automatically detects the mandibular cortex on panoramic radiographs and then measures its width requires fully trained evaluators and high-precision electronic instruments [5], but this level of training and digital instruments are not part of routine dental practice. Artificial intelligence might be a new perspective in the diagnosis of osteoporosis, making this easier and perhaps affordable in the future [24, 25].

Currently, there is a tendency to apply simplified visual methods for MCI and MCW analysis to identify patients with osteoporosis [4, 14]. In our study, 50 general dentists measured the MCW and MCI indices on a negatoscope by using the simplified method [14], mimicking usual clinical practice. Under these conditions, we obtained a sensitivity of 52.9% and a specificity of 64.0% between the dentists' opinions and the DXA results regarding osteoporosis. Depending on the author, the sensitivity of a dentist's evaluation of osteoporosis varies between 67 and 87%, and the specificity varies between 70 and 86% [23]. Compared with our results, the higher agreement obtained in studies conducted in the academic environment shows that, aside from being simple, the radiomorphometric analysis on panoramic radiographs requires a certain degree of expertise and experience to obtain consistency in the results. These competences cannot be acquired by a general dentist when evaluating routine panoramic radiographs after an online training course. Considering that dentists have an opportunity to make unique contributions by early identifying osteoporotic patients based on their oral and dental health problems, such as reduced jawbone density, destruction of periodontal tissue, tooth loss, and temporomandibular disorders, their acquisition of fundamental skills in osteoporosis assessment during their regular course of study is imperative. The same lack of familiarity with osteoporosis has also been observed among GPs in previous studies, and the results provide important information to guide new actions targeted to these physicians [11, 12].

The present study has some limitations. First, the majority of the panoramic radiographs belonged to patients being treated with bisphosphonates, which can result in changes to the mandibular cortical structure, thereby introducing bias [26, 27]. Second, the performance of the dentists might have be influenced by the effectiveness of the training method; and third, the radiographs were obtained by the same operator, which does not reflect daily practice. This research intended to motivate dentists to refer patients to medical evaluation and not to make the diagnosis of osteoporosis and is in line with the necessity to increase the interest of these professionals in health-related topics not restricted to dental specialties.

Conclusions

We observed that dentists in São Paulo city have insufficient knowledge about osteoporosis and that their performance in detecting patients with osteopenia and osteoporosis by using a simple visual method to evaluate the MCW and MCI on panoramic radiographs was lower than that described in the literature. As these indices are correlated with bone mineral density and can represent an appropriate instrument for decision making, greater educational efforts must be made to promote knowledge about osteoporosis among dentists. This perspective may motivate dentists to actively participate in the fight against and prevention of this silent and devastating disease.

Abbreviations

MCW: Mandibular cortical width; MCI: Mandibular cortical index; DXA: Dual-energy X-ray scans; GP: General practitioners; OSIRIS: Osteoporosis Index of Risk

Acknowledgments

We would like to express our gratitude to the dentists who participated in this study.

Authors' contributions

RVF contributed to conception, design, data analysis, and interpretation, drafted and critically revised the manuscript. SR contributed to conception, design, data acquisition, analysis, and interpretation, drafted and critically revised the manuscript; VLS contributed to conception and data acquisition, critically revised the manuscript. All authors gave final approval and agreed to be accountable for all aspects of the work.

Author details

[1]Rheumatology Division, Universidade Federal de Sao Paulo (UNIFESP), Sao Paulo, Brazil. [2]Department of Internal Medicine, Universidade Federal de Sao Paulo (UNIFESP), Rua Angelina Maffei Vita 670, Sao Paulo, SP CEP:01455070, Brazil.

References

1. Kanis JA, Glüer CC. An update on the diagnosis and assessment of osteoporosis with densitometry. Committee of Scientific Advisors, international Osteoporosis Foundation. Osteoporos Int. 2000;11(3):192–202. https://doi.org/10.1007/s001980050281.
2. López-López J, Estrugo-Devesa A, Jane-Salas E, et al. Early diagnosis of osteoporosis by means of orthopantomograms and oral X-rays: a systematic review. Med Oral Patol Oral Cir Bucal. 2011;16:e905–13. https://doi.org/10.4317/medoral.17304.
3. Tugnait A, Clerehugh V, Hirschmann PN. Radiographic equipment and techniques used in general dental practice: a survey of general dental practitioners in England and Wales. J Dent. 2003;31(3):197–203. https://doi.org/10.1016/S0300-5712(03)00013-7.
4. Lee K, Taguchi A, Ishii K, Suei Y, Fujita M, Nakamoto T, et al. Visual assessment of the mandibular cortex on panoramic radiographs to identify postmenopausal women with low bone mineral densities. Oral Surg Oral Med Oral Pathol Oral Radiol Endod. 2005;100(2):226–31. https://doi.org/10.1016/j.tripleo.2004.11.052.
5. Devlin H, Allen PD, Graham J, Jacobs R, Karayianni K, Lindh C, et al. Automated osteoporosis risk assessment by dentists: a new pathway to diagnosis. Bone. 2007;40(4):835–42. https://doi.org/10.1016/j.bone.2006.10.024.
6. Karayianni K, Horner K, Mitsea A, Berkas L, Mastoris M, Jacobs R, et al. Accuracy in osteoporosis diagnosis of a combination of mandibular cortical width measurement on dental panoramic radiographs and a clinical risk index (OSIRIS): the OSTEODENT project. Bone. 2007;40(1):223–9. https://doi.org/10.1016/j.bone.2006.07.025.
7. Liccardo D, Cannavo A, Spagnuolo G, Ferrara N, Cittadini A, Rengo C, et al. Periodontal disease: a risk factor for diabetes and cardiovascular disease. Int J Mol Sci. 2019;20(6):1414. https://doi.org/10.3390/ijms20061414

8. Voinescu I, Petre A, Burlibasa M, et al. Evidence of Connections Between Periodontitis and Ischemic Cardiac Disease - an Updated Systematic Review. Maedica (Buchar). 2019;14:384–90.
9. Khan AA, Morrison A, Hanley DA, Felsenberg D, McCauley LK, O'Ryan F, et al. Diagnosis and management of osteonecrosis of the jaw: a systematic review and international consensus. J Bone Miner Res. 2015;30(1):3–23. https://doi.org/10.1002/jbmr.2405.
10. Wan JT, Sheeley DM, Somerman MJ, Lee JS. Mitigating osteonecrosis of the jaw (ONJ) through preventive dental care and understanding of risk factors. Bone Res. 2020;8(1):14. https://doi.org/10.1038/s41413-020-0088-1.
11. Taylor JC, Sterkel B, Utley M, Shipley M, Newman S, Horton M, et al. Opinions and experiences in general practice on osteoporosis prevention, diagnosis and management. Osteoporos Int. 2001;12(10):844–8. https://doi.org/10.1007/s001980170035.
12. Szejnfeld VL, Jennings F, Castro CHM, et al. Conhecimento dos médicos clínicos do Brasil sobre as estratégias de prevenção e tratamento da osteoporose. Rev Bras Reumatol. 2007;47:251–7. https://doi.org/10.1590/S0482-50042007000400003 Available from: http://www.scielo.br/scielo.php?script=sci_arttext&pid=S0482-50042007000400003&lng=en&nrm=iso. ISSN 1809-4570. [cited 15 Oct 2020].
13. Pinheiro MM, Ciconelli RM, Jacques NO, et al. The burden of osteoporosis in Brazil: regional data from fractures in adult men and women - The Brazilian Osteoporosis Study (BRAZOS). Rev Bras Reumatol. 2010;50:113–20. https://doi.org/10.1590/S0482-50042010000200002 Available from: http://www.scielo.br/scielo.php?script=sci_arttext&pid=S0482-50042010000200002&lng=en&nrm=iso. ISSN 0482-5004. [cited 15 Oct 2020].
14. Leite AF, Figueiredo PTS, Guia CM, et al. Radiografia panorâmica: instrumento auxiliar no diagnóstico da osteoporose. Rev Bras Reumatol. 2008;48:226–33. https://doi.org/10.1590/S0482-50042008000400006 Available from: http://www.scielo.br/scielo.php?script=sci_arttext&pid=S0482-50042008000400006&lng=en&nrm=iso. ISSN 1809-4570. [cited 15 Oct 2020].
15. Alhussain A, Peel S, Dempster L, Clokie C, Azarpazhooh A. Knowledge, practices, and opinions of Ontario dentists when treating patients receiving bisphosphonates. J Oral Maxillofac Surg. 2015;73(6):1095–105. https://doi.org/10.1016/j.joms.2014.12.040.
16. Marcano Belisario JS, Jamsek J, Huckvale K, O'Donoghue J, Morrison CP, Car J, et al. Comparison of self-administered survey questionnaire responses collected using mobile apps versus other methods. Cochrane Database Syst Rev. 2015;7:MR000042. https://doi.org/10.1002/14651858.MR000042.pub2.
17. Blumenberg C, Barros AJD. Response rate differences between web and alternative data collection methods for public health research: a systematic review of the literature. Int J Public Health. 2018;63(6):765–73. https://doi.org/10.1007/s00038-018-1108-4.
18. Hartmann RC, Rossetti BR, Siqueira Pinheiro L, Poli de Figueiredo JA, Rossi-Fedele G, S. Gomes M, et al. Dentists' knowledge of dental trauma based on the International Association of Dental Traumatology guidelines: a survey in South Brazil. Dent Traumatol. 2019;35(1):27–32. https://doi.org/10.1111/edt.12450.
19. Sarkis-Onofre R, Pereira-Cenci T, Opdam NJ, Demarco FF. Preference for using posts to restore endodontically treated teeth: findings from a survey with dentists. Braz Oral Res. 2015;29:1–6. https://doi.org/10.1590/1807-3107bor-2015.vol29.0001.
20. Demarco FF, Baldissera RA, Madruga FC, et al. Anterior composite restorations in clinical practice: findings from a survey with general dental practitioners. J Appl Oral Sci. 2013;21(6):497–504. https://doi.org/10.1590/1679-775720130013.
21. Gullberg J, Lindh C, Axtelius B, Horner K, Devlin H, Povlsen L. Osteoporosis risk assessment in primary dental care - the attitudes of Swedish dentists, patients and medical specialists. Gerodontology. 2020;37(2):208–16. https://doi.org/10.1111/ger.12462.
22. Taguchi A, Tsuda M, Ohtsuka, et al. Use of dental panoramic radiographs in identifying younger postmenopausal women with osteoporosis. Osteoporos Int. 2006;17(3):387–94. https://doi.org/10.1007/s00198-005-2029-7.
23. Calciolari E, Donos N, Park JC, Petrie A, Mardas N. Panoramic measures for oral bone mass in detecting osteoporosis: a systematic review and meta-analysis. J Dent Res. 2015;94(3 Suppl):17S–27S. https://doi.org/10.1177/0022034514554949.
24. Aliaga I, Vera V, Vera M, García E, Pedrera M, Pajares G. Automatic computation of mandibular indices in dental panoramic radiographs for early osteoporosis detection. Artif Intell Med. 2020;103:101816. https://doi.org/10.1016/j.artmed.2020.101816
25. Tanaka R, Tanaka T, Yeung AWK, Taguchi A, Katsumata A, Bornstein MM. Mandibular radiomorphometric indices and tooth loss as predictors for the risk of osteoporosis using panoramic radiographs. Oral Health Prev Dent. 2020;18(1):773–82. https://doi.org/10.3290/j.ohpd.a45081.
26. Krimmel M, Ripperger J, Hairass M, Hoefert S, Kluba S, Reinert S. Does dental and oral health influence the development and course of bisphosphonate-related osteonecrosis of the jaws (BRONJ)? Oral Maxillofac Surg. 2014;18(2):213–8. https://doi.org/10.1007/s10006-013-0408-3.
27. Oyhanart SR, Escudero ND, Mandalunis PM. Effect of alendronate on the mandible and long bones: an experimental study in vivo. Pediatr Res. 2015;78(6):618–25. https://doi.org/10.1038/pr.2015.163.

13

Prevalence, demographics and clinical characteristics of Latin American patients with spondyloarthritis

Gustavo Citera[1*], Wilson Bautista-Molano[2], Ingris Peláez-Ballestas[3], Valderilio F. Azevedo[4], Risto A. Perich[5], José A. Méndez-Rodríguez[6], Mariel S. Cutri[7] and Cecilia E. Borlenghi[7]

Abstract

Large epidemiologic and clinical estimates of spondyloarthritis (SpA) in Latin America are not available. In this narrative review, our goal was to descriptively summarize the prevalence and features of SpA in Latin America, based on available small studies. A review of peer-reviewed literature identified 41 relevant publications. Of these, 11 (mostly based on Mexican data) estimated the prevalence of SpA and its subtypes, which varied from 0.28 to 0.9% (SpA), 0.02 to 0.8% (ankylosing spondylitis), 0.2 to 0.9% (axial SpA), and 0.004 to 0.08% (psoriatic arthritis). Demographic and/or clinical characteristics were reported in 31 of the 41 publications, deriving data from 3 multinational studies, as well as individual studies from Argentina, Brazil, Chile, Colombia, Costa Rica, Mexico, Peru, Uruguay, and Venezuela. Data relating to treatment, disease manifestations (articular and extra-articular), and comorbidities were summarized across the countries. Available data suggest that there is a variability in prevalence, manifestations, and comorbidities of SpA across Latin America. Basic epidemiologic and clinical data are required from several countries not currently represented. Data relating to current treatment approaches, patient outcomes, and socioeconomic impact within this large geographic region are also needed.

Keywords: Prevalence, Spondyloarthropathy, Ankylosing spondylitis, Psoriatic arthritis, Latin America

Introduction

Spondyloarthritis (SpA) comprises a group of inflammatory diseases of the sacroiliac and spinal joints. The Assessment in Spondyloarthritis International Society (ASAS) classification criteria [1] defines the clinical manifestations of SpA as axial, peripheral, and extra-articular. The group of interrelated diseases considered subtypes of SpA include ankylosing spondylitis (AS), psoriatic arthritis (PsA), reactive arthritis (ReA), inflammatory bowel disease (IBD)-related SpA (IBD-SpA), and undifferentiated SpA (uSpA) [1, 2]. Juvenile-onset SpA (JSpA) also falls under the same umbrella categorization [1], but as JSpA has its own distinct set of challenges [3], it is out of the scope of this review. These diseases are all associated with the presence of the HLA-B27 antigen and share a number of features, including inflammatory back pain, peripheral arthritis, enthesitis, and dactylitis. Other shared features include uveitis, psoriasis, and IBD [4].

In 2016, the regional pooled prevalence of SpA around the world was estimated to range from 0.20% (95% confidence interval [CI]: 0.00–0.66) in South-East Asia to 1.61% (95% CI: 1.27–2.00) in the Northern Arctic communities [2]. In South/Latin America, the prevalence of SpA was estimated at 0.52% (95% CI: 0.10–1.25), which was similar to Europe (0.54%; 95% CI: 0.36–0.78) [2]. However, the estimates for South/Latin America were based on a limited number of available data for SpA, AS, and PsA (2, 4, and 4 studies, respectively) [2]. Several of

* Correspondence: gustavocitera@gmail.com
[1]Instituto de Rehabilitación Psicofísica, Echeverría 955, Buenos Aires, Argentina

those studies were based on data from the 2 large Latin American SpA registries: Registro Ibero-Americano de Espondiloartritis (RESPONDIA, The Ibero-American Registry of Spondyloarthritis) and Registro Brasileiro de Espondiloartrites (RBE, Brazilian Registry of Spondyloarthritis). RESPONDIA represents the largest series of patients with SpA in the Americas (> 100 university centers from 8 Latin American countries [Argentina, Brazil, Chile, Costa Rica, Ecuador, Mexico, Peru, Uruguay, and Venezuela], plus Portugal and Spain), and the RBE covers the 5 Brazilian geographic macro-regions [5].

The objective of this narrative review is to summarize the available SpA prevalence data from Latin America. Specifically, we aimed to assess the demographic and clinical characteristics of Latin American patients with SpA, and to identify major gaps in the literature that could be the subject of further investigation.

Methods

A search of the literature from 2008 onwards was conducted on June 6, 2019. PubMed, the ACR and EULAR abstract archives, and the online PANLAR abstracts (from the 2018 and 2016 meetings), were searched using pre-defined search terms. PubMed searches used the thread: *(spondyloarthritis OR spondyloarthropath* OR ankylosing spondylitis OR psoriatic arthritis) AND (latin america* OR argentin* OR bolivia* OR brazil* OR chile* OR colombia* OR costa rica* OR cuba* OR dominica* OR dominican republic OR ecuador* OR guatemala* OR hondura* OR mexic* OR nicaragua* OR panama* OR peru* OR urugua* OR venezuela*) AND (population OR prevalen* OR epidemiolog* OR inciden*)*. This search was repeated using the Latin American and Caribbean Health Sciences Literature (LILACS) platform. Online abstract archives and published abstracts were searched using the terms "population", "prevalen*" "epidemiolog*" and "inciden*" and any abstract titles containing these terms were hand-searched for relevant data (disease and geographical location).

Publications were excluded for the following reasons: 1) no data on either prevalence of SpA in Latin America, or patient demographics, or only provided for sub-populations (e.g., male vs. female); 2) not including patients with non-radiographic axSpA (nr-axSpA), AS, or PsA; 3) unidentified patient nationality (author affiliation was not taken as indicative of patient nationality); 4) SpA was not primary diagnosis, or was reported in combination with other inflammatory conditions (e.g., rheumatoid arthritis); 5) focused exclusively on JSpA; 6) combined patients from Latin America with non-Latin American countries as a single group; or 7) review of previously published data. Congress abstracts that were superseded by a journal article were excluded in favor of the article. No language restrictions were imposed.

Selected publications were manually searched for data regarding prevalence and incidence of SpA, patient demographics and clinical characteristics, HLA-B27, disease manifestations, comorbidities, patient quality of life and impact of illness on work, and treatments and medication used. Data were summarized and presented descriptively; no quantitative data analysis was performed.

Results

Studies included in the analysis

A total of 228 full-length publications and 5 congress abstracts were identified using the search criteria above. Following manual review, 41 publications were selected for inclusion. Eleven publications estimated the prevalence of SpA in Latin American countries (Table 1) [6–16]. Thirty-one publications reported demographic or clinical characteristics (Tables 2 and 3) [12, 17–46].

Prevalence of SpA

Latin American prevalence estimates were summarized from epidemiology studies conducted in Mexico [9–15], Colombia [6, 7], Cuba [8], and Venezuela [16], and ranged from 0.28 to 0.9% (SpA), 0.02 to 0.8% (AS), 0.2 to 0.9% (axSpA), and 0.004 to 0.08% (PsA) (Table 1).

Demographics and clinical characteristics

Publications from Latin American countries with demographic and clinical characteristics fitting the search criteria included Argentina, Brazil, Chile, Colombia, Costa Rica, Mexico, Peru, Uruguay, and Venezuela; the majority were from Argentina and Brazil. There were also 3 multinational studies reporting data from multiple Latin American countries. Of these 31 studies, only 6 encompassed > 1000 patients: 5 were conducted in Brazil [26–30] and the other was a multinational study comparing Latin American patients with those from Europe [45].

In 23 of the studies, the majority (> 50%) of patients were men (Table 2). Mean or median patient age was < 50 years, except in 1 study conducted in Brazil [33], in which the mean patient age was 56 years. In 9 of the 14 studies that recorded race, more than half of the patients (57.7–96%) with SpA were white. At least 1 study from each country reported the proportion of patients with a family history of SpA (Table 2).

Most studies enrolled patients with various SpA subtypes. One study from Argentina [17] enrolled patients with AS only. Three studies from Argentina [20, 21, 24] and 1 from Brazil [33] enrolled only patients with PsA (Table 2). Of the studies that enrolled patients with multiple SpA subtypes, AS was the most common subtype in most of the studies. Mean age at disease onset ranged from 28 to 40 years (Table 2), which suggests that some studies included patients with JSpA [18 19 26 27 29

Table 1 Prevalence of SpA in Latin American countries

Country	Study	Setting/Population	*N*	Diagnosis	Diagnostic criteria	*n*	Prevalence (%)	95% CI
Colombia	Londoño et al., 2018 [6]	6 Colombian cities	6693	uSpA	ESSG	n/r	0.28	0.13–0.61
				AS	n/r	n/r	0.11	0.03–0.36
	Fernández-Ávila et al., 2018 (CA) [7]	Colombia	n/r	AS	n/r	84, 356	0.18	n/r
				PsA	n/r	1670	0.004	n/r
Cuba	Reyes-Llerena et al., 2009 [8]	Havana	3155	AS	n/r	6	0.1	0.07–0.4
		Male	1238	AS	n/r	4	0.3	n/r
		Female	1917	AS	n/r	2	0.1	n/r
Mexico	Peláez-Ballestas et al., 2011 [9]	5 Mexican regions	19, 213	AS	mNYC	n/r	0.1	0.1–0.2
		Mexico City	4059	AS	mNYC	n/r	0.09	0.02–0.2
		Nuevo León	4712	AS	mNYC	n/r	0.04	0.05–0.10
		Yucatán	3195	AS	mNYC	n/r	0.04	0.05–0.10
		Sinaloa	4879	AS	mNYC	n/r	0.2	0.1–0.40
		Chihuahua	1647	AS	mNYC	n/r	0.6	0.2–1.1
		Adjusted point prevalence, total	19, 213	AS	mNYC	n/r	0.15	0.09–0.20
		Male	7611	AS	mNYC	n/r	0.18	0.09–0.28
		Female	11, 602	AS	mNYC	n/r	0.11	0.05–0.17
	Rodriguez-Amado et al., 2011 [10]	Nuevo León	4713	PsA	n/r	4	0.08	0.02–0.2
				AS	mNYC	2	0.04	0.05–0.1
	Alvarez-Nemegyei et al., 2011 [11]	Yucatán	3195	AS	mNYC	1	0.02	–
				PsA	Surveying physician	1	0.02	–
	Peláez-Ballestas et al., 2013 [12]	Mexico City	4059	SpA	ESSG	28	0.6	0.4–0.9
				AS	mNYC	4	0.09	0.02–0.2
	Del Río Nájera et al., 2016 [13]	Raramuri community	380	AS	mNYC	3	0.8	0.0–1.8
	Julián-Santiago et al., 2016 [14]	Mixtec & Chontal communities	1061	AS	mNYC	1	0.09	0.002–0.5
		Mixtec	937	AS	mNYC	1	0.1	0.002–0.5
		Chontal	124	AS	mNYC	–	–	–
	Peláez-Ballestas et al., 2009 (CA) [15]	Mexico City	9269	SpA	ESSG	36	0.9	0.6–1.3
				axSpA	ASAS-1	39	0.9	0.7–1.3
				axSpA	ASAS-2	10	0.2	0.1–0.4
Venezuela	Granados et al., 2016 [16]	Warao, Kari'ña, and Chaima communities	1537	SpA	mNYC	7	0.4	0.1–0.9
		Warao	583	SpA	mNYC	–	–	–

Table 1 Prevalence of SpA in Latin American countries *(Continued)*

Country	Study	Setting/Population	*N*	Diagnosis	Diagnostic criteria	*n*	Prevalence (%)	95% CI
		Kari'ña	262	SpA	mNYC	2	0.7	0.09–2.7
		Chaima	692	SpA	mNYC	5	0.7	0.2–1.6

References are articles unless indicated as conference abstracts (CA)
AS ankylosing spondylitis, *ASAS* Assessment in Spondyloarthritis International Society, *CA* conference abstract, *CI* confidence interval, *ESSG* European Spondyloarthropathy Study Group, *mNYC* modified New York criteria, *N* number of patients in study, *n* number of patients with specified condition, *n/r* not reported, *SpA* spondyloarthritis, *uSpA* undifferentiated spondyloarthritis

34, 39, 41–43]. Mean disease duration ranged from 18 months [24] to 17 years [31] (Table 2).

The proportions of patients in single-country studies who were HLA-B27-positive ranged from 5% [21] to 71% [45] (Table 3). Only 3 such studies reported < 20% patients as HLA-B27-positive [12, 21, 24], which likely reflects procedural differences within practice. For example, the HLA-B27 positivity being 4% suggests that the HLA-B27 test was not performed in a representative subset of the study population (the number of patients who were tested for HLA-B27 in that study was not reported) [44]. None of the studies reporting low HLA-B27 rates reported patient race (Table 3). Eleven studies reported mean C-reactive protein levels but most did not specify measurement units (mg/dL or mg/L), which limits data interpretation.

Mean scores for Bath Ankylosing Spondylitis Disease Activity Index (BASDAI) and Bath Ankylosing Spondylitis Functional Index (BASFI) ranged from 3.3 to 6.1 and from 3.2 to 5.2, respectively (Table 3). Ankylosing Spondylitis Quality of Life (ASQoL) scores ranged from 6.5 to 8.7 (mean) and 5 to 10 (median). One study reported an ASAS Health Index score of 10 [35].

Disease manifestations

Disease manifestations were reported in 21 manuscripts [5, 12, 18, 24–27, 29–32, 34, 37, 39–46], 2 of which reported data from 3 and 4 Latin American countries [44' 46], resulting in 26 assessments of disease manifestations from 11 countries. At the country level, Brazil had the highest number of studies reporting disease manifestation ($n = 5$). Across all studies, 12 articular and 13 extra-articular manifestations (from 11 and 9 Latin American countries, respectively) were identified (Fig. 1 and Supplementary Tables 1 and 2).

Articular manifestations

The most commonly reported disease manifestations were enthesitis (24 publications), dactylitis (17 publications), inflammatory lumbar pain (15 publications), and peripheral arthritis (14). Those with the highest occurrence among patients with SpA within any 1 study were inflammatory lumbar pain (100%, Mexico) [12], and axial arthritis (100%, El Salvador) [44], followed by bilateral sacroiliitis (88%, El Salvador [44]), peripheral arthritis (83%, Guatemala [44]), and enthesitis and lower limb arthritis (both 79%, Mexico [40]). However, the occurrence of most articular manifestations varied substantially from study to study, ranging from 42% [42] to 79% [40] for lower limb arthritis and from 9% [24] to 100% [44] for axial arthritis.

Extra-articular manifestations

Uveitis was the most commonly reported extra-articular disease manifestation (20 publications), followed by nail involvement (13 publications), psoriasis (10 publications), and IBD (9 publications). The extra-articular manifestations most frequently experienced by patients with SpA within any 1 study were nail involvement (49%, Argentina [24]), psoriasis (33%, Argentina [46]), and uveitis (26%, Brazil [31] and Argentina [25]). All other extra-articular manifestations occurred at a rate of < 10%, regardless of study or country.

Comorbidities

Three studies reported SpA comorbidities [22, 33, 46], while 2 reported a history of infection without specifying the cause [27, 37]. The largest of the 3 studies reporting SpA comorbidities ($N = 390$), which was conducted in Argentina, Colombia, and Mexico, found that the most common comorbidities were arterial hypertension (25%), hypercholesterolemia (22%), osteoporosis (9%), and gastrointestinal ulcer (8%). Arterial hypertension in Colombia and Mexico occurred at a higher rate than was seen in the general population of those countries (21% vs. 13%). Prevalence of tuberculosis (TB), defined as historic or currently active TB, was 3%, which was 10 times that observed in the general population (0.3%). Prevalence of malignancies was 2.8%, which was similar to that observed in the general population (2.6%) [46]. The other 2 studies enrolled approximately 80 patients each. In the Argentinian study [22], the most common comorbidities reported in patients with axSpA were arterial hypertension (27%), gastritis (26%), dyslipidemia (24%), gallstone disease (13%), and nephrolithiasis (12%). Of these, only nephrolithiasis occurred at a higher frequency than that seen in the general population (4%). Mean age and disease duration were significantly greater

Table 2 Demographics of patients with SpA across Latin America

Country	Study	Patients with SpA (*n*)	Male (%)	Age (y)	Race (%)	Family history of SpA (%)	Diagnosis (%)					Age at disease onset (y)	Disease duration (y)
							AS	PsA	uSpA	ReA	IBD-SpA		
Argentina	Marengo et al., 2008 [17]	61	90.2	43*	n/r	n/r	100	0	0	0	0	n/r	n/r
	Bellomio et al., 2008 [18]	405	59	48.1	71 (W) 23 (WI)	16.4	30.3	46.7	12.4	6.3	0.7	38.4	9.7[a]
	Buschiazzo et al., 2011 [19]	402	59	48.3*	70.8 (W) 22.8 (WI)	16.8	21.4	60.2	8.2	6.2	2.5	n/r	8*
	Soriano et al., 2011 [20]	65	63.1	n/r	92–96 (W)[b] 2–4 (Asian)[b]	n/r	0	100	0	0	0	40.3	8.5
	Schneeberger et al., 2015 [21]	73	49.3	49*	n/r	n/r	0	100	0	0	0	43*	6*
	Sommerfleck et al., 2018a [22]	86	80	46*	n/r	n/r	n/r [c]	n/r [c]	n/r [c]	n/r [c]	n/r [c]	n/r	19*
	Sommerfleck et al., 2018b [23]	50	80	47*	n/r	n/r	70	28	0	0	0	n/r	13*
	Scarafia et al., 2016 (CA) [24]	92	46.7	47.7	n/r	n/r	0	100	0	0	0	n/r	3
	Capelusnik et al., 2018 (CA) [25]	231	75.3	46*	n/r	n/r	n/r [c]	n/r [c]	n/r [c]	n/r [c]	n/r [c]	n/r [c]	20.5*
Brazil	Sampaio-Barros et al., 2008 [26]	1036	73.6	43.7	59.5 (W) 25.9 (AB)	16.2	72.3	13.7	6.3	3.6	1.0	31	12.7[a]
	Skare et al., 2012a [27]	1318	71.9	n/r	65.0 (W) 31.3 (AB)	15.9	65.1	18.3	6.8	3.5	3.5	n/r	14.2
	Skare et al., 2012b [28]	1424	75.9 (< 40 y) 60.6 (≥40 y)	n/r	n/r	19.2 (< 40 y) 13.1 (≥40 y)	66.3	18	6.7	5.5	3.5	28.6	n/r
	Rodrigues et al., 2012 [29]	1472	n/r	n/r	n/r	n/r	65.4	18.4	6.7	3.3	3.3	n/r	n/r
	Duarte et al., 2014 [30]	1189	70.6	44.5	57.7 (W) 42.3 (NW)	n/r	n/r	n/r	n/r	n/r	n/r	n/r	n/r
	Ribeiro et al., 2018 [31]	202	64.2	48.6	62.4 (W) 37.6 (NW)	19.3	71.3[d]	28.7[d]	0	0	0	n/r	17.2
	Simioni et al., (2019) [32]	85	64.7%	49.3*	76.4% (W) 23.5% (AB)	n/r	61.1	21.1	5.8	1.1	0	n/r	14*
	Henrique et al., 2018 (CA) [33]	82	50	56	n/r	n/r	0	100	0	0	0	n/r	9.4
Chile	Gutiérrez et al., 2008 [34]	109	58.4	42	16.8 (W) 64.6 (WI)	13.3	58.7	25.6	7.3	0.9	5.5	35.3	7.1
	Ibáñez et al., 2019 (CA) [35]	472	36.7	42	n/r	n/r	n/r	n/r	n/r	n/r	n/r	n/r	n/r
Colombia	Valle-Onate et al., 2011 [36]	279	69.9	n/r	n/r	n/r	34.4	3.6	39.1	18.3	0.4	n/r	n/r
	Bautista-Molano et al., 2016 [37]	581	71.7	35	n/r	5.3	29.1	3.6	39.6	26.9	0.9	28	7.3
	Santos et al., 2017 [38]	189	63.8	35.9	n/r	n/r	46.0	0	35.5	18.5	0	n/r	n/r
Costa Rica	Sáenz Castro et al., 2008 [39]	33	57.6	41.3	21.2 (W) 66.7 (WI)	12.2	45.5	6.1	45.5	0	0	34.5	6.8[a]
Mexico	Casasola-Vargas et al.,	172	59.3	38.1	18.5 (W)	18.6	34.9	8.7	11.6	1.7	1.2	28.0	10.1[a]

Table 2 Demographics of patients with SpA across Latin America *(Continued)*

Country	Study	Patients with SpA (*n*)	Male (%)	Age (y)	Race (%)	Family history of SpA (%)	Diagnosis (%)					Age at disease onset (y)	Disease duration (y)
							AS	PsA	uSpA	ReA	IBD-SpA		
	2008 [40]				76.3 (WI)								
	Peláez-Ballestas et al., 2013 [12]	28	50	40.7	n/r	21.4	n/r	n/r	n/r	n/r	n/r	n/r	n/r
Peru	Chávez-Corrales et al., 2008 [41]	60	65	40.3	3.3 (W) 93.3 (WI)	18.6	53	6.7	13.3	1.7	0	30.6	9.7[a]
Uruguay	Palleiro and Spangenberg, 2008 [42]	53	66.0	41.2	86.8 (W) 11.3 (MR)	13.2	53	17	19	0	4	31.0	10.2[a]
Venezuela	Chacón et al., 2008 [43]	69	62.3	40.9	31.9 (W) 39.1 (MR)	27.5	55.1	21.7	11.6	0	4.3	29.4	11.5[a]
Multinational	García-Kutzbach et al., 2011 [44]	233	46	47.5*	n/r	n/r	10	9	33	47.2	0.8	n/r	n/r
	Benegas et al., 2012 [45]	1083	75	43	n/r	n/r	100	0	0	0	0	28	n/r
	Bautista-Molano et al., 2018 [46]	390	64	45	n/r	n/r	n/r	n/r	n/r	n/r	n/r	n/r	7.0

Continuous values are mean unless indicated (*) as median
References are articles unless indicated as conference abstracts (CA)
[a]Information not available in original RESPONDIA publication; data taken from Gallinaro et al., 2010 [5].
[b]Data for the 2 regional populations (Autonomous City of Buenos Aires, membership of the Hospital Italiano Medical Care Program) were presented separately.
[c]Patients were described as having axial spondyloarthritis.
[d]Patients were classified as having either axial SpA which was predominantly AS, or peripheral SpA which was predominantly PsA.
AB African-Brazilian (could include MR), *AS* ankylosing spondylitis, *CA* conference abstract, *I* Indigenous, *n* number of patients with specified condition, *MR* mixed race (white-black), *n/r* not reported, *NW* non-white, *O* Other; *PsA* psoriatic arthritis, *ReA* reactive arthritis, *SpA* spondyloarthritis, *T* total population, *uSpA* undifferentiated spondyloarthritis, *W* White, *WI* White-Indigenous, *y* years

($P < 0.05$) in patients with ≥3 comorbidities compared with patients who reported no comorbidities, as were mean BASDAI and BASFI scores (5.8 and 5.2 [≥3 comorbidities] vs. 3.3 and 3.2 [no comorbidities], respectively, $P < 0.05$) [22]. The most common comorbidities in patients with PsA from 2 hospitals in Southern Brazil were metabolic syndrome (54%), arterial hypertension (52%), and diabetes (20%); no comparisons were made with the general population [33].

Quality of life (QoL)

ASQoL or ASAS scores were presented in 9 single-country studies (Table 3). The highest mean/median ASQoL or ASAS score was 11.2 [23] and the lowest was 5 [17, 18]. The relationship between SpA status and QoL may have been impacted by factors such as employment status [17], ethnicity [27, 31], and treatment status [35], but their reporting was sporadic and interpreting the potential relationship is beyond the scope of this review.

Treatments

Data relating to SpA treatment were available from 14 studies [5, 18, 26, 27, 31, 32, 34, 39, 40, 42–46]. Nonsteroidal anti-inflammatory drugs (NSAIDs) were the most commonly used class of medication, with most studies reporting use in 68–98% of patients. However, the most recent study from Brazil reported a use rate of 32% [32]. Conventional synthetic disease-modifying antirheumatic drugs (csDMARDs) were the second-most commonly prescribed class of treatment (Fig. 2). Methotrexate (MTX) and sulfasalazine (SSZ) were more frequently used than leflunomide (LEF), although there was a wider range of prescription rates for MTX (19–67% [Brazil]) and SSZ (9% in Argentina to 87% in Mexico) than for LEF (4% in Chile to 29% Mexico). Corticosteroid (CS) use ranged from 5 to 50% of patients (both Brazil). Tumor necrosis factor inhibitor (TNFi) use ranged from 5 to 45% of the populations in which they were reported (Fig. 2 and Supplementary Table 3), with etanercept (ETN) being the most commonly prescribed agent (35% of patients in 1 Brazilian study).

Discussion

This manuscript represents a comprehensive overview of the prevalence and burden of SpA in Latin America. A 2014 systematic review of global AS prevalence found the rate in Latin America to be 10.2 per 10,000 [47]. This calculation was based on 4 studies included here [8–11]. The additional studies included in our review are generally consistent with that prevalence rate. However, the majority (60%) of the epidemiology studies included in this narrative review were from Mexico, with prevalence data largely unavailable for the majority of

Table 3 Clinical characteristics of patients with SpA across Latin America

Country	Study	# Patients	HLA-B27 positive (%)	CRP, mg/dL	BASDAI	BASFI	ASQoL
Argentina	Marengo et al., 2008 [17]	61	n/r	n/r	27.2* (Em) 57.7* (Un)	40.3* (Em) 53.1* (Un)	5* (Em) 8* (Un)
	Bellomio et al., 2008 [18]	405	46	1.9*[b]	4.0	3.3	5
	Buschiazzo et al., 2011 [19]	402	45.3	n/r	3.8*	2.6*	n/r
	Schneeberger et al., 2015 [21]	73	5	n/r	n/r	n/r	n/r
	Sommerfleck et al., 2018 [22]	86	n/r	n/r	3.3 (0 c-m) 4.3 (1–2 c-m) 5.8 (≥3 c-m)	3.2 (0 c-m) 4.5 (1–2 c-m) 5.2 (≥3 c-m)	n/r
	Sommerfleck et al., 2018 [23]	50	n/r	n/r	4.1*	4.2*	11.2* (PsAQoL)
	Scarafia et al., 2016 (CA) [24]	92	5.6	n/r	n/r	n/r	n/r
Brazil	Sampaio-Barros et al., 2008 [26]	1036	69.5	n/r	4.1	4.5	n/r
	Skare et al., 2012 [27]	1318	72.8 (W) 62.4 (AB) 35 (O)	9.3 (W)[b] 9.3 (AB)[b] 11.2 (O)[b]	4.0 (W) 4.3 (AB) 4.4 (O)	4.4 (W) 4.8 (AB) 4.7 (O)	7.1 (W) 8.6 (AB) 8.7 (O)
	Skare et al., 2012 [28]	1424	72.8 (< 40 y) 49.5 (≥40 y)	10.3 (< 40 y) 8.02 (≥40 y)	4.15 (< 40 y) 4.47 (≥40 y)	4.6 (< 40 y) 4.7 (≥40 y)	7.8 (< 40 y) 7.8 (≥40 y)
	Duarte et al., 2014 [30]	1189	67.9	n/r	4.3	4.7	7.9
	Ribeiro et al., 2018 [31]	202	64.2	3.6 (W)[b] 3.7 (NW)[b]	3.6 (W) 3.7 (NW)	4.5 (W) 4.1 (NW)	7.9 (W) 6.5 (NW)
	Simioni et al., 2019 [32]	85	69.2	8*	2.4*	5.1*	9.2*
Chile	Gutiérrez et al., 2008 [34]	109	66.4	16.2[b]	4.9	4.5	n/r
	Ibáñez et al., 2019 (CA) [35]	472	n/r	n/r	6.1	5	10[a]
Colombia	Bautista-Molano et al., 2016 [37]	581	43.9	11.7	5.4 (Ax) 5.3 (Pr)	n/r	n/r
	Santos et al., 2017 [38]	189	40.7	n/r	n/r	n/r	n/r
Costa Rica	Sáenz Castro et al., 2008 [39]	33	57.1	0.6	4.6	3.9	n/r
Mexico	Casasola-Vargas et al., 2008 [40]	172	n/r	12[b]	4.5	4.0	n/r
	Peláez-Ballestas et al., 2013 [12]	28	14.3	n/r	n/r	n/r	n/r
Peru	Chávez-Corrales et al., 2008 [41]	60	31	n/r	n/r	n/r	n/r
Uruguay	Palleiro and Spangenberg, 2008 [42]	53	approx. 50 (AS, uSpA) 14 (PsA)	6.2 mg/L	5.3	4.3	n/r
Venezuela	Chacón et al., 2008 [43]	69	n/r	8.4[b]	4.4	3.6	n/r
Multinational	García-Kutzbach et al., 2011 [44]	233	57.1 (Costa Rica) 29 (El Salvador) 4 (Guatemala)[c]	n/r	n/r	n/r	n/r
	Benegas et al., 2012 [45]	1083	71	10[b]	4.3	4.8	7
	Bautista-Molano et al., 2018 [46]	390	n/r	n/r	n/r	3.4	n/r

Continuous values are mean unless indicated (*) as median
References are articles unless indicated as conference abstracts (CA)
[a]ASAS Health Index.
[b]Units (mg/dL or mg/L) not given in publication.
[c]HLA-B27 test not routinely performed.
AB African-Brazilian, *AS* ankylosing spondylitis, *ASQoL* Ankylosing Spondylitis Quality of Life, *Ax* patients with axial SpA, *BASDAI* Bath Ankylosing Spondylitis Disease Activity Index, *BASFI* Bath Ankylosing Spondylitis Functional Index, *CA* conference abstract, *c-m* comorbidities, *Em* employed, *HLA* human leukocyte antigen, *I* indigenous, *n/r* not reported, *NW* non-white, *MR* mixed race (white-black), *Pr* patients with peripheral SpA, *PsA* psoriatic arthritis, *Un* unemployed, *uSpA* undifferentiated spondyloarthritis, *W* white, *y* years

countries. Therefore, these data may not be representative of Latin America as a whole.

Patient demographics were widely available. Sex and mean age of patients with SpA were consistently reported, whereas race, ethnicity, family history of SpA, age at disease onset, and disease duration were not. Most patients were male and, where reported, typically had disease onset before the age of 40. These values are consistent with previously reported global estimates [4]. The proportions of patients with AS and PsA varied between countries. Patients included in studies conducted in Argentina were more likely to have PsA than AS,

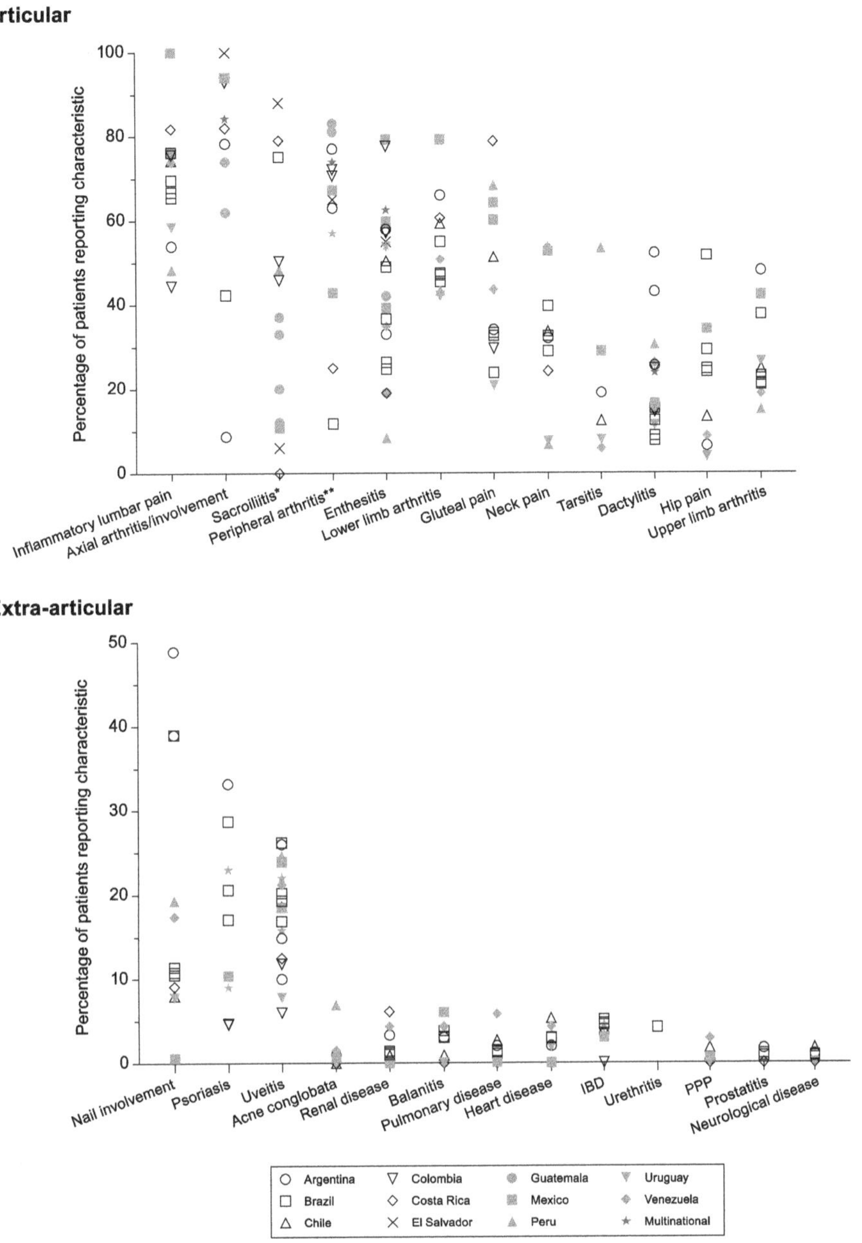

Fig. 1 Disease manifestations in Latin American patients with SpA: **a** articular; **b** extra-articular. * Sacroiliitis includes bilateral sacroiliitis, unilateral sacroiliitis, radiographic sacroiliitis, sacroiliitis assessed by MRI, and sacroiliac syndrome. ** Peripheral arthritis includes peripheral arthritis, oligoarthritis, asymmetrical oligoarthritis, and arthritis that is unspecified by the publication. Source data for this figure can be found in Supplementary Tables 1 and 2. IBD, inflammatory bowel disease; MRI, magnetic resonance imaging

while the opposite was the case in studies from Brazil. There were fewer patients with PsA than other SpA subtypes in studies from Colombia (4 studies), Costa Rica, Mexico, Peru, Uruguay, and Venezuela (1–3 studies each). However, the majority of studies in these countries were small (< 100 patients) and differences in the proportion of SpA subtypes may be due to potential differences in patient selection and the diagnostic criteria used, rather than representative of prevalence as a whole.

The majority of studies reporting clinical characteristics were conducted in Argentina and Brazil. One study reported HLA-B27 status by ethnicity [27] and 1 by age [28] (both Brazil). HLA-B27-positive status was more common in white than in black patients [28], and in older than younger patients [28], consistent with previously reported global estimates [4]. HLA-B27 is not common among indigenous communities in South America [48], but no studies

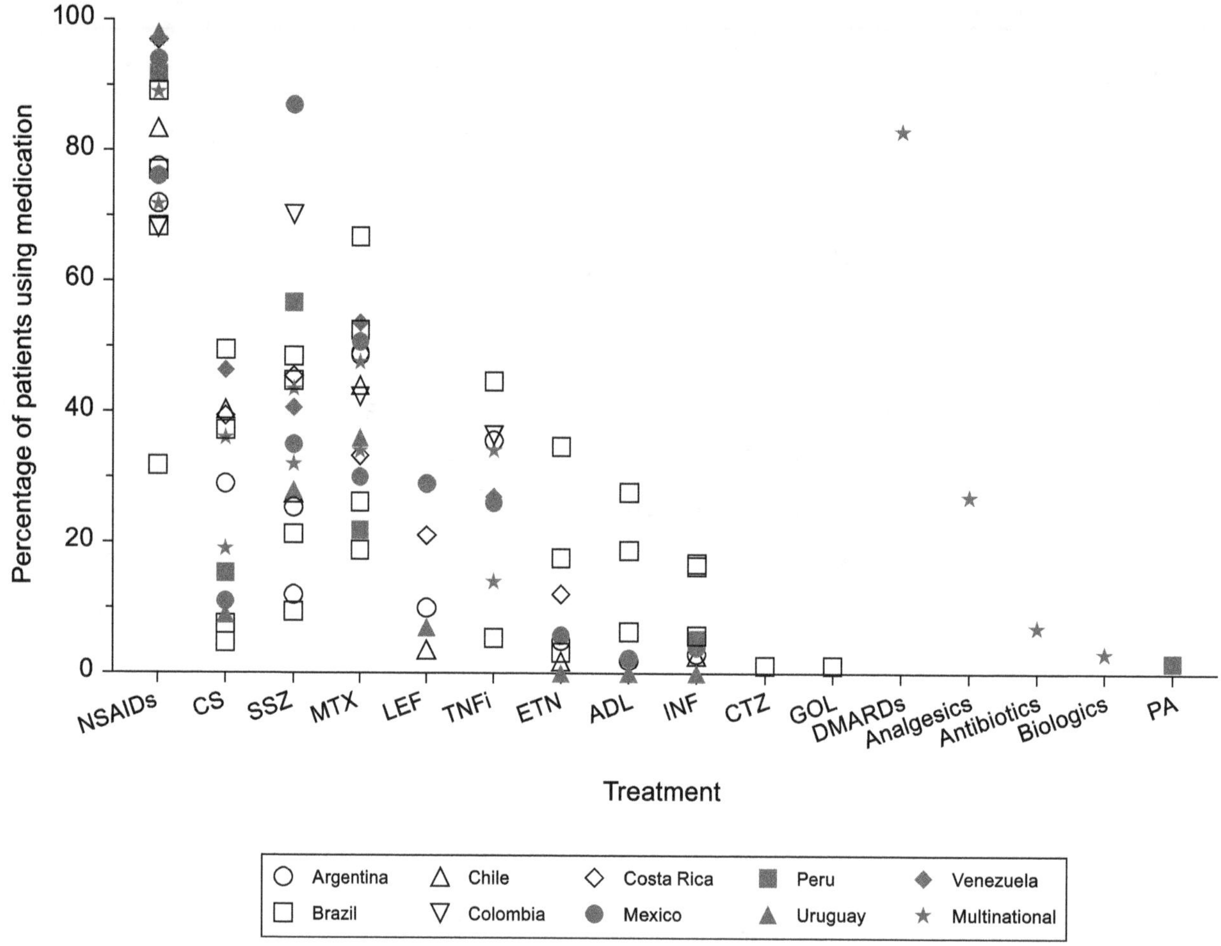

Fig. 2 Treatments utilized by Latin American patients with SpA. Source data for this figure can be found in Supplementary Table 3. ADL, adalimumab; CS, corticosteroids; CTZ, certolizumab pegol; DMARDs; disease-modifying anti-rheumatic drugs; ETN; etanercept; EU, European Union; GOL, golimumab; INF, infliximab; LEF, leflunomide; MTX, methotrexate; NSAIDs, non-steroidal anti-inflammatory drugs; PA, pamidronic acid; SSZ, sulfasalazine; TNFi, tumor necrosis factor inhibitor

collected for this review provided HLA-B27 data for these populations.

Consistent with the findings of the ASAS-COMOSPA study of patients from 22 countries [49], the prevalence ranges of disease manifestations reported here showed considerable variability. Peripheral articular involvement and enthesitis were similar in range between ASAS-COMOSPA and our study (3–82% vs. 12–73%, and 6–72% vs. 8–79%, respectively), whereas the study conducted in Latin America and the European Union (EU) reported higher prevalence of peripheral arthritis and enthesitis in Latin American than in EU patients [45]. We found a wider range of reported joint involvement (9–100%) and dactylitis (8–52%) than ASAS-COMOSPA (52–100% and 0–35%, respectively), whereas the range of reported extra-articular manifestations was generally lower in our study than in the ASAS-COMOSPA study.

Overall, there was a lack of data on impact of disease variables and comorbidities in Latin American patients with SpA. One study investigated the impact of variables such as disease duration or activity on QoL [17]. Other studies explored the relationship between QoL and employment status, treatment status [17, 35], or patients' age or age at disease onset [28, 45], but there were too few to make any meaningful conclusions. Only 3 studies presented data on comorbidities. Conditions such as osteoporosis, cardiovascular disease, cancer, and infections are key comorbidities in patients with SpA [50], yet only 1 study presented frequencies of malignancies and infections (TB) [46].

Treatment data were available from almost half of the studies reviewed, but for most countries, information was available from a single study only. The range of NSAID use across studies was largely comparable with that previously reported in the ASAS-COMOSPA study (32–98% vs. 46–98%, respectively). MTX use was higher in our review (19–67% vs. 2–51%), but SSZ (9–87% vs. 0–90%) and TNFi (5–45% vs. 44%) use was typically lower [49]. In the comparison study of Latin America and Europe, Latin American patients with AS had a significantly higher use of NSAIDs, CS, MTX, SSZ, and MTX-TNFi combination therapy than their EU counterparts ($P < 0.001$ for all comparisons); there was no significant difference in the use of TNFi monotherapy [45].

Although the literature surveyed was relatively recent (the past 10 years), most of the estimates of treatment data date back to the beginning of that period. Since then, most Latin American countries have adopted regulatory standards for biosimilars [51] and have allowed biosimilars into their markets, and new therapies are constantly being developed. Therefore, treatment options for patients with SpA in this region have changed and the estimates summarized here may not be representative of the current situation.

This review had some limitations. Overall, we found that, outside of the 8 RESPONDIA papers, study methodology and design varied widely, and the types of data collected (prevalence, disease manifestations, comorbidities, QoL, treatments) were not consistent between studies. Several areas covered had limited data. The possibility of assessing the true extent of disease manifestations was limited due to a lack of clarity regarding data collection. Fewer than one-quarter of studies listed disease manifestations that were reported by none of the enrolled patients [34, 37, 39, 40, 42, 44]. For other studies, it was not obvious if unreported disease manifestations were not found or if the data were not collected. Several treatment-related areas were not covered. For example, patient views on medication, including patient satisfaction with their treatment, were missing. Treatment adherence was not reported in any of the studies, even though poor adherence to treatments for inflammatory diseases is associated with poorer clinical outcomes [52]. Finally, study inclusion criteria for this review were specific to prevalence data or patient demographics. Consequently, studies with a sole focus on other aspects (e.g., disease manifestations) may not have been identified.

In summary, our review identified several gaps in the literature on SpA from Latin America. Prevalence studies outside Mexico are generally lacking. More than half the studies providing data on clinical characteristics came from Argentina and Brazil. There are insufficient data on comorbidities and QoL, particularly from countries other than Argentina and Brazil. Finally, data on treatment patterns are mostly out of date. Up-to-date reports on treatment adherence or patient views would add clarification to the literature. Future research efforts in this region should also focus on the need for standardized care, follow-up, and regular monitoring of disease, as well as characterizing the side effects of medications used for treatment.

Conclusions

A total of 41 publications relating to the prevalence and characteristics of SpA in Latin America were identified. Several gaps were evident in terms of the countries and data covered, particularly in terms of the treatment patterns and impact of SpA. More consistent methodologies between studies would help provide a more accurate picture of the disease burden in this region.

Abbreviations

ADL: Adalimumab; AS: Ankylosing spondylitis; ASAS: Assessment in Spondyloarthritis International Society; ASQoL: Ankylosing Spondylitis Quality of Life; BASDAI: Bath Ankylosing Spondylitis Disease Activity Index; BASFI: Bath Ankylosing Spondylitis Functional Index; CS: Corticosteroids; csDMARDs: Conventional synthetic disease-modifying anti-rheumatic drugs; CTZ: Certolizumab pegol; ETN: Etanercept; EU: European Union; GOL: Golimumab; IBD: Inflammatory bowel disease; INF: Infliximab; JSpA: Juvenile-onset SpA; LEF: Leflunomide; MRI: Magnetic resonance imaging; MTX: Methotrexate; nr-axSpA: Non-radiographic axSpA; NSAID: Non-steroidal anti-inflammatory drugs; PsA: Psoriatic arthritis; QoL: Quality of life; ReA: Reactive arthritis; SpA: Spondyloarthritis; SSZ: Sulfasalazine; TB: Tuberculosis; TNFi: Tumor necrosis factor inhibitor; uSpA: Undifferentiated SpA

Acknowledgements

Medical writing support was provided by Lorna Forse, PhD, of Engage Scientific Solutions and was funded by Pfizer.

Authors' contributions

All authors contributed to the design of the work, the analysis and interpretation of the data reviewed, revised each draft critically for important intellectual content, approved the final version to be published, and agreed to be accountable for all aspects of the work.

Author details

[1]Instituto de Rehabilitación Psicofísica, Echeverría 955, Buenos Aires, Argentina. [2]Universidad Militar Nueva Granada and University Hospital Fundación Santa Fe de Bogotá, Bogotá, Colombia. [3]Hospital General de México "Dr. Eduardo Liceaga", Mexico City, Mexico. [4]Universidade Federal do Paraná, Curitiba, Brazil. [5]Hospital Nacional Guillermo Almenara Irigoyen, Lima, Peru. [6]Hospital La Católica, Guadalupe, San José, Costa Rica. [7]Pfizer, Buenos Aires, Argentina.

References

1. Rudwaleit M, van der Heijde D, Landewe R, et al. The Assessment of SpondyloArthritis International Society classification criteria for peripheral spondyloarthritis and for spondyloarthritis in general. Ann Rheum Dis. 2011; 70:25–31.
2. Stolwijk C, van Onna M, Boonen A, van Tubergen A. Global prevalence of spondyloarthritis: a systematic review and meta-regression analysis. Arthritis Care Res. 2016;68:1320–31.
3. Burgos-Vargas R, Peláez-Ballestas I, Gutiérrez-Suárez R. Challenges in juvenile-onset spondyloarthritis. Int J Clin Rheumatol. 2010;5:229–39.
4. Stolwijk C, Boonen A, van Tubergen A, Reveille JD. Epidemiology of spondyloarthritis. Rheum Dis Clin N Am. 2012;38:441–76.
5. Gallinaro AL, Ventura C, Sampaio Barros PD, Goncalves CR. Spondyloarthritis: analysis of a Brazilian series compared with a large Ibero-American registry (RESPONDIA group). Rev Bras Reumatol. 2010;50:581–9.
6. Londono J, Pelaez Ballestas I, Cuervo F, et al. Prevalence of rheumatic disease in Colombia acording to the Colombian Rheumatology Association (COPCORD) strategy. Prevalence study of rheumatic disease in Colombian population older than 18 years. Rev Colomb Reumatol. 2018;25:245 56.

7. Fernández-Ávila DG, Bernal-Macías S, Rincón-Riaño DN, Gutiérrez-Dávila JM, Rosselli-Cock D. Prevalence of rheumatic diseases in Colombia: an approach from the ministry of health and social protection data (SISPRO). J Clin Rheumatol. 2018;24:S172.
8. Reyes-Llerena GA, Guibert-Toledano M, Penedo-Coello A, et al. Community-based study to estimate prevalence and burden of illness of rheumatic diseases in Cuba: a COPCORD study. J Clin Rheumatol. 2009;15:51–5.
9. Peláez-Ballestas I, Sanin LH, Moreno-Montoya J, et al. Epidemiology of the rheumatic diseases in Mexico. A study of 5 regions based on the COPCORD methodology. J Rheumatol Suppl. 2011;86:3–8.
10. Rodriguez-Amado J, Pelaez-Ballestas I, Sanin LH, et al. Epidemiology of rheumatic diseases. A community-based study in urban and rural populations in the state of Nuevo Leon, Mexico. J Rheumatol Suppl. 2011; 86:9–14.
11. Alvarez-Nemegyei J, Pelaez-Ballestas I, Sanin LH, Cardiel MH, Ramirez-Angulo A, Goycochea-Robles MV. Prevalence of musculoskeletal pain and rheumatic diseases in the southeastern region of Mexico. A COPCORD-based community survey. J Rheumatol Suppl. 2011;86:21–5.
12. Peláez-Ballestas I, Navarro-Zarza JE, Julian B, et al. A community-based study on the prevalence of spondyloarthritis and inflammatory back pain in Mexicans. J Clin Rheumatol. 2013;19:57–61.
13. Del Rio ND, Santana N, Pelaez-Ballestas I, Gonzalez-Chavez SA, Quinonez-Flores CM, Pacheco-Tena C. Prevalence of rheumatic diseases in Raramuri people in Chihuahua, Mexico: a community-based study. Clin Rheumatol. 2016;35(Suppl 1):43–52.
14. Julian-Santiago F, Garcia-Garcia C, Garcia-Olivera I, Goycochea-Robles MV, Pelaez-Ballestas I. Epidemiology of rheumatic diseases in Mixtec and Chontal indigenous communities in Mexico: a cross-sectional community-based study. Clin Rheumatol. 2016;35(Suppl 1):35–42.
15. Peláez-Ballestas I, Navarro-Zarza E, Julian B, et al. The prevalence of inflammatory back pain, spondyloarthritis, and axial spondyloarthritis in the community. Arthritis Rheum. 2009;60:1652–3.
16. Granados Y, Rosillo C, Cedeno L, et al. Prevalence of musculoskeletal disorders and rheumatic disease in the Warao, Kari'na, and Chaima indigenous populations of Monagas State, Venezuela. Clin Rheumatol. 2016; 35(Suppl 1):53–61.
17. Marengo MF, Schneeberger EE, Citera G, Cocco JA. Work status among patients with ankylosing spondylitis in Argentina. J Clin Rheumatol. 2008;14: 273–7.
18. Bellomio V, Berman A, Sueldo RR, et al. Registro Iberoamericano de Espondiloartritis (RESPONDIA): Argentina. Reumatol Clin. 2008;4:S23–9.
19. Buschiazzo E, Maldonado-Cocco JA, Arturi P, et al. Epidemiology of spondyloarthritis in Argentina. Am J Med Sci. 2011;341:289–92.
20. Soriano ER, Rosa J, Velozo E, et al. Incidence and prevalence of psoriatic arthritis in Buenos Aires, Argentina: a 6-year health management organization-based study. Rheumatology (Oxford). 2011;50:729–34.
21. Schneeberger EE, Citera G, Rodriguez Gil G, et al. Clinical and immunogenetic characterization in psoriatic arthritis patients. Clin Rheumatol. 2015;34:1413–8.
22. Sommerfleck F, Schneeberger E, Citera G. Comorbidities in Argentine patients with axial spondyloarthritis: Is nephrolithiasis associated with this disease? Eur J Rheumatol. 2018;5:169–72.
23. Sommerfleck FA, Schneeberger EE, Orozco MC, Zamora N, Landi M, Citera G. Validation and cultural adaptation of the qualisex questionnaire in patients with axial spondyloarthritis in Argentina. Rheumatol Int. 2018;38:2103–9.
24. Scarafia S, Duarte V, Romanini FE, et al. Prevalence of overweight and obesity in early psoriatic arthritis clinic. J Clin Rheumatol. 2016;22:139.
25. Capelusnik D, Cavalieri M, Rolón Campuzano R, et al. Prevalence and characteristics of uveitis in a large cohort of patients with axial spondyloarthritis. J Clin Rheumatol. 2018;24:S103–4.
26. Sampaio-Barros PD, Gonçalves CR, Braga da Silva JA, et al. Registro Iberoamericano de Espondiloartritis (RESPONDIA): Brasil. Informe del Registro Brasileño de Espondiloartritis. Reumatol Clin. 2008;4:S30 5.
27. Skare TL, Bortoluzzo AB, Goncalves CR, et al. Ethnic influence in clinical and functional measures of Brazilian patients with spondyloarthritis. J Rheumatol. 2012;39:141–7.
28. Skare TL, Leite N, Bortoluzzo AB, et al. Effect of age at disease onset in the clinical profile of spondyloarthritis: a study of 1424 Brazilian patients. Clin Exp Rheumatol. 2012;30:351–7.
29. Rodrigues CE, Vieira WP, Bortoluzzo AB, et al. Low prevalence of renal, cardiac, pulmonary, and neurological extra-articular clinical manifestations in spondyloarthritis: analysis of the Brazilian Registry of Spondyloarthritis. Rev Bras Reumatol. 2012;52:375–83.
30. Duarte AP, Marques CD, Bortoluzzo AB, et al. Epidemiologic profile of juvenile-onset compared to adult-onset spondyloarthritis in a large Brazilian cohort. Rev Bras Reumatol. 2014;54:424–30.
31. Ribeiro SLE, de Campos APB, Palominos PE, et al. Different ethnic background is associated with distinct clinical profiles in the spondyloarthritides in the North and South of Brazil. Clin Rheumatol. 2018; 383:195–203.
32. Simioni J, Skare TL, Campos APB, et al. Fecal calprotectin, gut inflammation and spondyloarthritis. Arch Med Res. 2019;50:41–6.
33. Henrique L, Mello A, Kohem C, et al. Psoriatic arthritis patients followed in university hospitals in southern Brazil have a high prevalence of metabolic syndrome, overweight/obesity, diabetes and hypertension. J Clin Rheumatol. 2018;24:S106.
34. Gutiérrez MA, Pérez C, Saavedra J, et al. Registro Iberoamericano de Espondiloartritis (RESPONDIA): Chile. Reumatol Clin. 2008;4:S41–7.
35. Ibanez S, van Bentum R, Valenzuela O, van der Horst-Bruisnsma I. Chilean axial spondyloarthritis patients report high disease burden and impaired work activity - an internet survey in 472 patients. Ann Rheum Dis. 2019;78:A477.
36. Valle-Onate R, Candia L, Romero-Sanchez C, et al. Epidemiology of spondyloarthritis in Colombia. Am J Med Sci. 2011;341:293–4.
37. Bautista-Molano W, Landewe RB, Londono J, Romero-Sanchez C, Valle-Onate R, van der Heijde D. Analysis and performance of various classification criteria sets in a Colombian cohort of patients with spondyloarthritis. Clin Rheumatol. 2016;35:1759–67.
38. Santos AM, Pena P, Avila M, et al. Association of human leukocyte A, B, and DR antigens in Colombian patients with diagnosis of spondyloarthritis. Clin Rheumatol. 2017;36:953–8.
39. Sáenz CR. Registro Iberoamericano de Espondiloartritis (RESPONDIA): Costa Rica. Reumatol Clin. 2008;4:S36–40.
40. Casasola-Vargas JC, Flores-Alvarado DE, Huerta-Sil G, et al. Registro Iberoamericano de Espondiloartritis (RESPONDIA): México. Reumatol Clin. 2008;4:S56–62.
41. Chávez-Corrales JE, Montero Jáuregui M, Alva Linares M, et al. Registro Iberoamericano de Espondiloartritis (RESPONDIA): Perú. Reumatol Clin. 2008;4: S63–7.
42. Palleiro DR, Spangenberg E. Registro Iberoamericano de Espondiloartritis (RESPONDIA): Uruguay. Reumatol Clin. 2008;4:S73–8.
43. Chacón R, Granados Y, Esteva MH, et al. Registro Iberoamericano de Espondiloartritis (RESPONDIA): Venezuela. Reumatol Clin. 2008;4:S79–86.
44. García-Kutzbach A, Montenegro A, Iraheta I, Bara C, Saenz R. Epidemiology of spondyloarthropathies in Central America. Am J Med Sci. 2011;341:295–7.
45. Benegas M, Munoz-Gomariz E, Font P, et al. Comparison of the clinical expression of patients with ankylosing spondylitis from Europe and Latin America. J Rheumatol. 2012;39:2315–20.
46. Bautista-Molano W, Landewé R, Burgos-Vargas R, et al. Prevalence of comorbidities and risk factors for comorbidities in patients with spondyloarthritis in Latin America: a comparative study with the general population and data from the ASAS-COMOSPA study. J Rheumatol. 2018;45: 206–12.
47. Dean LE, Jones GT, MacDonald AG, Downham C, Sturrock RD, Macfarlane GJ. Global prevalence of ankylosing spondylitis. Rheumatology (Oxford). 2014;53:650–7.
48. Khan MA. HLA-B27 and its subtypes in world populations. Curr Opin Rheumatol. 1995;7:263–9.
49. Molto A, Etcheto A, van der Heijde D, et al. Prevalence of comorbidities and evaluation of their screening in spondyloarthritis: results of the international cross-sectional ASAS-COMOSPA study. Ann Rheum Dis. 2016;75:1016–23.
50. Molto A, Nikiphorou E. Comorbidities in spondyloarthritis. Front Med (Lausanne). 2018;5:62.
51. Azevedo VF, Babini A, Caballero-Uribe CV, Castaneda-Hernandez G, Borlenghi C, Jones HE. Practical guidance on biosimilars, with a focus on Latin America: what do rheumatologists need to know? J Clin Rheumatol. 2019;25:91–100.
52. Contreras-Yanez I, Ponce De Leon S, Cabiedes J, Rull-Gabayet M, Pascual-Ramos V. Inadequate therapy behavior is associated to disease flares in patients with rheumatoid arthritis who have achieved remission with disease-modifying antirheumatic drugs. Am J Med Sci. 2010;340:282–90.

14

Psoriatic Arthritis Quality of Life Questionnaire: Translation, cultural adaptation and validation into Brazilian Portuguese language

Rafaela Silva Guimaraes Gonçalves[1*], Alice Heaney[2], Stephen P. McKenna[2,3], Jonas Braynner Carvalho[1], Maria Eduarda Lima Vidal[1], Marina Coelho Mores de Brito[1] and Angela Luzia Branco Pinto Duarte[1]

Abstract

Introduction: Psoriatic arthritis (PsA) is a multifaceted inflammatory disease that can cause joint destruction and impair quality of life. The Psoriatic Arthritis Quality of Life Questionnaire (PsAQoL) was the first disease-specific tool for determining the impact of the disease on the quality of life of people with PsA.

Objectives: The primary objective was to develop and validate a Brazilian Portuguese version of the PsAQoL.

Methods: The UK PsAQoL was translated into Brazilian Portuguese using two translation panels. This translation then checked for face validity and construct validity with new samples of patients. Finally, a test-retest validation study was conducted with 52 patients with PsA. The survey included the Nottingham Health Profile (NHP) as a comparator instrument.

Results: Internal consistency and reproducibility were both excellent for the new adaptation (0.91 and 0.90 respectively Scores on the PsAQoL were found to correlate as expected with the comparator measure and the instrument was able to detect differences in score related to perceived severity of PsA, general health status and presence of a flare.

Conclusion: The Brazilian PsAQoL was found easy to understand and complete and has excellent reliability and construct validity. The new measure will be a valuable new tool for use in routine PsA practice and clinical trials.

Keywords: Psoriatic arthritis, Quality of life, Validation, Translation

Introduction

Psoriatic arthritis (PsA) is a chronic inflammatory disease that is part of the group of spondyloarthropathies, affecting up to 1% of the population [1]. It is a complex diseasewhich, in addition to the cutaneous involvement, the patient presents musculoskeletal problems (related to the spine, enthesis and peripheral joints) and may also present extra-muscular manifestations including the intestine or the eye [1]. PsA is the most prevalent extra-cutaneous manifestation in patients with psoriasis, affecting between 8 and 42% of psoriatic patients [2].

PsA has been shown to have a negative impact on patients' quality of life (QoL) [3]. It is therefore important to able to assess the extent to which an individual's life is affected by their condition and to evaluate the value gained by patients from new and existing treatment strategies. The articular condition (arthritis, tenosynovitis, enthesitis and/or dactylitis) may significantly limit functional ability, including activities of daily living and employment. This may well lead to important socioeconomic impacts [4].

* Correspondence: rafa_sgg@hotmail.com
[1]Hospital das Clinicas da Universidade Federal de Pernambuco, Recife, Brazil

One of the measures available for assessing outcome is the Health Assessment Questionnaire (HAQ) [5]. However, The HAQ assesses health status rather than QoL. The latter has become an important outcome for both physicians and patients. It is now necessary for clinical studies to show the impact on patient-reported outcomes, such as QoL, in addition to efficacy and safety [6].

McKenna et al. developed and validated the Psoriatic Arthritis Quality of Life (PsAQoL) questionnaire [3]. Rather than measuring symptoms and functional limitations, the PsAQoL assesses the degree to which patients are able to meet their fundamental human needs [7]. The PsAQoL is the only patient-centric outcome measure that is able to assess the true impact of PsA and its treatment on the overall lives of patients. The aim of the present study was to produce a Brazilian Portuguese version of the PsAQoL for use in clinical practice, international trials and research settings.

Methods

The adaptation of the PsAQoL consisted of three stages: translation; assessment of face and content validity; psychometric evaluation.

Translation of the PsAQoL

The dual-panel methodology [8] was adopted to translate the UK English PsAQoL into Brazilian Portuguese. This involves running two independent panels – a bilingual panel and a lay panel. An initial translation of the PsAQoL was produced by the bilingual panel. This consisted of a group of professional individuals who were native speakers of Brazilian Portuguese and also fluent in English. Their role was to work together to produce conceptually equivalent translations of the questionnaire items, instructions and response options. The translated version was then presented to a lay panel for consideration. This consisted of a group of monolingual Portuguese-speakers with an average educational level. These individuals were invited to comment on the comprehension of the translations and suggest changes, where necessary, to ensure the final wording of items was easy to understand and expressed in natural, everyday language.

Both panels were led by the same moderator who encouraged the panel members to work as a team and ensured the original meaning of each item was maintained in the final translation. A representative from the team that developed the UK English questionnaire also attended both panels to ensure the precise conceptual meaning of the items was conveyed to the moderator. Individuals with PsA were not invited to take part in the panels as the purpose of this stage was to produce an appropriate translation of the questionnaire, not to test the suitability of the content.

Assessment of face and content validity

Cognitive debriefing interviews (CDIs) were conducted with PsA patients to assess the extent to which the translated questionnaire was relevant, comprehensive and easy to complete. The interviews took the form of a one-to-one semi-structured approach. Respondents were asked to complete the questionnaire while an interviewer observed and noted any obvious difficulties or hesitations. Respondents were then asked to provide feedback on the questionnaire, including whether all important aspects of their experience of PsA had been covered.

Psychometric evaluation

A postal survey was conducted to establish the psychometric properties of the Brazilian Portuguese PsAQoL. Individuals who satisfied the Classification Criteria for Psoriatic Arthritis (CASPAR) were recruited from the outpatient rheumatology department at the Hospital das Clínicas, UFPE. The PsAQoL was administered to participants on two occasions, with 14 days between administrations. The measure consists of 20 items with a dichotomous response format (True/Not True). The number of 'True' responses is summed to produce a total score ranging from 0 to 20, with a higher score indicating poorer quality of life. At the first administration, – the Nottingham Health Profile was included in the postal survey as a comparator questionnaire (NHP) [9]. The NHP is a generic measure of perceived distress consisting of 38 items covering six sections: physical mobility, pain, energy level, emotional reactions, sleep and social isolation. For each section, scores range from 0 to 100, with higher scores indicative of greater perceived distress. Demographic and disease information was also collected from participants. An ID number was allocated to all participants to ensure anonymity and to allow the data collected at each administration to be matched.

The following analyses were conducted on the survey data.

Descriptive statistics for the PsAQoL at both time points and NHP scores at baseline were calculated. PsAQoL scores were also compared by age group (above median versus below median) and gender. Internal consistency is a measure of the extent to which items in a scale are inter-related. This was assessed using Cronbach's alpha coefficients. An alpha value above 0.7 indicates that the items are sufficiently related to form a scale. Test-retest reliability is an estimate of reproducibility over time, assuming no change in condition has occurred. This was assessed by correlating PsAQoL cores obtained on the two administrations, using Spearman's rank correlation coefficients. A value of 0.85 or above indicates that the instrument produces low levels of random measurement error.

Convergent validity was assessed by measuring the association between scores on one scale and those on a comparator measure that measures the same or related constructs. PsAQoL scores were correlated with scores on the NHP sections using Spearman rank correlation coefficients. Known group validity was demonstrated by testing the ability of the PsAQoL to distinguish between groups of people that differed according to their perceived general health (poor/fair/good/excellent), perceived disease severity (mild/moderate/quite severe/very severe) and whether they were currently experiencing a flare (yes/no). Mann-Whitney U tests were used to investigate whether there were differences in PsAQoL scores between these groups.

The statistical analyses were conducted using SPSS (version 25.0). Non-parametric tests were employed due to the data collected measuring at the ordinal level.

Results

Translation of the PsAQoL

The bilingual panel consisted of four female and two male participants aged between 19 and 25 years. Overall, the panel found the questionnaire items and instructions easy to translate. There was discussion concerning the 'True/Not true' response options, in which the panel suggested 'Yes/No' (Sim/Não) as this was considered more natural in Brazilian Portuguese. The item 'I take it out on people close to me' was considered particularly difficult to translate because it is a colloquial expression in English. After much discussion, the panel was able to find an appropriate translation that captured the intended meaning.

The lay panel consisted of three male and two female patients aged between 48 and 60 years. Only minor changes were made to three items, including the removal of pronouns and replacing 'the disease' with 'my disease' to improve immediacy and clarity. All panel members agreed that the final translations were easy to understand and sounded natural in Brazilian Portuguese.

Assessment of face and content validity

Ten CDIs were conducted with PsA patients, of whom eight were female. The mean time taken to complete the questionnaire was 4 min (range = 3–6 min). Overall, the questionnaire was considered clear and easy to understand and complete. All patients felt that the items reflected their own situation well and they could relate to the ideas expressed. No items were thought to be irrelevant or inappropriate, resulting in no changes being made to the questionnaire following this stage.

Psychometric evaluation

Fifty-two participants took part in the validation study and completed the PsAQoL on two occasions.

Demographic and disease information of the sample is provided in Table 1.

Scores obtained on the PsAQoL and NHP are shown in Table 2. The median score for the Brazilian Portuguese PsAQoL did not change between administrations of the postal survey. No floor or ceiling effects were observed for the PsAQoL. In contrast, half of the NHP sections (energy level; sleep; social isolation) demonstrated

Table 1 Demographic and disease information of postal survey sample ($n = 52$)

Age (years)	
Mean (SD)	54.7 (11.8)
Range	24.5–78.6
Gender (%)	
Male	17 (32.7)
Female	35 (67.3)
Marital Status (%)	
Married/Living as Married	31 (59.6)
Divorced	4 (7.7)
Widowed	4 (7.7)
Single	13 (25.0)
Work Status (%)	
Full-time	10 (19.2)
Part-time	4 (7.7)
Retired	14 (26.9)
Long term sick leave	10 (19.2)
Homemaker	7 (13.5)
Unemployed	7 (13.5)
Perceived disease severity (%)	
Mild	16 (30.8)
Moderate	19 (36.5)
Quite Severe	14 (26.9)
Very Severe	3 (5.8)
Perceived general health (%)	
Excellent	2 (3.8)
Good	14 (26.9)
Fair	30 (57.7)
Poor	6 (11.5)
Flare (%)	
Yes	14 (26.9)
No	38 (73.1)
Disease Duration (years)	
Mean (SD)	8.9 (6.6)
Range	0.5–30

Table 2 Descriptive statistics for the PsAQoL and NHP sections

	n	Median (IQR)	Min - Max	% scoring minimum	% scoring maximum
PsAQoL (Time 1)	52	9.0 (3.0–14.0)	0.0–19.0	7.7	0.0
PsAQoL (Time 2)	52	9.0 (2.0–13.8)	0.0–20.0	11.5	1.9
NHP					
Energy level	52	33.3 (0.0–91.7)	0.0–100.0	36.5	25.0
Pain	52	56.3 (25.0–75.0)	0.0–100.0	13.5	5.8
Emotional reactions	52	44.4 (22.2–77.8)	0.0–100.0	13.5	3.8
Sleep	52	40.0 (0.0–80.0)	0.0–100.0	32.7	13.5
Social isolation	52	20.0 (0.0–40.0)	0.0–100.0	36.5	3.8
Physical mobility	52	50.0 (25.0–62.5)	0.0–87.5	9.6	0.0

PsAQoL Psoriatic Arthritis Quality of Life sale, *NHP* Nottingham Health Profile, *IQR* Inter-quartile range

large floor effects. Respondents scored highest on the pain and physical mobility NHP sections.

The PsAQoL demonstrated high internal consistency. Cronbach's alpha coefficients for the PsAQoL were 0.91 and 0.93 at Time 1 and 2, respectively, indicating that the items are sufficiently inter-related. A correlation coefficient of 0.90 was found for test-retest reliability, suggesting the questionnaire will produce low levels of random measurement error.

Correlation coefficients between scores on the PsAQoL and NHP sections are presented in Table 3.

PsAQoL scores correlated most strongly with the emotional reactions section of the NHP. Strong correlations were observed between PsAQoL scores and those obtained on the energy level, physical mobility and social isolation NHP sections.

Table 4 shows PsAQoL scores for patients grouped by gender and age (above versus below median age). No significant difference in PsAQoL scores was found between older and younger patients. However, a significant difference in PsAQoL scores between males and females was observed, with females scoring significantly higher than males. A chi-square test of independence was performed to explore whether females had worse general health or disease severity compared to males. No significant association was found between gender and perceived disease severity (χ^2 (52) = 0.12, $p = 0.73$) or between gender and perceived general health, (χ^2 (52) = 0.24, $p = 0.62$).

Due to the relatively small number in each group, the categories for perceived disease severity were grouped into 'mild/moderate' and 'quite severe/very severe' for the known group analyses. The categories for perceived general health were grouped into 'excellent/good' and 'fair/poor' for the same reason.

Mann Whitney U tests demonstrated significant differences in PsAQoL scores between patients who differed according to their perceived disease severity (Fig. 1), perceived general health (Fig. 2) and whether they were experiencing a flare (Fig. 3).

Discussion

The dual-panel methodology resulted in a Brazilian Portuguese version of the PsAQoL that was comprehensible, natural and reflected the same concepts as the original UK English. Cognitive debriefing interviews confirmed that the content of the measure was appropriate to Brazilian patients. The PsAoL was considered relevant, comprehensive and easy for local respondents to complete. The new language version demonstrated excellent internal consistency, test-retest reliability and was capable of detecting meaningful differences between PsA

Table 3 Association between PsAQoL and NHP section scores ($n = 52$)

	PsAQoL
NHP	
Energy level	0.75
Pain	0.69
Emotional reactions	0.89
Sleep	0.65
Social isolation	0.71
Physical mobility	0.75

All correlations significant at the 0.01 level (2-tailed)

Table 4 Median PsAQoL scores by demographic factors

	n	Median (IQR)
Gender		
Male	17	3 (1–10.5)
Female	35	11 (5–15)
p		< 0.05
Age		
Below Median	25	8 (1–15)
Above Median	26	9 (4.8–13.3)
p		0.41

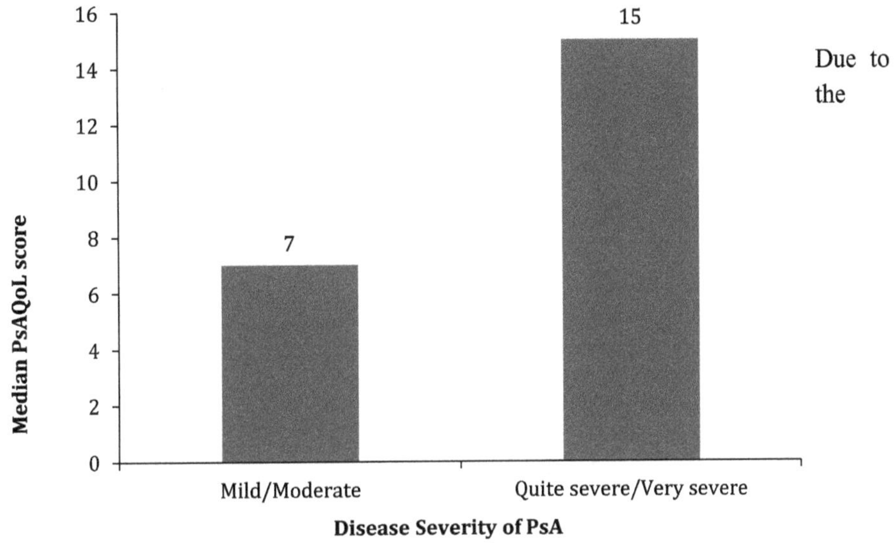

Fig. 1 PsAQoL scores by perceived disease severity ($p < 0.01$)

patients in terms of perceived ratings of disease severity, general health and presence of flare.

Cronbach's Alpha coefficients for at both administrations of the PsAQoL were above 0.9, suggesting the items are adequately related to form a measure. The high value obtained for test-retest reliability indicates that the Brazilian Portuguese PsAQoL will produce low levels of random measurement error. This means that smaller samples are required to detect changes in QoL resulting from treatment. The PsAQoL correlated as expected with NHP sections, demonstrating that QoL is largely influenced by pain and physical mobility. However, the PsAQoL was also capable of detecting the impact of emotional and social issues associated with PsA, suggesting QoL is dependent on multiple factors in this patient group. Findings to support known group validity were in line with the results of other studies that have validated new language versions of the PsAQoL [10–12].

The PsAQoL is a widely used measure of QoL specific to PsA patients. It is one of several disease-specific

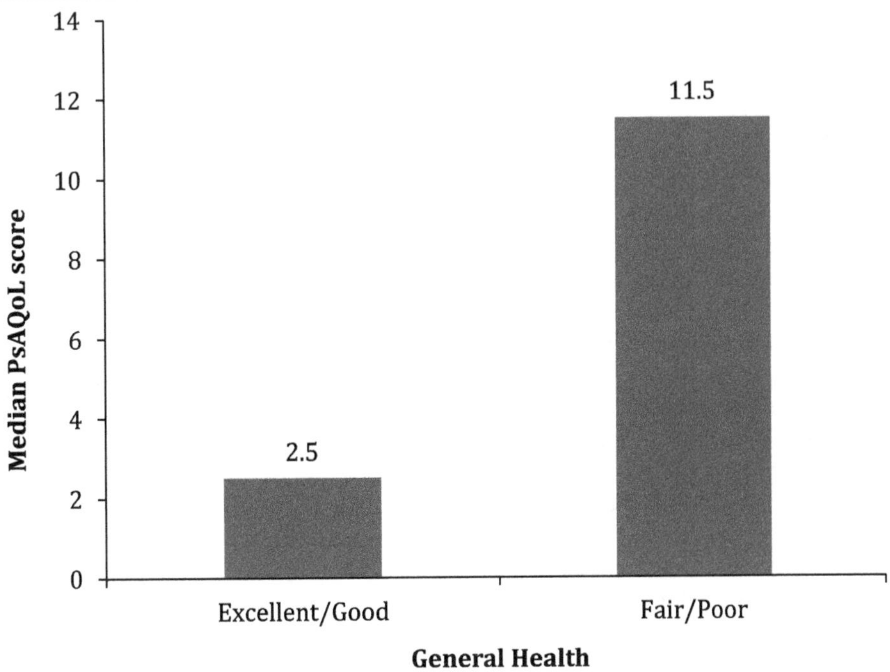

Fig. 2 PsAQoL scores by perceived general health ($p < 0.001$)

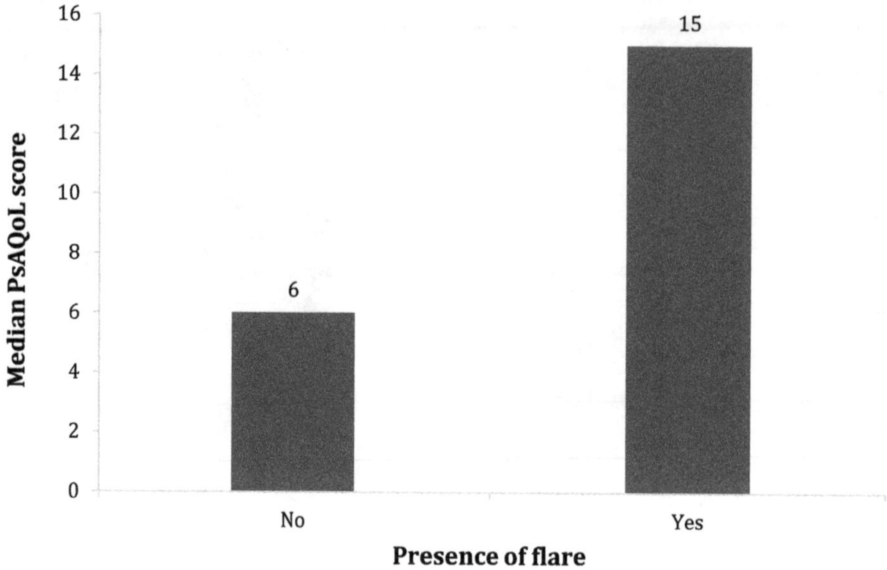

Fig. 3 PsAQoL scores by presence of flare ($p < 0.001$)

instruments based on the needs-based model of QoL that are used in rheumatology [13, 14]. These instruments differ from traditional patient-reported outcome measures, which predominantly assess HRQL. Whereas HRQL collects information that is primarily of interest to clinicians, needs-based questionnaires cover relevant issues that are important to the lives of patients and are truly patient-based. Because the PsAQoL assesses a different type of outcome to other available PROMS, it can be used in combination with measures such as the HAQ and NHP.

Differences in QoL scores between males and females were found, in contrast to other adaptations studies of the PsAQoL and the original UK English version [3, 12, 15]. An additional adaptation of the Cambridge Pulmonary Hypertension Outcome Review (CAMPHOR; a measure of HRQL and needs-based QoL) [16] was recently conducted for use with Pulmonary Hypertension patients in Brazil [17]. Significant differences in scores between males and females were found on all CAMP HOR scales, which appeared to be caused by gender differences in ratings of perceived general health. However, research conducted across 14 countries suggested that despite having similar levels of disease activity, female PsA patients demonstrated worse patient-reported outcomes across quality of life, level of disability and impact of disease [18]. This finding that the impact of PsA seems to be greater in women is one possible explanation for the gender differences in QoL scores that were found in the current sample.

The availability of a Brazilian Portuguese version of the PsAQoL provides a valid and reliable means of evaluating QoL as well as determining the value gained by patients from both clinical and non-clinical interventions. The new language version can also be incorporated in international clinical trials, which are increasingly including South American countries.

The main limitation of the present study is the relatively small sample size. Further research is required to evaluate the responsiveness of the new language version.

Conclusion

The Brazilian Portuguese version of the PsAQoL demonstrated excellent psychometric properties. The new language version will prove to be a valuable addition to the PsA community, offering a means of evaluating QoL in routine clinical practice, research studies and international clinical trials in Brazil.

Acknowledgements

The authors would like to acknowledge all participants who took part in the study.

Authors, contributions

Study concept and design: SPM and AH. Data collection: RSGG, JBC, MELV, MCMB, GAP, ALBPD. Statistical analysis and data interpretation: AH and SPM. RSGG prepared the first version of the manuscript and all authors contributed to critical revision of the manuscript. All authors gave final approval of the version to be published.

Author details

[1]Hospital das Clinicas da Universidade Federal de Pernambuco, Recife, Brazil. [2]Galen Research Ltd, Manchester, UK. [3]School of Health Sciences, University of Manchester, Manchester, UK.

References

1. Ritchlin CT, Colbert RA, Gladman DD. Psoriatic arthritis. N Engl J Med. 2017; 376(10):957–70.

2. Taylor W, Gladman D, Helliwell P, Marchesoni A, Mease P, Mielants H, et al. Classification criteria for psoriatic arthritis: development of new criteria from a large international study. Arthritis Rheum. 2006;54(8):2665–73.
3. McKenna SP, Doward LC, Whalley D, Tennant A, Emery P, Veale DJ. Development of the PsAQoL: a quality of life instrument specific to psoriatic arthritis. Ann Rheum Dis. 2004;63(2):162–9.
4. Turan Y, Duruoz MT, Cerrahoglu L. Relationship between enthesitis, clinical parameters and quality of life in spondyloarthritis. Joint Bone Spine. 2009; 76(6):642–7.
5. Bruce B, Fries JF. The Stanford Health Assessment Questionnaire: dimensions and practical applications. Health Qual Life Outcomes. 2003; 1:20.
6. U.S. Department of Health and Human Services FDA Center for Drug Evaluation and Research; U.S. Department of Health and Human Services FDA Center for Biologics Evaluation and Research; U.S. Department of Health and Human Services FDA Center for Devices and Radiological Health. Guidance for industry: patient-reported outcome measures: use in medical product development to support labeling claims: draft guidance. Health Qual Life Outcomes. 2006;4:79. https://doi.org/10.1186/1477-7525-4-79.
7. McKenna SP. Measuring patient-reported outcomes: moving beyond misplaced common sense to hard science. BMC Med. 2011;9:86.
8. Hunt SM, Alonso J, Bucquet D, Niero M, Wiklund I, McKenna S. Cross-cultural adaptation of health measures. European Group for Health Management and Quality of Life Assessment. Health Policy. 1991;19(1):33–44.
9. Hunt SM, McKenna SP, McEwen J, Williams J, Papp E. The Nottingham health profile: subjective health status and medical consultations. Soc Sci Med A. 1981;15(3 Pt 1):221–9.
10. Billing E, McKenna SP, Staun M, Lindqvist U. Adaptation of the Psoriatic Arthritis Quality of Life (PsAQoL) instrument for Sweden. Scand J Rheumatol. 2010;39(3):223–8.
11. Wink F, Arends S, McKenna SP, Houtman PM, Brouwer E, Spoorenberg A. Validity and reliability of the Dutch adaptation of the Psoriatic Arthritis Quality of Life (PsAQoL) Questionnaire. PLoS One. 2013;8(2): e55912.
12. Barcelos A, Ambrosio C, Pereira da Silva JA, McKenna S, Wilburn J, Lopes Ferreira P. Psoriatic Arthritis Quality of Life questionnaire: translation, cultural adaptation and validation into Portuguese language. Rheumatol Int. 2018; 38(2):249–54.
13. Keenan AM, McKenna SP, Doward LC, Conaghan PG, Emery P, Tennant A. Development and validation of a needs-based quality of life instrument for osteoarthritis. Arthritis Rheum. 2008;59(6):841–8.
14. Doward LC, Spoorenberg A, Cook SA, Whalley D, Helliwell PS, Kay LJ, et al. Development of the ASQoL: a quality of life instrument specific to ankylosing spondylitis. Ann Rheum Dis. 2003;62(1):20–6.
15. Heaney A, Stepanous J, McKenna SP, Athanassiou P, Vidalis AA. Translation and validation of the greek psoriatic arthritis quality of life scale. Psychiatriki. 2017;28(3):219.
16. McKenna SP, Doughty N, Meads DM, Doward LC, Pepke-Zaba J. The Cambridge Pulmonary Hypertension Outcome Review (CAMPHOR): a measure of health-related quality of life and quality of life for patients with pulmonary hypertension. Qual Life Res. 2006;15(1):103–15.
17. Correa RA, Pereira MC, Bizzi MF, de Oliveira RWR, Rezende CF, de Oliveira B, et al. Adaptation and validation of the quality of life assessment of the Cambridge pulmonary hypertension outcome review (CAMPHOR) for Brazil. J Patient Rep Outcomes. 2020;4(1):43.
18. Orbai AM, Perin J, Gorlier C, Coates LC, Kiltz U, Leung YY, Palominos PE, Cañete JD, Scrivo R, Balanescu A, Dernis E, Tälli S, Ruyssen-Witrand A, Soubrier M, Aydin S, Eder L, Gaydukova I, Lubrano E, Kalyoncu U, Richette P, Husni ME, Smolen JS, de Wit M, Gossec L. Determinants of Patient-Reported Psoriatic Arthritis Impact of Disease: An Analysis of the Association With Sex in 458 Patients From Fourteen Countries. Arthritis Care Res (Hoboken). 2020; 72(12):1772–79. https://doi.org/10.1002/acr.24090.

15

Association of homocysteine with ankylosing spondylitis

Hui-hui Li[1,2†], Xue-quan Li[3†], Lin-tao Sai[4], Yi Cui[5], Jia-hui Xu[6], Chi Zhou[7], Jing Zheng[2], Xing-fu Li[8], Hua-xiang Liu[8*] and Ying-jie Zhao[2,8*]

Abstract

Background: Hyperhomocysteinemia is associated with autoimmune diseases such as ankylosing spondylitis (AS), systemic lupus erythematosus (SLE), and rheumatoid arthritis (RA). Current findings regarding plasma/serum homocysteine (HCY) levels in AS patients are inconsistent. This study aims to systematically evaluate the association between circulating HCY levels and AS.

Methods: Online electronic databases (PubMed, Web of Science, Embase, ScienceDirect, China National Knowledge Infrastructure (CNKI), and Wanfang data) were used to retrieve all relevant articles published up to May 7, 2020. The pooled standardized mean difference (SMD) with 95% confidence interval (CI) was calculated using the random-effect model, Stata16 software.

Results: Nine articles containing 778 AS patients and 522 controls were included in this meta-analysis. No significant differences in HCY levels were found between AS and control groups (pooled SMD = 0.46, 95% CI = −0.30 to 1.23, $P = 0.23$). However, subgroup analysis suggested that HCY levels were significantly higher ($P < 0.05$) in the AS group treated with methotrexate (MTX) compared with the control group. In contrast, HCY levels were significantly ($P < 0.05$) lower in the AS group receiving anti-TNF-α treatment compared with the control group. No significant differences were detected between HCY levels and disease activity scores (Bath AS disease activity index, BASDAI), and methylenetetrahydrofolate reductase (MTHFR) C677T genotype.

Conclusion: This meta-analysis indicates that HCY levels are similar between AS and controls, and do not correlate with disease activity. However, different medical treatments cause fluctuations of circulating HCY levels in AS patients. Further and larger-scale studies are needed to confirm these findings.

Trial registration: This study was registered at international prospective register of systematic reviews (PROSPERO), registration number: CRD42020184426.

Keywords: Homocysteine, Meta-analysis, Ankylosing spondylitis, Controls

* Correspondence: lzzlhx63@163.com; yzhaoqilu@sdu.edu.cn
†Hui-hui Li and Xue-quan Li contributed equally to this work.
[8]Department of Rheumatology, Qilu Hospital, Cheeloo College of Medicine, Shandong University, Jinan 250012, Shandong, China
[2]Department of Obstetrics and Gynecology, University of Wisconsin-Madison, Madison, WI 53715, USA

Background

Ankylosing spondylitis (AS) is an immune-associated systemic inflammatory rheumatic disease characterized primarily by progressive inflammation of the spine, sacroiliitis, and various extra-articular manifestations such as anterior uveitis, inflammatory bowel disease, subclinical inflammation of the gut, psoriasis, airway disease, and interstitial lung abnormalities [1–6]. Increasing evidence indicates that AS increases cardiovascular morbidity and mortality as compared with the general population [7].

Homocysteine (HCY) is a sulfur-containing amino acid formed during the metabolism of methionine to cysteine [8]. HCY levels are elevated in many acquired disorders such as cardiovascular disease, cerebrovascular disease, dementia-type disorders, osteoporosis-associated fractures, chronic renal disease, autoimmune diseases, inflammatory diseases, deficiency of vitamins B6, B12, or folic acid, as well as during anti-folate drug therapy [9–19] Elevated HCY may trigger autoimmune reactions through binding and structurally modifying specific proteins, resulting in the formation of neoantigens that are potentially relevant either in the onset of specific autoimmune diseases or in the progression of the associated cardiovascular damage [20].

HCY could modify Human Leukocyte Antigens-B27 (HLA-B27) through forming a disulfide bond with an unpaired cysteine residue at position 67 (Cys67) of the HLA-B27 heavy chain [21], and subsequently, be destroyed by the abnormal autoimmunological reactions [21]. An in vitro study has shown HCY could induce specific cytotoxic T lymphocytes (CTLs), and HLA-B27-restricted HCY-specific CTLs are more often found in B27-positive patients [21]. HCY-treated B cells can be specifically lysed by CTLs in patients with AS and reactive arthritis (ReA) [21]. Evidence also suggests that Salmonella infection could lead to the modification of HLA antigens and such modified HLA antigens can be recognized by HCY-specific CTLs [21]. Collectively, these findings support the notion that HCY may be involved in the mechanism underlying HLA-B27-associated AS.

Previous studies have shown both pro-inflammatory and anti-inflammatory properties of HCY [22–25]. An association between hyperhomocysteinemia and inflammation has been identified in human and experimental animal models [17, 26]. In vitro, HCY induces mRNA and protein expression of the inflammatory cytokines including tumor necrosis factor (TNF)-α, Interleukin (IL)-1β, IL-6, IL-8, and IL-12 in human monocytes [27]. Correlations of HCY with soluble 75-kDa TNF-receptor (sTNF-R75) has also been found in RA patients [28]. HCY may activate nuclear factor-kappaB (NF-κB) activation [29], which may lead to increased chemokine expression in vascular smooth muscle cells (VSMCs) and macrophages [30, 31]. HCY, at the range of physiologic concentrations, enhances monocyte proliferation in vitro [27]. HCY may also be involved in corona virus disease-19 (COVID-19) infection via transsulfuration pathway [32], which is catalyzed by cystathionine β-synthase and cystathionine γ-lyase (CSE) and serves as a modulator of inflammation [33]. Nevertheless, HCY significantly ameliorates cholesterol-induced inflammation in an in vivo hypercholesterolemic rat model possibly by acting on the tissue plasminogen activator (tPA)-induced process [24].

Based on the facts that AS is associated with increased cardiovascular morbidity and mortality, the high level of HCY is considered a well-known risk factor for cardiovascular disease [7, 8], it is necessary to define the association between HCY and AS. However, the conclusions of HCY levels reported in AS patients are inconsistent. Several studies reported high levels of serum/plasma HCY levels in AS patients [34–38]. In contrast, others claimed that HCY levels in AS patients were similar or lower compared with control patients [16, 39–41]. Therefore, in this meta-analysis, we aim to determine HCY levels in AS and investigate the correlation between HCY levels and disease activity and medical treatments.

Methods

Search strategy

We performed electronic literature searches in PubMed, Web of Science, Embase, ScienceDirect, China National Knowledge Infrastructure (CNKI), and Wanfang data up to May 7, 2020 with keywords including Homocysteine, Hyperhomocysteinemia, Ankylosing, and Spondylitis.

Inclusion criteria and exclusion criteria

The article inclusion criteria were as follows: (1) a case-control or cross-sectional study; (2) based on adults; (3) AS patients must conform to the American College of Rheumatology (ACR) criteria [42] or European Spondyloarthropathy Study Group (ESSG) criteria for classification of spondylarthropathies [43]; and (4) serum or plasma HCY concentrations of both patients and controls were available. Articles were not limited to geographic location or language of publication. Articles excluded in this meta-analysis were as follows: (1) reviews; (2) animal studies; and (3) lack of controls. A detailed flow chart of article inclusion and exclusion process was presented in Fig. 1. All articles obtained electronically were examined independently by two researchers.

Data extraction and quality assessment

Each of the enrolled articles was extracted by two researchers independently for the following information: first author's name, year of publication, study design, the

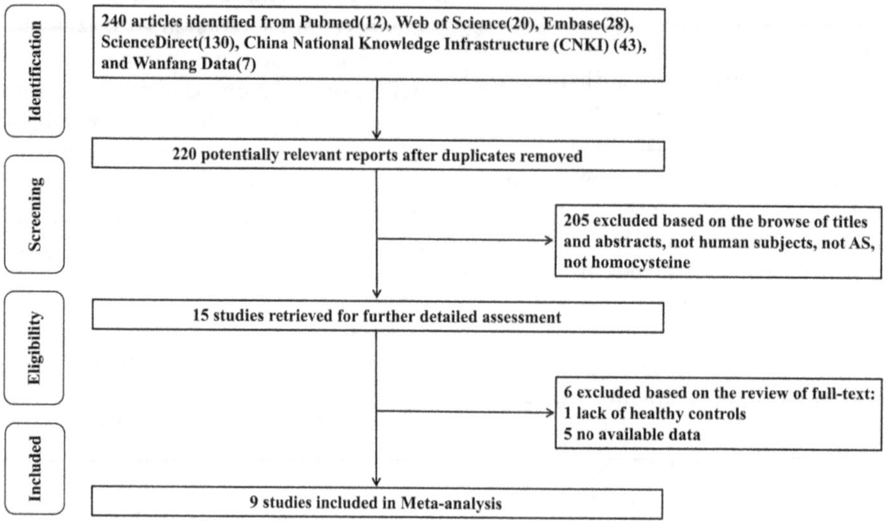

Fig. 1 Flow chart of selected articles

language of the article, region, participants' characteristics (age and gender), disease activity score (Bath AS disease activity index, BASDAI) [44], disease duration, mean ± SD or mean ± SEM of the plasma/serum HCY levels in AS and control groups, measurement method, sample type, and any other relevant information. Meta-analysis was performed according to the Preferred Reporting Items for Systematic Reviews and Meta-Analysis (PRISMA) guidelines [45]. Any disagreement on study inclusion or data extraction was discussed with a third reviewer to reach a consensus. The Newcastle-Ottawa quality assessment scale (NOS) was used to assess the methodological quality of eligible studies [46].

Statistical analysis

The extracted results that were presented in median, standard error, range, and interquartile range were converted to mean and standard deviation (SD) [47, 48]. The mean and SD (mean ± SD) were extracted or estimated in each study. For each study, the standardized mean difference (SMD) and 95% confidence intervals (95% CI) were elaborately shown by the forest plot. Cochrane *Q* statistics (chi-square test, χ2) were employed to evaluate statistical heterogeneity. The *I*-square (I^2) statistics was used to further assess the extent of heterogeneity ($I^2 = ([Q - df]) \times 100\%$) [49]. Based on the Cochrane Handbook for Systematic Reviews' recommendations, we interpreted I^2 statistic between 0 and 40% as representing an insignificant amount of heterogeneity; 30 to 60% as moderate heterogeneity; 50 to 90% as substantial heterogeneity; and 75 to 100% as considerable heterogeneity [50]. When $P < 0.05$ for the Q test or $I^2 > 50$, it indicated that heterogeneity was significant in the study. Assuming that the heterogeneity is significant, the random-effects model was adopted to pool the SMD value; or else, the fixed-effect model was adopted. Subgroup analysis was performed to discover the sources of heterogeneity. Sensitivity analysis was also executed to detect studies that extremely contributed to the observed heterogeneity. This was done by omitting each study one after the other to measure its impact on the summary estimate. To evaluate the publication bias, Egger's and Begg's tests were used. Stata 16 software was used in this meta-analysis to perform statistical analysis.

Results

Publication search and study characteristics

Out of a total of 15 relevant studies found, 9 original studies met our inclusion criteria and were selected for this meta-analysis. These 9 studies were published between 2005 and 2020 and included 778 AS patients and 522 controls [16, 34–41]. Of the 9 studies, 4 were conducted in Asia, 3 in Asia-Europe (Turkey), 1 in Europe, and 1 in South America. As of the controls, 1 study included non-inflammatory low back pain [39], 1 included osteoarthritis or soft tissue rheumatism [41], and the other 7 included healthy controls [16, 34–38, 40]. Our methodological quality assessment showed the NOS scores of included studies ranged from 7 to 8. The characteristics of the included studies are summarized in Table 1. Extracted data on circulating HCY levels were presented in Table 2.

Results of meta-analysis

Publication bias was assessed by Egger's regression test ($t = -0.74$, $P = 0.48$) and Begg's test ($z = -0.31$, $P = 1.25$), suggesting no publication bias present. Among the enrolled studies, significant heterogeneity was observed

Table 1 Characteristics of individual studies included

First author, year	Region	AS					Control						
		Age (year) (mean ± sd)	BMI	Sex ratio (M/F)	BASDAI	Duration (year) (mean ± sd)	Age (year) (mean ± sd)	BMI	Sex ratio (M/F)	Assay method, sample	Study type	Criteria for the classification	NOS
Shu JL, 2020 [16]	Mainland China	41.6 ± 8.6	NA	30/5	NA	NA	39.7 ± 14.4	NA	36/5	NA	CS	ACR	7
Geçene M, 2013 [39]	Turkey	36.7 ± 4.8	24.9 ± 3.1	50/0	2.4 ± 1.7	NA	36.3 ± 4.7	25.0 ± 3.0	50/0	HPLC, plasma	CS	ACR	7
Mao N, 2012 [34]	Mainland China	NA	NA	NA	NA	NA	NA	NA	NA	ELISA, plasma	CS	ACR	7
Capkin E, 2012 [40]	Turkey	36.4 ± 11.2	NA	88/20	3.7 ± 1.6	8.4 ± 5.6	38.2 ± 13.0	NA	49/16	ELISA, plasma	CS	ACR	7
Başkan BM, 2009 [35]	Turkey	40.1 ± 11.0	NA	NA	4.2 ± 1.7	10.0 ± 7.7	38.1 ± 0.6	NA	NA	NA	CS	ACR	7
Gonzalez-Lopez L, 2008 [36]	Mexico	39.9 ± 8.4	26.0 ± 2.8	73/24	5.4 ± 2.1	7.8 ± 6.0	38.9 ± 7.8	25.8 ± 4.2	73/24	FPIA, Serum	CSS	ACR	8
Wei JC, 2007 [37]	Taiwan, China	NA	NA	NA	NA	NA	NA	NA	NA	ELISA, plasma	CSS	ACR	7
Malesci D, 2007 [41]	Italy	47.6 ± 11.8	29.5 ± 4.4	21/3	2.7 ± 1.8	18.5 ± 10.8	49.6 ± 6.0	NA	16/3	NA	CS	ACR&ESSG	8
Xu XY, 2005 [38]	Mainland China	32.1 ± 13.7	NA	44/16	NA	NA	30.8 ± 19.7	NA	30/32	FPIA, plasma	CS	ACR	7

AS Ankylosing spondylitis, *BMI* Body mass index, *BASDAI* Bath AS disease activity index, *NOS* Newcastle-Ottawa Scale, *NA* Not available, *HPLC* High performance liquid chromatography, *ELISA* Enzyme-linked immunosorbent assays, *FPIA* Fluorescence polarization immunoassay, *CS* Case control, *CSS* Cross-sectional study, *ACR* American College of Rheumatology, *ESSG* European Spondyloarthropathy Study Group

($I^2 = 97.3\%$, $P < 0.01$). Sensitivity analysis by sequentially omitting individual studies did not significantly change the pooled results, suggesting that these results were stable (Fig. 2).

HCY levels and subgroup analysis

The random-effect model was used for the analysis of results in this study based on the result that significant heterogeneity was observed among the enrolled studies ($P < 0.01$). There were no significant differences in circulating HCY levels between AS patients and controls (pooled SMD = 0.46, 95% CI = − 0.30 to 1.23, $P = 0.23$) (Fig. 3). Subgroup analysis stratified by region, sample size, disease activity, smoker or not, methylenetetrahydrofolate reductase (MTHFR) C677T genotype, and medication treatment were performed (Table 3). As of disease activity, 1 study defined that patients with BASDAI values ≥4 were regarded as active AS group [40]. Two studies defined that patients with BASDAI values > 3 and ESR > 20 mm/h were regarded as active AS group [35, 37]. To conduct medication treatment subgroup analysis, we analyzed four subgroups: nonsteroidal anti-inflammatory drugs (NSAIDs), sulfasalazine (SSZ), SSZ + methotrexate (MTX), and anti-TNF-α. In SSZ + MTX treatment subgroup, HCY levels in AS patients were significantly higher than those in controls (pooled SMD = 0.915, 95% CI = 0.312 to 1.518, $P = 0.003$). In anti-TNF-α treatment subgroup, HCY levels in AS patients were significantly lower than in controls (pooled SMD = − 0.774, 95% CI = − 1.163 to − 0.385, $P < 0.001$). Meanwhile, no significant differences of HCY levels between AS patients and controls were detected in NSAIDs or SSZ treatment subgroup. In particular, no significant correlation between HCY levels and disease activity, and MTHFR C677T genotype, as well as in region, sample size, and smoking subgroups was detected.

Table 2 Extracted data on HCY levels of 9 studies included

First author, year	AS (μmol/L)			Control (μmol/L)		
	N	Mean	SD	*N*	Mean	SD
Shu JL, 2020 [16]	35	12.27	7.52	41	13.94	3.73
Geçene M, 2013 [39]	50	14.26	9.96	50	11.81	5.53
Mao N, 2012 [34]	200	18.71	2.42	120	10.97	2.93
Capkin E, 2012 [40]	108	18.90	8.70	65	23.80	5.80
Başkan BM, 2009 [35]	92	17.18	12.47	58	13.16	4.09
Gonzalez-Lopez L, 2008 [35]	97	11.35	5.39	97	9.61	2.33
Wei JC, 2007 [37]	112	9.91	3.47	10	8.60	1.20
Malesci D, 2007 [41]	24	8.70	2.00	19	9.10	1.20
Xu XY, 2005 [38]	60	16.47	6.50	62	12.24	3.58

HCY Homocysteine, *N* Number, *SD* Standard deviation

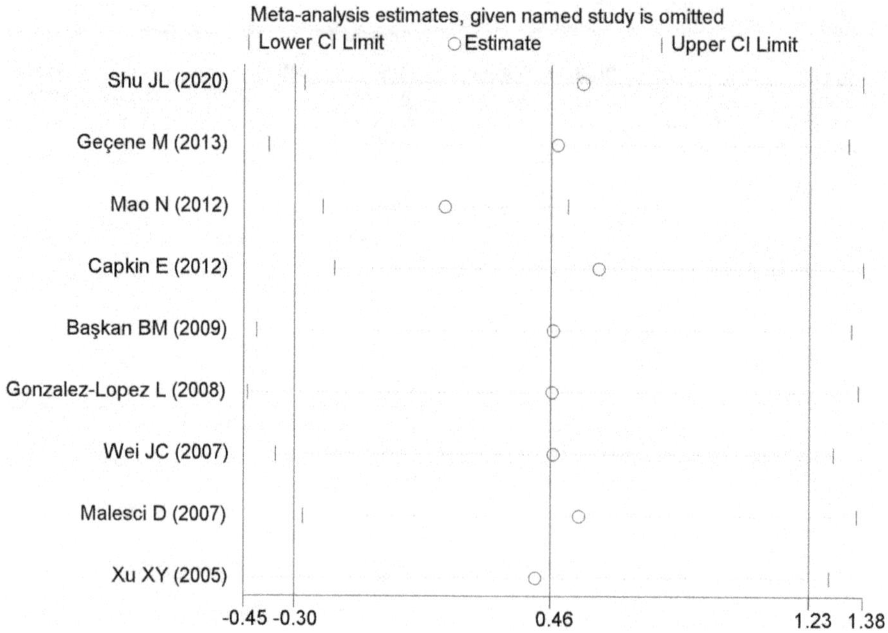

Fig. 2 Sensitivity analysis of the included studies. The two vertical axes, vertical middle axis, hollow circles, and two ends of the dotted lines respectively represent 95% confidence interval, overall odd ratio, pooled odd ratios, and 95% confidence interval

Discussion

A positive relationship was reported between circulating HCY levels and certain clinical features of rheumatoid arthritis (RA), such as higher disease activity [51] and higher radiological damage [52]. A significant correlation also exists between HCY levels and the various indexes of disease activity of systemic lupus erythematosus (SLE), such as erythrocyte sedimentation rate, anti-double-stranded DNA, complement levels in patients of SLE [15]. Intensive steroid therapy in RA patients results in significant HCY reduction [53]. In contrast, Shu et al. has reported that HCY levels are not associated with C-

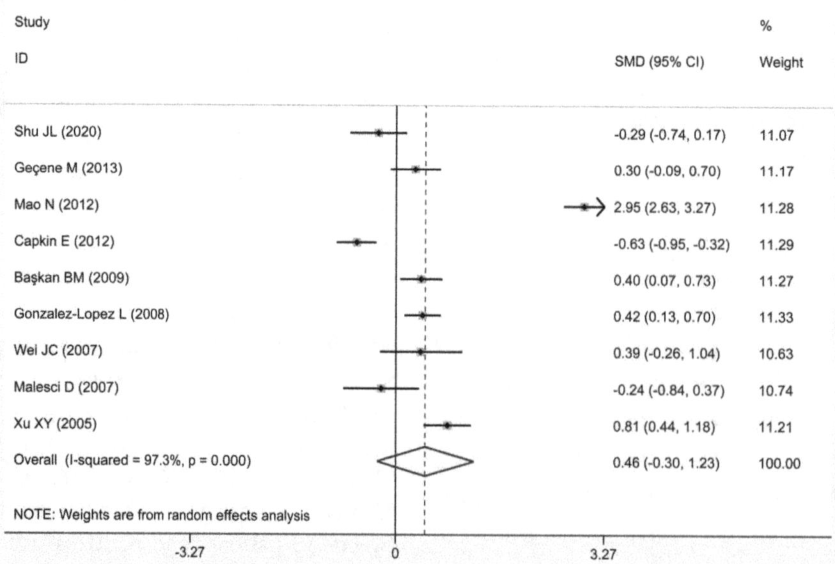

Fig. 3 Forest plot of 9 studies in HCY levels for AS patients versus controls, based on random effects model

Table 3 Subgroup analysis of HCY levels in AS

Subgroups		*N*	SMD (95% CI)	*Z*	*P*	Heterogeneity test	
						P	I^2 (%)
Region	Asia	4	0.974 (−0.573, 2.521)	1.23	0.217	< 0.001	98.1%
	Asia + Europe (Turkey)	3	0.018 (− 0.661, 0.698)	0.05	0.958	< 0.001	91.4%
	Europe/America	2	0.148 (−0.484, 0.780)	0.46	0.646	0.055	73.0%
	Combined	9	0.463 (−0.300, 1.226)	1.19	0.234	< 0.001	97.3%
Sample size	≥ 50	6	0.708 (−0.283, 1.700)	1.40	0.162	< 0.001	98.1%
	< 50	2	−0.269 (− 0.632, 0.093)	1.46	0.145	0.891	0.0%
	Combined	8	0.471 (−0.355, 1.298)	1.12	0.264	< 0.001	97.6%
Disease activity	active	3	0.048 (−0.904, 1.000)	0.10	0.921	< 0.001	92.0%
	inactive	3	0.078 (−0.733, 0.889)	0.19	0.851	< 0.001	89.0%
	Combined	6	0.059 (−0.488, 0.606)	0.21	0.833	< 0.001	88.5%
Smoking	Smoker	1	0.497 (−0.066, 1.060)	1.73	0.084	NA	NA
	Non-smoker	1	0.201 (−0.355, 0.757)	0.71	0.478	NA	NA
	Combined	2	0.347 (−0.048, 0.743)	1.72	0.085	0.464	0.0%
MTHFR C677T genotype	CC	2	1.599 (−0.864, 4.062)	1.27	0.203	< 0.001	98.1%
	CT	2	1.693(−1.256, 4.642)	1.13	0.260	< 0.001	97.7%
	TT	2	2.771(−1.141, 6.682)	1.39	0.165	< 0.001	92.2%
	Combined	6	1.992 (0.663, 3.320)	2.94	0.003	< 0.001	95.7%
Treatment	NSAIDs	2	−0.365(− 1.020, 0.291)	1.09	0.275	0.092	64.8%
	SSZ	2	0.024 (−0.872, 0.920)	0.05	0.958	0.003	88.7%
	SSZ + MTX	1	0.915 (0.312, 1.518)	2.97	0.003	NA	NA
	Anti-TNF-α	1	−0.774 (−1.163, − 0.385)	3.90	< 0.001	NA	NA
	Combined	6	−0.094 (− 0.634, 0.445)	0.34	0.732	0.000	87.7%

HCY Homocysteine, *NA* Not available, *MTHFR* Methylenetetrahydrofolate reductase, *NSAIDs* Non-steroidal anti-inflammatory drugs, *SSZ* Sulfasalazine, *MTX* Methotrexate, *TNF* Tumor necrosis factor

reactive protein (CRP), erythrocyte sedimentation rate (ESR), rheumatoid factor (RF), and anti-citrullinated protein antibody (ACPA) in RA [16]. Our study indicates no significant correlation between HCY levels and AS disease activity. However, subgroup analysis suggests that elevated HCY levels are associated with the AS group treated with MTX. This association may be attributed to the inhibitory effect of MTX on the levels of folate [19, 40]. Specifically, MTX treatment influences folate metabolism in RA patients, leading to a decrease in serum folate levels and a rise in HCY levels [54]. However, while MTX increases plasma HCY levels, folate supplementation decreases HCY concentrations, protecting against potential cardiovascular risks in RA patients [55]. In clinical practice, folate supplement is used to reduce side-effect incidence of MTX in RA patients, suggesting that folate supplement should be considered for AS patients treated with MTX. Of the 9 studies included in this analysis, 4 recruited AS patients on MTX [35–37, 41], 2 of which used folate supplementation [35, 36]. Of the other 5 studies, 3 didn't use MTX [38–40] and 2 didn't mention any treatment method [16, 34].

SSZ has also been reported to have anti-folate properties [56], implying SSZ may increase HCY levels in patients. This is supported by the observation that plasma HCY levels was increased significantly in AS patients under SSZ, and SSZ/MTX combination treatment [37]. However, our subgroup analysis showed no significant differences in HCY levels in AS patients treated with SSZ compared with controls. In addition, HCY levels were significantly lower in AS group treated with anti-TNF-α regimen. These findings support the note that different medical treatments may influence HCY levels. However, the reasons attributed to the above results remain unknown. In this meta-analysis, two studies contain HCY levels and treatment methods in AS patients (n = 198) [35, 40]. The above findings might be a result of the small sample size employed in the individual studies. Further studies are needed to confirm these findings.

HCY levels are known to be controlled by methylenetetrahydrofolate reductase (MTHFR), which is a key enzyme in HCY metabolism [57]. MTHFR C677T polymorphism causes a thermolability of MTHFR, reducing its enzymatic activity [57]. Such a reduction inhibits the formation of 5-methyltetrahydrofolate, which serves as a methyl donor during the remethylation of HCY to methionine [57]. Studies indicated that the TT genotype of the MTHFR C677T polymorphism exhibits higher plasma HCY concentrations than CT heterozygotes and CC homozygotes [58, 59]. Besides, Mao et al. reported that high plasma HCY levels are associated with MTHF R 677TT polymorphism as compared with the CC or CT genotype in AS patients [34]. In this meta-analysis, subgroup analysis showed no significant correlation between all 3 genotypes of the MTHFR C677T polymorphism and HCY levels in AS. This result agrees with the previous report which showed no association between MTHFR 677TT polymorphism and plasma HCY levels in obese children and adolescents [60] and no statistically significant differences according to the frequency of MTHFR C677T polymorphism between AS patients and controls [39].

As a well-known risk factor for cardiovascular disease, HCY can mediate the development of the cardiovascular disease by acting adversely on vascular endothelium and smooth muscle cells [61]. Elevated HCY levels may also enhance oxidative stress and inflammation of vascular endothelial cells and reduce the production and bioavailability of nitric oxide (a strong relaxing factor) by endothelium [62]. HCY stimulates the proliferation of vascular smooth muscle cells, synthesis of collagen, and deterioration of arterial wall elastic material [61]. AS also significantly increases risks of myocardial infarction and stroke [63]. Multiple factors contribute to such increased cardiovascular risk. In this regard, systemic inflammation and high disease activity play pivotal roles in the process [64]. Another possible factor is the proatherogenic profile of AS patients who were smokers and/or hypertensive with a poor atherogenic lipid profile [64]. Recommendations from EULAR pointed out that disease activity should be controlled optimally to lower CVD risk in all patients with AS, RA or psoriatic arthritis (PsA) [65]. In addition, MTX treatment decreases the acute myocardial infarction (AMI) among RA patients [66], suggesting that MTX plays a role in protecting patients from CVD risk, possibly via controlling the inflammatory process although MTX elevates HCY levels.

To our knowledge, this is the first meta-analysis that provides evidence of HCY levels in AS patients compared with controls. We are able to extract valid and accurate results from the individual articles and use a sample size of 778 patients of AS and 522 of controls for HCY levels to increase the statistical power and resolution of our analysis compared with the individual studies. However, several limitations are recognized. First, the significant heterogeneity in our meta-analysis may restrict the generalization of the pooled result. Second, due to the lack of sufficient data to perform more exhaustive subgroup analysis and meta-regression, the origin of heterogeneity could not be fully revealed.

Conclusions

This meta-analysis suggests that HCY may partially participate in the pathogenesis of AS, although it is not a major contributing factor. Further and larger studies are needed to confirm these findings.

Acknowledgements

Not applicable.

Authors' contributions

HHL performed literature search and prepared the draft of the paper. XQL performed literature search and prepared the draft of the paper. LTS participated in manuscript preparation. YC draw the figures. JHX participated in manuscript preparation and designed the Table. CZ read the manuscript critically. JZ developed the main idea and read the manuscript critically. XFL developed the main idea and read the manuscript critically. HXL developed the main idea, designed the work, and read the manuscript critically. YJZ developed the main idea, designed the work, and read the manuscript critically. All authors read and approved the final manuscript.

Author details

[1]Department of Obstetrics and Gynecology, Qilu Hospital, Cheeloo College of Medicine, Shandong University, Jinan 250012, Shandong, China. [2]Department of Obstetrics and Gynecology, University of Wisconsin-Madison, Madison, WI 53715, USA. [3]Department of Gastroenterology, Shouguang People's Hospital, Shouguang 262700, Shandong, China. [4]Department of Infectious Diseases, Qilu Hospital, Cheeloo College of Medicine, Shandong University, Jinan 250012, Shandong, China. [5]Department of Intensive Care Unit, Qilu Hospital, Cheeloo College of Medicine, Shandong University, Jinan 250012, Shandong, China. [6]Shandong First Medical University & Shandong Academic of Medical Sciences, Jinan 250000, Shandong, China. [7]School of Animal and Comparative Biomedical Sciences, University of Arizona, Tucson, AZ, USA. [8]Department of Rheumatology, Qilu Hospital, Cheeloo College of Medicine, Shandong University, Jinan 250012, Shandong, China.

References

1. Braun J, Baraliakos X, Listing J, Sieper J. Decreased incidence of anterior uveitis in patients with ankylosing spondylitis treated with the anti-tumor necrosis factor agents infliximab and etanercept. Arthritis Rheum. 2005;52(8): 2447–51.
2. Brophy S, Calin A. Ankylosing spondylitis: interaction between genes, joints, age at onset, and disease expression. J Rheumatol. 2001;28(10):2283–8.
3. Leirisalo-Repo M, Turunen U, Stenman S, Helenius P, Seppälä K. High frequency of silent inflammatory bowel disease in spondylarthropathy. Arthritis Rheum. 1994;37(1):23–31.
4. Souza AS Jr, Müller NL, Marchiori E, Soares-Souza LV, de Souza Rocha M. Pulmonary abnormalities in ankylosing spondylitis: inspiratory and expiratory high-resolution CT findings in 17 patients. J Thorac Imaging. 2004;19(4):259–63.
5. El Maghraoui A, Chaouir S, Abid A, Bezza A, Tabache F, Achemlal L, et al. Lung findings on thoracic high-resolution computed tomography in patients with ankylosing spondylitis. Correlations with disease duration, clinical findings and pulmonary function testing. Clin Rheumatol. 2004;23(2): 123–8.
6. Shimabuco AY, Gonçalves CR, Moraes JCB, Waisberg MG, Ribeiro ACM,

Sampaio-Barros PD, et al. Factors associated with ASDAS remission in a long-term study of ankylosing spondylitis patients under tumor necrosis factor inhibitors. Adv Rheumatol. 2018;58(1):40.
7. Peters MJ, van der Horst-Bruinsma IE, Dijkmans BA, Nurmohamed MT. Cardiovascular risk profile of patients with spondylarthropathies, particularly ankylosing spondylitis and psoriatic arthritis. Semin Arthritis Rheum. 2004; 34(3):585–92.
8. Kumar A, Palfrey HA, Pathak R, Kadowitz PJ, Gettys TW, Murthy SN. The metabolism and significance of homocysteine in nutrition and health. Nutr Metab (Lond). 2017;14:78.
9. Shenoy V, Mehendale V, Prabhu K, Shetty R, Rao P. Correlation of serum homocysteine levels with the severity of coronary artery disease. Indian J Clin Biochem. 2014;29(3):339–44.
10. Homocysteine Studies Collaboration. Homocysteine and risk of ischemic heart disease and stroke: a meta-analysis. Jama. 2002;288(16):2015–22.
11. Loscalzo J. Homocysteine and dementias. N Engl J Med. 2002;346(7):466–8.
12. Herrmann M, Peter Schmidt J, Umanskaya N, Wagner A, Taban-Shomal O, Widmann T, et al. The role of hyperhomocysteinemia as well as folate, vitamin B (6) and B (12) deficiencies in osteoporosis: a systematic review. Clin Chem Lab Med. 2007;45(12):1621–32.
13. Long Y, Nie J. Homocysteine in Renal Injury. Kidney Dis (Basel). 2016;2(2):80–7.
14. Capelli I, Cianciolo G, Gasperoni L, Zappulo F, Tondolo F, Cappuccilli M, et al. Folic acid and vitamin B12 administration in CKD, why not? Nutrients. 2019;11(2):383.
15. Sam NB, Zhang Q, Li BZ, Li XM, Wang DG, Pan HF, et al. Serum/plasma homocysteine levels in patients with systemic lupus erythematosus: a systematic review and meta-analysis. Clin Rheumatol. 2020;39(6):1725–36.
16. Shu J, Sun X, Li J, Li F, Tang J, Shi L. Serum homocysteine levels and their association with clinical characteristics of inflammatory arthritis. Clin Rheumatol. 2020;39(11):3295–302.
17. Phelip JM, Ducros V, Faucheron JL, Flourie B, Roblin X. Association of hyperhomocysteinemia and folate deficiency with colon tumors in patients with inflammatory bowel disease. Inflamm Bowel Dis. 2008;14(2):242–8.
18. Wakkee M, Thio HB, Prens EP, Sijbrands EJ, Neumann HA. Unfavorable cardiovascular risk profiles in untreated and treated psoriasis patients. Atherosclerosis. 2007;190(1):1–9.
19. Refsum H, Helland S, Ueland PM. Fasting plasma homocysteine as a sensitive parameter of antifolate effect: a study of psoriasis patients receiving low-dose methotrexate treatment. Clin Pharmacol Ther. 1989; 46(5):510–20.
20. Lazzerini PE, Capecchi PL, Selvi E, Lorenzini S, Bisogno S, Galeazzi M, et al. Hyperhomocysteinemia, inflammation and autoimmunity. Autoimmun Rev. 2007;6(7):503–9.
21. Gao XM, Wordsworth P, McMichael AJ, Kyaw MM, Seifert M, Rees D, et al. Homocysteine modification of HLA antigens and its immunological consequences. Eur J Immunol. 1996;26(7):1443–50.
22. Elsherbiny NM, Sharma I, Kira D, Alhusban S, Samra YA, Jadeja R, et al. Homocysteine induces inflammation in retina and brain. Biomolecules. 2020;10(3):393.
23. Wang S, Huang Z, Li W, He S, Wu H, Zhu J, et al. IL-37 expression is decreased in patients with hyperhomocysteinemia and protects cells from inflammatory injury by homocysteine. Mol Med Rep. 2020;21(1):371–8.
24. Pirchl M, Ullrich C, Sperner-Unterweger B, Humpel C. Homocysteine has anti-inflammatory properties in a hypercholesterolemic rat model in vivo. Mol Cell Neurosci. 2012;49(4):456–63.
25. Morimoto M, Shivappa N, de Souza GP, Martini LA, Schuch NJ, Hebert JR, et al. Lack of association between dietary inflammatory index and low impact fractures in the Brazilian population: the Brazilian osteoporosis study (BRAZOS). Adv Rheumatol. 2019;59(1):16.
26. Liu Z, Luo H, Zhang L, Huang Y, Liu B, Ma K, et al. Hyperhomocysteinemia exaggerates adventitial inflammation and angiotensin II-induced abdominal aortic aneurysm in mice. Circ Res. 2012;111(10):1261–73.
27. Su SJ, Huang LW, Pai LS, Liu HW, Chang KL. Homocysteine at pathophysiologic concentrations activates human monocyte and induces cytokine expression and inhibits macrophage migration inhibitory factor expression. Nutrition. 2005;21(10):994–1002.
28. Schroecksnadel K, Frick B, Kaser S, Wirleitner B, Ledochowski M, Mur E, et al. Moderate hyperhomocysteinaemia and immune activation in patients with rheumatoid arthritis. Clin Chim Acta. 2003;338(1–2):157–64.
29. Au-Yeung KK, Woo CW, Sung FL, Yip JC, Siow YL, O K. Hyperhomocysteinemia activates nuclear factor-kappaB in endothelial cells via oxidative stress. Circ Res. 2004;94(1):28–36.
30. Wang G, Siow YL, O K. Homocysteine stimulates nuclear factor kappaB activity and monocyte chemoattractant protein-1 expression in vascular smooth-muscle cells: a possible role for protein kinase C. Biochem J. 2000; 352 Pt 3(Pt 3):817–26.
31. Wang G, Siow YL, O K. Homocysteine induces monocyte chemoattractant protein-1 expression by activating NF-kappaB in THP-1 macrophages. Am J Physiol Heart Circ Physiol. 2001;280(6):H2840–7.
32. Singh Y, Gupta G, Kazmi I, Al-Abbasi FA, Negi P, Chellappan DK, et al. SARS CoV-2 aggravates cellular metabolism mediated complications in COVID-19 infection. Dermatol Ther. 2020;33:e13871.
33. Li JJ, Li Q, Du HP, Wang YL, You SJ, Wang F, et al. Homocysteine triggers inflammatory responses in macrophages through inhibiting CSE-H2S signaling via DNA hypermethylation of CSE promoter. Int J Mol Sci. 2015; 16(6):12560–77.
34. Mao N, Chen JW, Peng WF, Chen LX, Xie X. The relationship of plasma homocysteine levels and the methylenetetrahydrofolate reductase C677T gene polymorphism to Ankylosing spondylitis in a Chinese population. Turk J Rheumatol. 2012;27(3):174–8.
35. Baskan BM, Sivas F, Aktekin LA, Dogan YP, Ozoran K, Bodur H. Serum homocysteine level in patients with ankylosing spondylitis. Rheumatol Int. 2009;29(12):1435–9.
36. Gonzalez-Lopez L, Sanchez-Hernandez JD, Aguilar-Chavez EA, Cota-Sanchez AR, Lopez-Olivo MA, Villa-Manzano AI, et al. Hyperhomocysteinemia in ankylosing spondylitis: prevalence and association with clinical variables. Rheumatol Int. 2008;28(12):1223–8.
37. Wei JC, Jan MS, Yu CT, Huang YC, Yang CC, Tsou HK, et al. Plasma homocysteine status in patients with ankylosing spondylitis. Clin Rheumatol. 2007;26(5):739–42.
38. Xu XY, Zhou WH, Xiao CS, Li XF, Wang LY. A clinical study of hyperhomocysteinemia in rheumatological diseases. Zhonghua Nei Ke Za Zhi. 2005;44(2):111–4.
39. Geçene M, Tuncay F, Borman P, Yücel D, Senes M, Yılmaz BK. Atherosclerosis in male patients with ankylosing spondylitis: the relation with methylenetetrahydrofolate reductase (C677T) gene polymorphism and plasma homocysteine levels. Rheumatol Int. 2013;33(6):1519–24.
40. Capkin E, Karkucak M, Akyüz A, Alver A, Turkyilmaz AK, Zengin E. The relationship between plasma homocysteine level and different treatment modalities in patients with ankylosing spondylitis. Rheumatol Int. 2012;32(8): 2349–53.
41. Malesci D, Niglio A, Mennillo GA, Buono R, Valentini G, La Montagna G. High prevalence of metabolic syndrome in patients with ankylosing spondylitis. Clin Rheumatol. 2007;26(5):710–4.
42. van der Linden S, Valkenburg HA, Cats A. Evaluation of diagnostic criteria for ankylosing spondylitis. A proposal for modification of the New York criteria. Arthritis Rheum. 1984;27(4):361–8.
43. Dougados M, van der Linden S, Juhlin R, Huitfeldt B, Amor B, Calin A, et al. The European Spondylarthropathy study group preliminary criteria for the classification of spondylarthropathy. Arthritis Rheum. 1991;34(10):1218–27.
44. Garrett S, Jenkinson T, Kennedy LG, Whitelock H, Gaisford P, Calin A. A new approach to defining disease status in ankylosing spondylitis: the bath ankylosing spondylitis disease activity index. J Rheumatol. 1994;21(12):2286–91.
45. Moher D, Liberati A, Tetzlaff J, Altman DG. Preferred reporting items for systematic reviews and meta-analyses: the PRISMA statement. PLoS Med. 2009;6(7):e1000097.
46. Stang A. Critical evaluation of the Newcastle-Ottawa scale for the assessment of the quality of nonrandomized studies in meta-analyses. Eur J Epidemiol. 2010;25(9):603–5.
47. Luo D, Wan X, Liu J, Tong T. Optimally estimating the sample mean from the sample size, median, mid-range, and/or mid-quartile range. Stat Methods Med Res. 2018;27(6):1785–805.
48. Wan X, Wang W, Liu J, Tong T. Estimating the sample mean and standard deviation from the sample size, median, range and/or interquartile range. BMC Med Res Methodol. 2014;14:135.
49. Higgins JP, Thompson SG, Deeks JJ, Altman DG. Measuring inconsistency in meta-analyses. BMJ. 2003;327(7414):557–60.
50. Deeks JJ, Higgins JP, Altman DG, Group obotCSM. Analysing data and undertaking meta-analyses. Cochrane Handb Syst Rev Intervent. 2019. p. 241–84.

51. Wållberg-Jonsson S, Cvetkovic JT, Sundqvist KG, Lefvert AK, Rantapää-Dahlqvist S. Activation of the immune system and inflammatory activity in relation to markers of atherothrombotic disease and atherosclerosis in rheumatoid arthritis. J Rheumatol. 2002;29(5):875–82.
52. Lopez-Olivo MA, Gonzalez-Lopez L, Garcia-Gonzalez A, Villa-Manzano AI, Cota-Sanchez AR, Salazar-Paramo M, et al. Factors associated with hyperhomocysteinaemia in Mexican patients with rheumatoid arthritis. Scand J Rheumatol. 2006;35(2):112–6.
53. Lazzerini PE, Capecchi PL, Bisogno S, Galeazzi M, Marcolongo R, Pasini FL. Reduction in plasma homocysteine level in patients with rheumatoid arthritis given pulsed glucocorticoid treatment. Ann Rheum Dis. 2003;62(7): 694–5.
54. Hornung N, Ellingsen T, Stengaard-Pedersen K, Poulsen JH. Folate, homocysteine, and cobalamin status in patients with rheumatoid arthritis treated with methotrexate, and the effect of low dose folic acid supplement. J Rheumatol. 2004;31(12):2374–81.
55. van Ede AE, Laan RF, Blom HJ, Boers GH, Haagsma CJ, Thomas CM, et al. Homocysteine and folate status in methotrexate-treated patients with rheumatoid arthritis. Rheumatology (Oxford). 2002;41(6):658–65.
56. Selhub J, Dhar GJ, Rosenberg IH. Inhibition of folate enzymes by sulfasalazine. J Clin Invest. 1978;61(1):221–4.
57. Wan L, Li Y, Zhang Z, Sun Z, He Y, Li R. Methylenetetrahydrofolate reductase and psychiatric diseases. Transl Psychiatry. 2018;8(1):242.
58. Fowler B. Disorders of homocysteine metabolism. J Inherit Metab Dis. 1997; 20(2):270–85.
59. Goyette P, Sumner JS, Milos R, Duncan AM, Rosenblatt DS, Matthews RG, et al. Human methylenetetrahydrofolate reductase: isolation of cDNA, mapping and mutation identification. Nat Genet. 1994;7(2):195–200.
60. Gallistl S, Sudi K, Mangge H, Erwa W, Borkenstein M. Insulin is an independent correlate of plasma homocysteine levels in obese children and adolescents. Diabetes Care. 2000;23(9):1348–52.
61. Ganguly P, Alam SF. Role of homocysteine in the development of cardiovascular disease. Nutr J. 2015;14:6.
62. Zhang S, Bai YY, Luo LM, Xiao WK, Wu HM, Ye P. Association between serum homocysteine and arterial stiffness in elderly: a community-based study. J Geriatr Cardiol. 2014;11(1):32–8.
63. Schieir O, Tosevski C, Glazier RH, Hogg-Johnson S, Badley EM. Incident myocardial infarction associated with major types of arthritis in the general population: a systematic review and meta-analysis. Ann Rheum Dis. 2017; 76(8):1396–404.
64. Mathieu S, Soubrier M. Cardiovascular events in ankylosing spondylitis: a 2018 meta-analysis. Ann Rheum Dis. 2019;78(6):e57.
65. Agca R, Heslinga SC, Rollefstad S, Heslinga M, McInnes IB, Peters MJ, et al. EULAR recommendations for cardiovascular disease risk management in patients with rheumatoid arthritis and other forms of inflammatory joint disorders: 2015/2016 update. Ann Rheum Dis. 2017;76(1):17–28.
66. Suissa S, Bernatsky S, Hudson M. Antirheumatic drug use and the risk of acute myocardial infarction. Arthritis Rheum. 2006;55(4):531–6.

16

Depressive symptoms are associated with impaired sleep, fatigue and disease activity in women with rheumatoid arthritis

Fernando Henrique Azevedo Lopes[1], Max Victor Carioca Freitas[2], Veralice Meireles Sales de Bruin[1] and Pedro Felipe Carvalhedo de Bruin[1*]

Abstract

Objectives: To investigate the associations between sleep quality, fatigue, disease activity and depressive symptoms in women with rheumatoid arthritis (RA).

Methods: Female patients with previous diagnosis of RA from a Rheumatology Outpatient Clinic at a tertiary referral centre, in Fortaleza, Brazil, were consecutively recruited into the study. Sleep quality was assessed by the Pittsburgh Sleep Quality Index (PSQI); fatigue by the Fatigue Severity Scale (FSS); daytime sleepiness by the Epworth Sleepiness Scale (ESS); and depressive symptoms by the Beck Depression Inventory II (BDI-II). RA activity was measured by the disease activity score (DAS28).

Results: One hundred ten women (mean age $\pm$ SD $= 51.1 \pm 13.0$ y) were included in the study. On average, patients with depressive symptoms (BDI-II > 13), as compared to those without, showed poorer sleep quality (PSQI: 10.09 ± 4.1 vs 7.33 ± 3.55; $p = 0.001$ respectively), more fatigue (FSS: 4.69 ± 1.89 vs 3.34 ± 1.8; $p = 0.001$) and higher disease activity level (DAS28: 4.36 ± 1.53 vs 3.7 ± 1.39; $p = 0{,}047$). The logistic regression analysis showed that sleep quality is an independent predictor of depressive symptom severity.

Conclusion: Depressive symptoms, impaired sleep and fatigue are common in women with RA. Poor sleep is associated with greater frequency and severity of depressive symptoms in these patients, suggesting that screening for sleep and mood problems may be relevant both in clinical research and routine patient care. Future studies investigating the impact of measures to promote healthy sleep on depressive symptom control in this patient population are warranted.

Keywords: Rheumatoid arthritis, Sleep, Fatigue, Sleepiness, Depression

Introduction

Rheumatoid arthritis (RA) is a chronic, autoimmune disease, with overall prevalence estimated at 0.24% [1]. Women are three times more affected than men and usually report more symptoms and greater disability [1, 2]. Although RA primarily involves the joints, it may also cause important systemic manifestations [3]. Approximately 20–30% of RA patients become unable to work within a period of 3 years after diagnosis [4].

Depressive symptoms are common in RA [5]. Frequency of major depression in these patients has been reported to be almost 17%, considerably higher than that of the general population [6]. In clinical practice, diagnosis of depression in patients with RA is usually complicated by the fact that somatic symptoms of depression can overlap with symptoms of RA [7]. Fatigue, a common feature of depression, can affect 41% of RA patients [8]. Depressive symptoms in RA have been associated with increased pain [9], physical disability [10] and

* Correspondence: pedrobruin@gmail.com
[1]Laboratory of Sleep and Biological Rhythms, Department of Medicine, Federal University of Ceara, Rua Prof. Costa Mendes 1608 – 4° andar, CEP 60430-971 Fortaleza, Ceara, Brazil

comorbidities [11], reduced quality of life [12] and higher mortality levels [13]. Recently, it has been reported that baseline and persistent depressive symptoms are associated with worse response to treatment and poorer long-term health outcomes [14]. The mechanism for the relationship between mood problems and RA outcomes remains incompletely understood [15]. The association between quality of sleep and depressive symptoms has not been adequately investigated in patients with RA in Brazil.

More than half of RA patients report sleep problems, including difficulty falling asleep, nocturnal awakenings, nonrestorative sleep and fatigue, a frequency that is three times higher than that of the general population [16]. It has been previously suggested that impaired sleep in RA is mainly secondary to joint pain, disease activity and altered mood [17–19]. On the other hand, there is evidence that disturbed sleep can be involved in the genesis of inflammatory disorders [20] and poor sleep quality has been shown to exacerbate pain perception in RA patients [21]. Additionally, sleep problems are recognized as an important risk factor for depression. Individuals suffering from insomnia are twice as likely to develop depression compared to those who do not have difficulty in sleep [22].

Fatigue is major symptom in patients with RA and has been associated with sleep problems, pain and depression. There is evidence that fatigue, poor sleep quality, pain, depression may be associated with greater disability in these patients [23].

The main purpose of this study was to assess the presence of depressive symptoms and its associations with sleep quality, fatigue, and disease activity in patients with RA.

Methods

This was a cross-sectional study of women with established RA, regularly attending an outpatient clinic at Dr. César Cals General Hospital, a tertiary referral centre in Fortaleza, Brazil, between April 2014 and December 2015. Female patients older than 18 years, who met the internationally-set RA diagnosis criteria [24], and whose therapeutic regimen had not been changed in the previous 3 months, were asked to take part in the study.

Disease activity was measured using the Disease Activity Score in 28 joints (DAS28), which comprises four scoring components, namely: number of swollen joints (0 to 28); number of painful joints (0 to 28); erythrocyte sedimentation rate (ESR); and general health visual analogue scale (VAS). DAS28 final score ranges from 0 to 10 and scores ≤2.6 were interpreted as remission; between 2.6 and 3.2, as low disease activity; between 3.2 and 5.1, as moderate activity; and > 5.1 as high activity [24].

Additionally, patients answered the following questionnaires, which have been previously translated and validated for use in Brazil: Beck Depression Inventory (BDI-II) [25]; Pittsburgh Sleep Quality Index (PSQI) [26]; Epworth Sleepiness Scale (ESS) [27]; Fatigue severity Scale (FSS) [28].

Depressive symptoms were assessed by the Beck Depression Inventory (BDI-II). This instrument consists of 21 sets of statements about the occurrence of depressive symptoms in the 15 days preceding the test application. Statements are classified in a Likert scale ranging from 0 to 3, to produce scores ranging from 0 to 63. Patients with BDI-II score > 13 were classified as positive for depressive symptoms [25, 29].

Sleep quality was assessed by the PSQI, a self-report questionnaire that consists of 19 items, creating seven components, each one dealing with a major aspect of sleep: subjective sleep quality, sleep latency, sleep duration, habitual sleep efficiency, sleep disturbances, use of sleeping medication and daytime dysfunctions. These components are weighted equally on a 0–3 scale, providing a global score ranging from 0 to 21 [26]. In the present study, scores higher than 5 were considered indicative of poor sleep quality. This cut-off point has shown satisfactory sensitivity (89.6%) and specificity (86.5%) to differentiate good from poor sleep quality [30].

Daytime sleepiness was evaluated by the Epworth Sleepiness Scale (ESS), a widely used instrument that infers the patient's likelihood of sleeping or dozing in eight daily life situations. This likelihood may range from zero (none) to three (high) for each situation. The final score corresponds to the sum of the values attributed to each individual question. Values higher than or equal to 10 were considered indicative of excessive daytime sleepiness [31].

Fatigue level was measured by the Fatigue Severity Scale (FSS), which consists of a sequence of 9 statements about the possible impact of fatigue on the responder's daily activities. For each statement, the subjects are asked to attribute a value from 1 to 7, depending on how appropriate they felt the statement applied to them over the previous 7 days. A low value indicates that the statement is not very appropriate whereas a high value indicates agreement. The final score represents the mean value calculated for the 9 items. Values higher than 4 indicate significant fatigue levels [32].

Additional socio-demographic and clinical data, including age, gender, time from diagnosis, and therapeutic regimen were gathered through interview and chart review.

Statistical analysis

Data are presented as mean ± standard deviation (SD) or frequency, as appropriate. Normality of the numerical data was assessed by the Kolmogorov-Smirnov test. Unpaired Student's t-test was used for variables with normal distribution. The Mann-Whitney test was used for non-normal variables. Categorical variables were analysed by the Fisher exact test. For comparative analysis, participants were allocated into two categories, according to the presence (BDI-II > 13) or absence of depressive symptoms. Spearman's correlation coefficients were calculated to examine possible correlations between BDI-II and other variables. Logistic regression analysis was performed to identify independent predictors for the occurrence of depressive symptoms using a forward stepwise approach. The Statistical Package for Social Science (SPSS) v22.0 (IBM CO., Armonk, NY, USA) was used for data analysis. A p-value < 0.05 was considered significant.

Results

One hundred and ten female patients, aged from 19 to 79 years, were included in the study. Depressive symptoms were present in 31.8% of the participants and were classified as mild (13 < BDI-II ≤ 19) in 14, moderate (19 < BDI-II ≤ 28) in 13 and severe (28 < BDI-II ≤ 63) in 6. Ten patients (9.1%) were on antidepressants (Amitriptyline: n = 05; Fluoxetine n = 02; Duloxetine: n = 1; Nortriptyline: n = 1; Amitriptyline + Fluoxetine: n = 1]. Poor quality sleep (PSQI > 5) was observed in 70.9% of the patients; fatigue (FSS > 4) in 41.8%; and excessive daytime sleepiness (ESS ≥ 10) in 39%. Disease activity level was calculated in 84 (76.4%) patients, for whom the erythrocyte sedimentation rate was available at the time they were included in the study and was classified as moderate / high (DAS28 > 3.2) in 59.5%. There was no significant difference in age, time from diagnosis and questionnaire results between the 26 patients with missing DAS28 results and other study participants.

On average, patients with depressive symptoms (BDI-II > 13), as compared to those without, showed poorer sleep quality (PSQI: 10.09 ± 4.1 vs 7.33 ± 3.55; p = 0.001), more fatigue (FSS: 4.69 ± 1.89 vs 3.34 ± 1.8; p = 0.001) and higher disease activity level (DAS28: 4.36 ± 1.53 vs 3.7 ± 1.39; p = 0.047). Daytime sleepiness was not significantly different between the two groups (Table 1). Analysis of the seven PSQI components showed that patients with depressive symptoms had poorer subjective sleep quality and more sleep disturbances and use of sleep medication (Fig. 1). Patients with moderate/ high disease activity (DAS28 > 3.2) showed poorer sleep quality (PSQI global score: 9.91 ± 4.08 vs 7.0 ± 3.67; p < 0.01) than those in remission/ low disease activity.

Sixty-nine (62.7%) patients were on regular use of glucocorticoids, 90 (81.8%) on traditional disease-modifying antirheumatic drugs; and 23 (20.9%) on biologic disease-modifying antirheumatic drugs.

The occurrence of depressive symptoms (BDI-II > 13) was positively correlated with sleep impairment (r = 0.378; p < 0.001), fatigue (r = 0.307; p = 0.001) and disease activity (r = 0.333; p = 0.002). Stepwise multiple regression analysis, with age, disease duration, PSQI, DAS28, FSS, and ESS scores as independent variables, showed that the PSQI global score was an independent predictor for the occurrence of depressive symptoms (Table 2).

Table 1 Demographic and clinical characteristics, quality of sleep, fatigue, and daytime sleepiness in 110 RA female patients

	Total n = 110	BDI-II ≤ 13 n = 74	BDI-II > 13 n = 36	p
Age, years (mean ± SD)	51.2 ± 8.1	52.3 ± 13.3	48.6 ± 12.15	0.054[b]
Disease duration, years (mean ± SD)	8.1 ± 7.8	8.9 ± 8.5	6.4 ± 5.7	0.147[b]
DAS28 score[a] (mean ± SD)	3.89 ± 1.45	3.7 ± 1.4	4.36 ± 1.53	0.047[b]
Moderate / high activity disease (DAS28 > 3,2), n (%)[a]	50(59.5)	31(53.4)	19(73.1)	0.100[c]
PSQI global score (mean ± SD)	8.21 ± 3.93	7.33 ± 3.55	10.09 ± 4.1	0.001[b]
Poor sleep, n (%)	78(70.9)	48(64)	30(85.7)	0.024[c]
FSS (mean ± SD)	3.77 ± 1.93	3.34 ± 1.8	4.69 ± 1.89	0.001[b]
Fatigue, n (%)	47(42.7)	26(34.7)	21(60)	0.014[c]
ESS (mean ± SD)	8.73 ± 5.41	8.39 ± 5.04	9.46 ± 6.15	0.450
EDS, n (%)	43(39.1)	28(37.3)	15(42.9)	0.676[c]
BDI-II (mean ± SD)	10.84 ± 9.11	5.55 ± 3.94	21.89 ± 6.65	< 0.01[b]

p values are for comparisons between groups of patients with (BDI-II > 13) and without depressive symptoms

Definition of abbreviations - *BDI-II* Beck Depression Inventory II, *DAS28* disease activity score in 28 joints, *PSQI* Pittsburgh Sleep Quality Index, *FSS* Fatigue Severity Scale, *ESS* Epworth Sleepiness Scale, *EDS* Excessive daytime sleepiness

[a]DAS28 values for 84 patients

[b]Mann-Whitney

[c]Fisher exact test

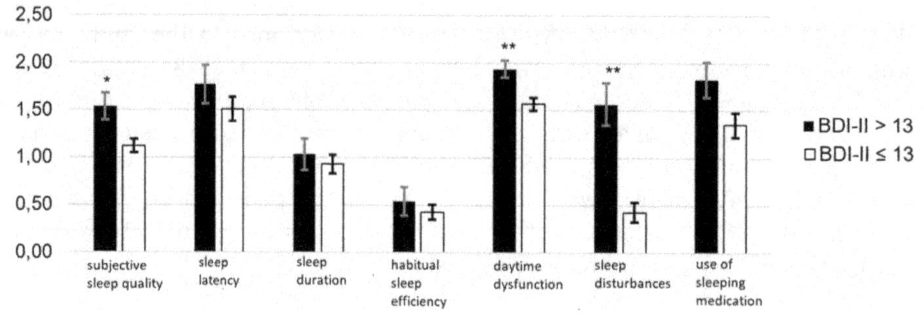

Fig. 1 Pittsburgh Sleep Quality Index components subjective sleep quality, sleep disturbances, use of sleep medication and daytime dysfunction were significantly impaired in RA patients with depressive symptoms as compared to those without depressive symptoms. Definition of abbreviations - BDI-II: Beck Depression Inventory. * $p < 0{,}05$; ** $p < 0{,}01$

Discussion

This study shows that depressive symptoms, sleep impairment and fatigue are very common in Brazilian women with RA. Importantly, poor sleep quality was found to be an independent predictor of depressive symptoms in these patients.

Almost one third of the study participants had depressive symptoms. Retrospective studies comprising large numbers of subjects also found a high prevalence of depressive symptoms in RA [5, 33]. A strong relationship between RA diagnosis and risk of depression was reported in 3698 newly diagnosed patients with RA. The incidence of depression in the RA cohort was 1.74-fold higher than in non-RA subjects [34]. In a retrospective study of a matched cohort of 18,285 participants it was found that RA patients were two times more likely to develop depression [35].

The present results show that the presence of depressive symptoms in patients with RA is associated with higher levels of disease activity, as previously reported [36]. In a study of 87 older women with RA, initially evaluated for depression and weekly assessed for 12 to 20 weeks for pain, depressive symptoms were found to be related to elevations in pain [37]. The effects of depression on markers of immune activation were evaluated in another study of 45 women with RA and 106 controls with no autoimmune disease. A greater CD4 activation was found among RA patients who were depressed as compared to other groups. Depressed RA patients under stress showed the highest levels of IL-6. Those results suggest that depression plays a significant role in autoimmune processes associated with RA [38]. It has also been previously reported that baseline depression in patients with RA can predict disease activity and disability after a two-year follow-up period [14].

In this study, poor-quality sleep was found in more than two thirds of the participants and was related to disease activity. This finding is in agreement with previous reports of a high prevalence of disturbed sleep in RA, particularly, in the more active cases [17–19, 38, 39]. Cytokines, including TNF-α and IL-6, which also play a significant pathogenetic role in RA, could be involved in the genesis of the sleep problems observed in these patients [40]. It has been previously reported that sleep deprivation can increase the concentration of Toll-like receptor 4 (TLR-4) which, in turn, stimulates the production of interleukin-6 (IL-6) and tumour necrosis factor - alpha (TNF-α), two proinflammatory cytokines directly involved in RA [41]. Additionally, sleep deprivation can lead to greater expression of genes related to these cytokines through nuclear factor - kappa B (NF-κB) activation, which is the main gene-transcription regulatory pathway in the inflammatory signalling cascade [20].

This study confirms previous reports of a high frequency of fatigue in RA [8]. Although it is generally recognized that inflammation plays a significant role in the development of fatigue in RA, there is also evidence that non-inflammatory pathways could be involved [42]. It is likely that fatigue in patients with RA has a multifactorial origin, probably involving a wide range of factors, which may include obesity, sedentary lifestyle, sleep disturbances, loss of muscle mass and depression [43].

Table 2 Results of the stepwise multiple regression analyses using depressive symptoms as the dependent variable

Independent variables	B	SE	Wald	p	OR	95% CI for OR	
						Lower	Higher
Age	−0.007	0.023	0.102	0.749	0.993	0.949	1.039
Disease duration	−0.019	0.046	0.160	0.690	0.982	0.896	1.075
DAS28	0.271	0.201	1.819	0.177	1.312	0.884	1.945
PSQI	0.199	0.082	5.837	0.016	1.22	1.038	1.434
FSS	0.024	0.019	1.685	0.194	1.025	0.988	1.063
ESS	−0.013	0.049	0.072	0.789	0.987	0.897	1.086
Constant	−4.320	1.724	6.277	0.012	0.013		

Definition of Abbreviations: *BDI-II* Beck Depression Inventory, *DAS28* Disease activity score in 28 joint, *PSQI* Pittsburgh Sleep Quality Index, *FSS* Fatigue Severity Scale, *B* coefficients, *OR* Odds ratio, *CI* Confidence interval

More than a third of the subjects in this study reported excessive daytime sleepiness, a frequency much higher than that found in the general adult population [44, 45]. No difference in daytime somnolence was observed between participants with and without depressive symptoms. A previous study in RA patients described a negative correlation between disease activity and subjective daytime sleepiness. Further studies are needed to clarify the relation between somnolence, disease activity, and depressive symptoms in RA [19].

The present results confirm that RA patients with depressive symptoms, on average, show higher disease activity than patients without these symptoms. Previously, an association between baseline depression symptom status and disease activity was found in a prospective study of 18,421 RA patients receiving biologic treatment. Depressive symptoms contributed to increased DAS28 over a 12-month follow-up period, and had an impact in changes in DAS28 in response to treatment. Interestingly, depression was associated with both subjective and objective aspects of disease activity, as assessed by specific components of the DAS28. It was suggested that these findings could be secondary to the negative impact of depression on health-related behaviours, particularly, medication adherence. They could also be related to biological factors, such as, systemic inflammation and elevated cytokines typically associated with disease severity in RA, which are also present in people with depressive disorder, or both [46].

An important finding of the present study is an independent association between poor-quality sleep and depressive symptoms. Disrupted sleep is generally recognized as a major feature of depression [47]. However, the relationship between poor sleep and depressive symptoms is probably bidirectional and may involve several factors [48]. Previous studies have shown a significant correlation between subjective sleep quality, as assessed by the global PSQI score, and measures of depression [49]. Additionally, depressed subjects present significantly higher PSQI scores than normal controls [30]. It has been suggested that the PSQI is better than objective measures of sleep for the detection of negative perceptions of sleep commonly found in patients with depression [50].

This study has limitations that must be considered. No male patients were included, so these results cannot be extrapolated to the entire RA population, mostly because of previously described effects of gender on disease activity measures as well as possible differences in cut-off values for some of the questionnaires that were used. Moreover, the presence of depressive symptoms assessed by the BDI-II is not sufficient for the diagnosis of depressive disorder, which requires a clinical structured interview. Besides, due to the cross-sectional design, causality cannot be implied, and prospective studies should be conducted to further investigate the associations between sleep quality, disease activity, fatigue, daytime sleepiness and depressive symptoms in RA patients.

Conclusions

This study shows a high frequency of impaired sleep, fatigue, and depressive symptoms in RA patients. Poor-quality sleep, found in the majority of cases, is associated with a higher frequency and severity of depressive symptoms. These findings highlight the importance of screening for sleep and mood disorders in RA patients both in clinical trials and in clinical practice. Future studies examining the impact of measures to promote healthy sleep on depressive symptom control in this patient population are warranted.

Acknowledgements

The authors wish to thank Dr. Francisco J. F. Vieira, Dr. Leonardo O. Cavalcante and Dr. Priscila D. Evangelista for their assistance in recruiting our patients, and Mr. Antonio Brazil Viana Jr. for providing technical assistance. We thank Coordenação de aperfeiçoamento de pessoal de nível superior (Capes) for the financial support.

Authors' contributions

FHAL: acquisition of subjects and data, interpretation of data, preparation of manuscript. MVCF: Screening and clinical evaluation of the subjects. VMSB: critical review of manuscript. PFCB: study concept and design, analysis and interpretation of data, preparation of manuscript. The author(s) read and approved the final manuscript.

Authors' information

Not applicable.

Author details

[1]Laboratory of Sleep and Biological Rhythms, Department of Medicine, Federal University of Ceara, Rua Prof. Costa Mendes 1608 – 4° andar, CEP 60430-971 Fortaleza, Ceara, Brazil. [2]Dr. Cesar Cals General Hospital, Fortaleza, Ceara, Brazil.

References

1. Hoy D, March L, Brooks P, Blyth F, Woolf A, Bain C, et al. The global burden of rheumatoid arthritis: estimates from the global burden of disease 2010 study. Ann Rheum Dis. 2014;73(6):968–74.
2. Sokka T, Toloza S, Cutolo M, Kautiainen H, Makinen H, Gogus F, et al. Women , men , and rheumatoid arthritis : analyses of disease activity , disease characteristics , and treatments in the QUEST-RA Study. Arthritis Res Ther. 2009;11(1):1–12.
3. Smolen JS, Aletaha D, McInnes IB. Rheumatoid arthritis. Lancet. 2016; 388(10055):2023–38.
4. Sokka T. Work disability in early rheumatoid arthritis. Ann Rheum Dis. 2003; 21(31):S71–4.
5. Matcham F, Rayner L, Steer S, Hotopf M. The prevalence of depression in rheumatoid arthritis: a systematic review and meta-analysis. Rheumatology (Oxford). 2013;52(12):2136–48.
6. Ferrari AJ, Somerville AJ, Baxter AJ, Norman R, Patten SB, Vos T, et al. Global variation in the prevalence and incidence of major depressive disorder: a

systematic review of the epidemiological literature. Psychol Med. 2013;43(3):471–81.
7. Zyrianova Y, Kelly BD, Gallagher C, McCarthy C, Molloy MG, Sheehan J, et al. Depression and anxiety in rheumatoid arthritis: the role of perceived social support. Ir J Med Sci. 2006;175(2):32–6.
8. Overman CL, Kool MB, Da Silva JAP, Geenen R. The prevalence of severe fatigue in rheumatic diseases: an international study. Clin Rheumatol. 2016; 35(2):409–15.
9. Brandstetter S, Riedelbeck G, Steinmann M, Ehrenstein B, Loss J, Apfelbacher C. Pain, social support and depressive symptoms in patients with rheumatoid arthritis: testing the stress-buffering hypothesis. Rheumatol Int. 2017;37(6):931–6.
10. El-Miedany YM, El Rasheed AH. Is anxiety a more common disorder than depression in rheumatoid arthritis? Jt Bone Spine. 2002;69(3):300–6.
11. Katz P, Yelin E. Prevalence and correlates of depressive symptoms among persons with rheumatoid arthritis. J Rheumatol. 1993;20(5):790–6.
12. Mikuls T, Saag K, Criswell L, Merlino L, Cerhan JR. Health related quality of life in women with elderly onset rheumatoid arthritis. J Rheumatol. 2003; 30(5):952–7.
13. Ang D, Choi H, Kroenke K, Wolfe F. Comorbid depression is an independent risk factor for mortality in patients with rheumatoid arthritis. J Rheumatol. 2005;32(6):1013–9.
14. Matcham F, Norton S, Scott DL, Steer S, Hotopf M. Symptoms of depression and anxiety predict treatment response and long-term physical health outcomes in rheumatoid arthritis: secondary analysis of a randomized controlled trial. Rheumatology. 2016;55(2):268–78.
15. Sheehy C, Murphy E, Barry M. Depression in rheumatoid arthritis: underscoring the problem. Rheumatol. 2006;45(11):1325–7.
16. Sariyildiz M, Batmaz I, Bozkurt M. Sleep quality in rheumatoid arthritis: relationship between the disease severity, depression, functional status and the quality of life. J Clin Med. 2014;6(1):44–52.
17. Westhovens R, Van Der Elst K, Matthys A, Tran M, Gilloteau I. Sleep problems in patients with rheumatoid arthritis. J Rheumatol. 2014;41(1):31–40.
18. Nicassio PM, Ormseth SR, Custodio MK, Olmstead R, Weisman MH, Irwin MR. Confirmatory factor analysis of the Pittsburgh sleep quality index in rheumatoid arthritis patients. Behav Sleep Med. 2014;12(1):1–12.
19. Grabovac I, Haider S, Berner C, Lamprecht T, Fenzl K, Erlacher L, et al. Sleep quality in patients with Rheumatoid Arthritis and associations with pain, disability, disease duration, and activity. J Clin Med. 2018;7(10):336.
20. Irwin MR, Wang M, Ribeiro D, Cho HJ, Ph D, Breen EC, et al. Sleep loss activates cellular inflammatory signaling. Biol Psychiatry. 2008;64(6):538–40.
21. Irwin MR, Olmstead R, Carrillo C, Sadeghi N, Fitzgerald JD, Ranganath VK, et al. Sleep loss exacerbates fatigue, depression, and pain in rheumatoid arthritis. Sleep. 2012;35(4):537–43.
22. Baglioni C, Battagliese G, Feige B, Spiegelhalder K, Nissen C, Voderholzer U, et al. Insomnia as a predictor of depression: a meta-analytic evaluation of longitudinal epidemiological studies. J Affect Disord. 2011;135(1–3):10–9.
23. Luyster FS, Chasens ER, Wasko MCM, Dumbar-Jacob J. Sleep Quality and Functional Disability in Patients with Rheumatoid Arthritis. J Clin Sleep Med. 2011;7(1):49–55.
24. Aletaha D, Neogi T, Silman AJ, Funovits J, Felson DT, Bingham CO, et al. 2010 rheumatoid arthritis classification criteria: an American College of Rheumatology/European league against rheumatism collaborative initiative. Arthritis Rheum. 2010;62(9):2569–81.
25. Gomes-Oliveira MH, Gorenstein C, Neto FL, Andrade LH, Wang YP. Validation of the Brazilian Portuguese version of the Beck depression inventory-II in a community sample. Rev Bras Psiquiatr. 2012;34(4):389–94.
26. Bertolazi AN, Fagondes SC, Hoff LS, Dartora EG, da Silva Miozzo IC, de Barba MEF, et al. Validation of the Brazilian Portuguese version of the Pittsburgh sleep quality index. Sleep Med. 2011;12(1):70–5.
27. Naimaier Bertolazi A, Chaves Fagondes S, Santos Hoff L, Dallagasperina Pedro V, Saldanha Menna Barreto S, Johns MW, et al. Portuguese-language version of the Epworth sleepiness scale: validation for use in Brazil* , ** Validação da escala de sonolência de Epworth em português para uso no Brasil. J Bras Pneumol. 2009;35(9):877–83.
28. Mendes MF, Pavan K, Marangoni BEM, Schmidt KB. Adaptação transcultural da escala de gravidade de fadiga para a língua portuguesa. Med Reabil. 2008;27(3):69–71.
29. Beck AT, Steer RA, Ball R, Ranieri W. Comparison of Beck Depression Inventories -IA and -II in psychiatric outpatients. J Pers Assess. 1996;67:588–97.
30. Buysse DJ, Reynolds CF, Monk TH, Berman SR, Kupfer DJ, III CFR, et al. The Pittsburgh sleep quality index: a new instrument for psychiatric practice and research. Psychiatry Res. 1989;28(2):193–213.
31. Johns MW. A new method for measuring daytime sleepiness: the Epworth sleepiness scale. Sleep. 1991;14(6):540–5.
32. Krupp LB, La Rocca NG, Muir-Nash J, Steinberg AD. The fatigue severity scale. Application to patients with multiple sclerosis and systemic lupus erythematosus. Arch Neurol. 1989;46(10):1121–3.
33. Isik A, Koca SS, Ozturk A, Mermi O. Anxiety and depression in patients with rheumatoid arthritis. Clin Rheumatol. 2007;26(6):872–8.
34. Lin M-C, Guo H-R, Lu M-C, Livneh H, Lai N-S, Tsai T-Y. Increased risk of depression in patients with rheumatoid arthritis: a seven-year population-based cohort study. Clinics (Sao Paulo). 2015;70(2):91–6.
35. Wang S-L, Chang C-H, Hu L-Y, Tsai S-J, Yang AC, You Z-H. Risk of developing depressive disorders following rheumatoid arthritis: a nationwide population-based study. PLoS One. 2014;9(9):e107791.
36. Rathbun AM, Reed GW, Harrold LR. The temporal relationship between depression and rheumatoid arthritis disease activity, treatment persistence and response: a systematic review. Rheumatology. 2013;52:1785–94.
37. Zautra A, Smith B. Depression and reactivity to stress in older women with rheumatoid arthritis and osteoarthritis. Psychosom Med. 2001;63(4):687–96.
38. Zautra A, Yocum D, Villanueva I, Smith B, Davis M, Attrep J, et al. Immune activation and depression in women with rheumatoid arthritis. J Rheumatol. 2004;31(3):457–63.
39. Austad C, Kvien TK, Olsen IC, Uhlig T. Sleep disturbance in patients with rheumatoid arthritis is related to fatigue, disease activity, and other patient-reported outcomes. Scand J Rheumatol. 2016;9742(June):1–9.
40. Taylor-Gjevre RM, Gjevre JA, Nair BV, Skomro RP, Lim HJ. Improved sleep efficiency after anti-tumor necrosis factor α therapy in rheumatoid arthritis patients. Ther Adv Musculoskelet Dis. 2011;3(5):227–33.
41. Irwin MR, Wang M, Campomayor CO, Collado-Hidalgo A, Cole S. Sleep deprivation and activation of morning levels of cellular and genomic markers of inflammation. Arch Intern Med. 2006;166(16):1756–62.
42. van Steenbergen HW, Tsonaka R, Huizinga TWJ, Boonen A, Mil AHM van der H. Fatigue in rheumatoid arthritis; a persistent problem: a large longitudinal study. RMD Open. 2015;1(1):e000041.
43. Katz P, Margaretten M, Trupin L, Schmajuk G, Yazdany J, Yelin E. Role of sleep disturbance, depression, obesity, and physical inactivity in fatigue in rheumatoid arthritis. Arthritis Care Res (Hoboken). 2016;68(1):81–90.
44. Ford ES, Cunningham TJ, Giles WH, Croft JB. Trends in insomnia and excessive daytime sleepiness among US adults from 2002 to 2012. Sleep Med. 2016;16(3):372–8.
45. Santos-Silva R, Bittencourt LRA, Pires MLN, de Mello MT, Taddei JA, Benedito-Silva AA, et al. Increasing trends of sleep complaints in the city of Sao Paulo, Brazil. Sleep Med. 2010;11(6):520–4.
46. Matcham F, Davies R, Hotof M, Hyrich K, Norton S, Steer S, et al. The relationship between depression and biologic treatment responsein rheumatoid arthritis: an analysis of the British Society for Rheumatology biologics register. Rheumatology. 2018;57(5):835–43.
47. Baglioni C, Spiegelhalder K, Lombardo C, Riemann D. Sleep and emotions: a focus on insomnia. Sleep Med Rev. 2010;14(4):227–38.
48. Barclay NL, Gregory AM. Quantitative genetic research on sleep: a review of normal sleep, sleep disturbances and associated emotional, behavioural, and health-related difficulties. Sleep Med Rev. 2013;17(1):29–40.
49. Carpenter JS, Andrykowski MA. Psychometric evaluation of the Pittsburgh sleep quality index. J Psychosom Res. 1998;45(1):5–13.
50. Grandner MA, Kripke DF, Yoon I, Youngstedt SD. Criterion validity of the Pittsburgh sleep quality index : investigation in a non-clinical sample. Sleep Biol Rhythms. 2006;4(June):129–36.

17

Chronic osteo-articular changes in patients with sickle cell disease

Taciana Fernandes Araújo Ferreira[1*], Ana Paula Teixeira dos Santos[2], Alexandra Silva Leal[3], Gilberto de Araújo Pereira[3], Sheila Soares Silva[3] and Helio Moraes-Souza[3]

Abstract

Background: Sickle cell disease (SCD) is an autosomal recessive genetic disease in which a mutation occurs in the β-globin chain gene, resulting in abnormal hemoglobin levels. In an environment with reduced oxygen concentration, red blood cells change their conformation, resulting in chronic hemolysis and consequent anemia and vaso-occlusive crises with injuries to several organs, with a significant impairment of the osteoarticular system. This study aimed to verify the chronic osteoarticular alterations and their association with clinical and laboratory characteristics of patients with SCD with a more severe phenotype (SS and Sβ^0), on a steady-state fasis.

Methods: Fifty-five patients were referred to a medical consultation with a specialized assessment of the locomotor system, followed by laboratory tests and radiographic examinations.

Results: In total, 74.5% patients had hemoglobinopathy SS; 67.3% were female; and 78.2% were non-whites. The mean patient age was 30.5 years. Most patients (61.8%) reported up to three crises per year, with a predominance of high-intensity pain (65.5%). Radiographic alterations were present in 80% patients. A total of 140 lesions were identified, most which were located in the spine, femur, and shoulders. Most lesions were osteonecrosis and osteoarthritis and were statistically associated with the non-use of hydroxyurea.

Conclusions: There was a high prevalence of chronic osteoarticular alterations, which was statistically associated only with the non-regular use of hydroxyurea.

Keywords: Osteonecrosis, Osteoarthritis, Osteopenia, Sickle cell disease, Hydroxyurea

Introduction

Hemoglobinopathies are a group of diseases of genetic origin in which mutations in the genes encoding hemoglobin (Hb) can result in changes in their synthesis. Most of them comprise qualitative defects that result in the production of different Hb molecules with abnormal structure, resulting in sickle cell disease (SCD), and quantitative defects that affect the synthesis of globin chains, resulting thalassemias [1].

Hemoglobin S (HbS) is caused by a mutation in the β-chain gene due to the replacement of the amino acids glutamate with valine at position 6 of chromosome 11. Hemoglobinopathies in which at least one of the mutant hemoglobin is HbS are known as SCD. Hemoglobin S in homozygosis (HbSS), is called sickle cell anemia (SCA), which is the most severe form of SCD. HbS may also be associated with other abnormal hemoglobins, such as HbC, HbD, and β-thalassemia, leading to hemoglobinopathies SC, SD, Sβ^0, and Sβ^+, while the combination of HbS and HbA is called sickle cell trait, in which the carrier does not develop the disease [2]. The most severe SCD phenotypes are associated with the SS and Sβ^0 genotypes, with similar clinical manifestations [3].

Since 1998 in Minas Gerais, Brazil, SCD is diagnosed at birth using the "little foot test," and children diagnosed with SCD are referred early for specialized follow-up.

* Correspondence: taciferreira@yahoo.com.br
[1]Clinical Hospital of Federal University Triângulo Mineiro, Functional Units Rom, Av. Getúlio Guaritá, 130, B. Nossa Senhora da Abadia, CEP 38.025-440, Uberaba, MG, Brazil

The clinical manifestations of SCD are due to two main phenomena—hemolysis and consequent chronic anemia as well as vaso-occlusion by red blood cells, followed by infarction in various organs and tissues. The vaso-occlusive phenomenon manifest acutely with severe pain crisis and chronically with lesions in various organs and tissues such as the lungs, heart, kidneys, liver, retina, skin, joints, and bones [4].

Osteoarticular manifestations occur in different forms of SCD and are more severe in SCA [5]. Acute lesions include hand-foot syndrome (sickle cell dactylitis), pain crises, osteomyelitis, infectious and inflammatory arthritis, stress fractures, bone infarctions, vertebral collapse secondary to osteonecrosis (ON) with a typical "fish mouth" appearance, dental changes, and orbital compression [6]. Chronic changes include avascular necrosis or ON, vertebral collapse due to low bone mass (fragility fractures), inflammatory chronic arthritis, osteoarthritis (OA), bone marrow hyperplasia triggering morphological changes and growth disorders, osteopenia, and osteoporosis [7].

Acute osteoarticular changes determine a severe clinical picture with generally intense events such as sickle cell dactylitis. In contrast, chronic changes can develop silently or after an acute event, determining functional limitations and symptoms of varying degrees of intensity. They are often underdiagnosed, although with an important impact on the morbidity and mortality of these patients, requiring accurate knowledge of the different manifestations to provide correct diagnosis and appropriate treatment.

Therapeutic approaches capable of modifying the natural history of SCD include hypertransfusion, use of hydroxyurea (HU), and hematopoietic stem cell transplantation (HSCT). Currently, HU is the only drug capable of altering the natural history of SCD. Its use in Brazil is guided by hematological clinical indications according to the Clinical Protocol and Therapeutic Guidelines of the Ministry of Health [8].

In addition to increasing the fetal hemoglobin (HbF) concentration, HU increases the total concentration of Hb and causes a reduction in the number of neutrophils, monocytes, and reticulocytes. Furthermore, HU affects the red blood-endothelium interaction and acts as a nitric oxide donor. Although HU treatment is effective, there is variability in patients' response to HU. In 10–25% cases, treatment with HU is not effective, perhaps due to genetic variation, bone marrow exhaustion, variation in drug metabolism, and possibly lack of adherence to treatment [9].

Objective

This study aimed to verify chronic osteoarticular alterations and their association with clinical and laboratory characteristic of patients with SCD of the more severe phenotype (SS and Sβ^0) who were followed up at Regional Blood Center of Uberaba (RBCU) and Clinical Hospital of Federal University of Triângulo Mineiro (CH-FUTM) on a steady-state fasis.

Methods

A cross-sectional study was conducted from May 2017 to January 2018 at RBCU. The sample size was maximized. All eligible patients who attended routine consultations were invited to participate and were included in the study according to their consent and compliance with the evaluation protocols. Of the 67 eligible patients (SS and Sβ^0, 14 years or older, non-pregnant women), 12 did not accept participation or did not complete the evaluation protocol, resulting in 55 participants (non-probabilistic sampling).

After signing the free and informed consent term and/or the informed consent form, the patients were referred for medical consultation with a rheumatologist, consisting of a clinical interview and physical examination with specialized assessment of the locomotor system, followed by laboratory and radiographic examinations. Data on patient's past history were collected from the medical records provided by the Medical File Service of RBCU and CH-FUTM.

Regarding age, the participants were divided into two groups according to the United Nations (UN) classification [10], with individuals aged 14–24 years being considered young patients and individuals aged > 25 years being considered adult patients. The skin color was classified as white, brown, or black based on self-reported data. However, for analysis, white and brown patients were included in the same subgroup since all non-black patients reported no black ancestry.

Prolonged use of HU was defined as use for at least 1 year without interruption.

The participants were asked about the average number of painful crises presented per year and classified into mild, moderate, or high groups according to the Pain Analog Scale scores [11].

The laboratory tests included those for ferritin, reticulocytes, C-reactive protein (CRP), and lactic dehydrogenase (LDH). We retrieved the values of fetal hemoglobin and basal hemoglobin (BHb) from the medical records.

For radiographic screening, the following were examined: the hand and wrist, shoulders, cervical, thoracic and lumbar spine, pelvis, and skull. When changes in physical examination were observed, the knees, ankle, feet, and long bones were examined.

The data were arranged in an Excel spreadsheet, from which descriptive statistical analysis and association were performed using the chi-square test. Statistical Package for Social Science for Windows (SPSS) version 22.1.1.1

was used for statistical analysis. The level of statistical significance set at 5% ($p < 0.05$).

Results

Among the 55 individuals, 41 (74.5%) had SS hemoglobinopathy, 14 (25.5%) had Sβ^0 hemoglobinopathy, 37 (67.3%) were female, 27 (49.1%) were black, and 28 (50.9%) were non-black. The mean (± standard deviation [SD]) patient age was 30.5 (± 11.5) years (range: 15–54 years). In total, 21 patients were categorized as young patients (age: 14–24 years; 38.2%), and 34 patients were categorized as adult patients (age: ≥25 years; 61,8%). Thirty-five (63.6%) participants used HU for at least 1 year uninterruptedly.

The mean (± SD) values of the various laboratory parameters evaluated were as follows: FHb, 11.3 (± 6.7) g/dL; BHb, 7.9 (± 1.2) g/dL; ferritin, 743.2 (± 1159.7) ng/mL; reticulocytes, 6.6% (± 2.9%); CRP, 0.7 (± 0.9) mg/L; and LDH, 472.9 (± 166.8) U/L.

The distribution of participants according to the frequency and intensity of pain crises is shown in Table 1. We observed that most participants reported up to three attacks per year (61.8%), and the pain was high in 65.8% painful episodes.

Regarding radiographic alterations, 140 lesions were identified, most of which occurred in the spine (62.1%), followed by the femur (16.4%) and the shoulders (7.1%). The most frequent alteration was ON (55%), followed by OA (21.4%) (Table 2). ON was identified in 29.1% patients, OA was identified in 25.4% patients. Most patients had several lesions simultaneously (Table 2).

Regarding the number of radiographic lesions per patient, most patients had 1–4 lesions (63.6%), with a variation of zero (20.0%) to nine (1.8%), with mean and SD of 2.61 and ± 2.22, respectively.

The association between laboratory and clinical parameters and the number of radiographic lesions was not statistically significant, except for the use of HU ($p = 0.0038$) (Table 3).

Among people with ≥5 injuries, most were women (21.6%), non-black (17.9%), adults (20.6%), with ≥4 attacks in 1 year (19.9%) and with high pain intensity (16.7%); however, the difference was not statistically significant (Table 3).

Of the 35 individuals who used HU regularly for > 1 year, only 8.6% had ≥5 injuries, while of the 20 individuals who did not use it regularly, 30.0% had ≥5 injuries ($p = 0.0038$) (Table 3).

Table 1 Distribution of the participants according to the frequency and intensity of painful crises

Variables	N	%
Number of crises per year		
0–3	34	61.8
≥ 4	21	38.2
Intensity of pain in crises		
Mild and moderate	19	34.5
High	36	65.5

Table 2 Distribution of radiographic lesions according to location and type of alteration

Radiographic Changes	N	%
Location of lesions		
Spine	74	52.8
Proximal femur/hip	23	16.4
Shoulders/humerus	10	7.1
Skull	7	5.0
Hands and wrists	4	2.8
Other[a]	22	15.7
Total	140	100.0
Types of alterations		
Osteonecrosis	77	55.0
Osteoarthritis	30	21.4
Other SCD-related changes[b]	17	12.2
Non-specific changes[c]	16	11.4
Total	140	100.0

Other[a]: tibia, fibula, knees, distal femur, ulna, ankle, and feet
Other changes related to SCD [b]: thickening of the diploe, sequelae of osteomyelitis, pyogenic arthritis, dactylitis, and discitis, consolidated fractures
Non-specific changes [c]: Non-specific lytic lesions, flexion deformity, clinodactyly, tendinopathy, kyphosis, scoliosis, transition vertebra, omovertebral bone, trigone bone, and equine foot

Discussion

The patients' profiles in this study are compatible with those described in the literature, with a predominance of homozygous disease (SS), female sex, non-white individuals, and young individuals [9, 12, 13]. However, most patients in this study reported a low frequency of pain crises, which is different from that reported in previous studies [9, 14, 15].

Platt and colleagues has suggested that people with SCD with HbF values > 8% have a higher survival rate [11], which may indicate a better prognosis for our patients, but with cumulative damage to the osteoarticular system.

The bone is the second most affected organ by SCD after the spleen [16]. We found 140 osteoarticular lesions in our cohort (mean: 2.61/participant). However, 20% participants did not present any radiographic lesions.

Previous studies have evaluated osteoarticular involvement in patients with SCD in the acute phase. However, our study evaluated lesions in patients on a steady-state fasis, which explains the low incidence of infectious and inflammatory changes, which were highly prevalent in past studies [17–19], and a high incidence of OA and ON.

Table 3 Evaluation of the number of lesions according to epidemiological and clinical characteristics

Number of injuries									
Clinical data	**0**		**1–4**		**≥5**		**Total**		***p* value***
	N	%	N	%	N	%	N	%	
Sex									
Male	6	33.3	11	61.1	1	5.6	18	100	0.1156
Female	5	13.6	24	64.8	8	21.6	37	100	
Total	11	20.0	35	63.6	9	16.4	55	100	
Skin color									
Black	4	14.8	19	70.4	4	14.8	27	100	0.5575
Non-black	7	25.0	16	57.1	5	17.9	28	100	
Total	11	20.0	35	63.6	9	16.4	55	100	
Age									
Young	7	33.3	12	57.1	2	9.6	21	100	0.1215
Adults	4	11.7	23	67.6	7	20.6	34	100	
Total	11	20.0	35	63.6	9	16.4	55	100	
Number of crises per year									
0–3	5	14.7	24	70.6	5	14.7	34	100	0.3546
≥ 4	6	28.6	11	52.4	4	19.0	21	100	
Total	11	20.0	35	63.6	9	16.4	55	100	
Intensity of crises									
Mild and moderate	4	21.1	12	63.2	3	15.8	19	100	0.9886
High	7	19.4	23	63.9	6	16.7	36	100	
Total	11	20.0	35	63.6	9	16.4	55	100	
HU use ≥ 1 years									
Yes	4	11.4	28	72.8	3	8.6	35	100	0.0038**
No	7	35.0	7	35.0	6	30.0	20	100	
Total	11	20.0	35	63.6	9	16.4	55	100	

* X^2 test; ** statistically significant

The main sites of bone involvement were the spine, followed by the femur and the shoulders and the most frequent changes were ON, followed by OA, as classically described [6].

The prevalence of ON in people with SCA ranges from 3.2 to 26.7% [19–22]. In our study, this complication affected approximately one-third of the patients. However, like other studies, we observed that the prevalence of ON increases with age, which may be a consequence of recurrent episodes of bone infarctions. Globally, SCD is probably the most common cause of avascular necrosis that most commonly affecting the femoral and humeral heads [23].

Patients with SCD may develop OA, usually secondary to ON, which progresses to OA in 86% patients when not properly treated [24, 25]. These data justify the high prevalence of this type of lesion verified in the evaluation of patients in an outpatient setting on a steady-state basis.

The occurrence of radiographic alterations did not present a statistically significant association with sex, skin, age, number, and intensity of pain attacks; however, we observed that despite the higher percentage of individuals without radiographic lesions in the young group, painful crises were of high intensity in this group. In the group of people with ≥5 injuries, the majority were adults and females. Radiographic changes are secondary to injuries suffered by patients throughout their lives, which may explain the higher incidence of young patients among those without identifiable radiographic injuries and adults with a higher incidence of radiographic damage.

Individuals who regularly used HU had a lower incidence of multiple lesions than those who did not use it, statistically significant result.

Treatment with HU is associated with a significant reduction in the incidence of hospitalization, acute chest crisis, stroke, and vaso-occlusive crises, however, the impact of the use of this drug on the prevention and treatment of chronic osteoarticular lesions needs further investigation.

There is only one study published thus far regarding the osteoarticular alterations of SCD, which has cited high-dose HU significantly reduced the incidence of ON in white and non-white patients aged > 18 years with ßS/ßS and ßS/ß$^+$ treated for 10 years [26].

A review article on the role of HU in SCD describes the importance of this medication in reducing the morbidity and mortality in these individuals [27]. Because of the effects of HU in reducing the sickling of red blood cells, elevating HbF, reducing oxidative stress and vaso-occlusive crisis consequently, we infer that HU also has a positive impact on osteoarticular lesions, as reinforced by the findings of the present study.

SCD is a disease that has a great impact on the osteoarticular system of affected patients, which can lead to functional limitations and low quality of life, requiring special care by a health team. Until new drugs are available, HU should always be considered an important therapeutic option in patients with SCD.

The main limitations of the study were the small sample size, its heterogeneity, the limitation in the recording of data in medical records, and the difficulty in performing some tests in our hospital.

Future studies with a larger sample, including other hemoglobinopathies, control group and nuclear magnetic resonance exams may bring further clarifications on this topic.

Conclusions

In patients whith SCD SS e Sβ^0 followed at RBCU and CH-FUTM, we observed a high prevalence of chronic osteoarticular alterations, being statistically associated, as a protective measure, only with regular use of HU.

Acknowledgements

Not applicable.

Authors' contributions

Calculations and nutritional assessments: Alexandra Silva Leal; Conducting and reporting the imaging exams: Ana Paula Teixeira dos Santos; Conception and design of the research: Taciana Fernandes Araújo Ferreira, Gilberto de Araújo Pereira, Sheila Soares Silva, Helio Moraes-Souza. The author(s) read and approved the final manuscript.

Authors' information

Taciana Fernandes Araújo Ferreira: Master's student of the Master's Program in Health Sciences of the Federal University of Triângulo Mineiro, Uberaba, MG, Brazil.
Ana Paula Teixeira dos Santos: Resident Physician specialized in Radiology and Diagnostic Imaging at the Clinical Hospital of Federal University of Triângulo Mineiro, Uberaba, MG, Brazil.
Alexandra Silva Leal: PhD in Health Sciences from the Federal University of Triângulo Mineiro, Uberaba, MG, Brazil.
Gilberto de Araújo Pereira: Associate Professor at the Institute of Health Sciences, Professor of the Professional Master's Graduate Programs in Technological Innovation and Public Management at the Federal University of Triângulo Mineiro, Uberaba, MG, Brazil.
Sheila Soares Silva: Associate Professor of the Discipline of Hematology and Hemotherapy, Federal University of Triângulo Mineiro, Uberaba, MG, Brazil.
Helio Moraes-Souza: Full Professor of the Discipline of Hematology and Hemotherapy, Federal University of Triângulo Mineiro, Uberaba, MG, Brazil.

Author details

[1]Clinical Hospital of Federal University Triângulo Mineiro, Functional Units Rom, Av. Getúlio Guaritá, 130, B. Nossa Senhora da Abadia, CEP 38.025-440, Uberaba, MG, Brazil. [2]Clinical Hospital of Federal University Triângulo Mineiro, Uberaba, MG, Brazil. [3]Federal University of Triângulo Mineiro, Uberaba, MG, Brazil.

References

1. Batista GA, Santos NA, Marquetti VB, Mota WB, Silvério ASD. Hemoglobinopatias: investigação em sangue periférico de acadêmicos de uma universidade de Alfenas - MG. Rev Med (São Paulo). 2020;99(3):246–50.
2. Brasil. Ministério da Saúde. Agência Nacional de Vigilância Sanitária. Manual de diagnóstico e tratamento de doenças falciformes. 1st ed. Brasília; 2002. p. 142.
3. Shayeb AM, Smeltzer MP, Kaste SC, Brown A, Estepp JH, Nottage KA. Vaso-occlusive crisis as a predictor of symptomatic avascular necrosis in children with sickle cell disease. Pediatric Blood Cancer. 2018;65(12):e27435.
4. Reed W, Vichinsky EP. New considerations in the treatment of sickle cell disease. Annu Rev Med. 1998;49:461–74.
5. Souza HM, Valize PCB, Souza LRMF. Manifestações reumáticas das hemoglobinopatias. In: Cecin HA, Ximenes AC, editors. Tratado Brasileiro de Reumatologia. São Paulo: Atheneu; 2015.
6. Almeida A, Roberts I. Bone involvement in sickle cell disease. Br J Haematol. 2005;129(4):482–90.
7. Claster S, Vichinsky EP. Managing sickle cell disease. Br Med J. 2003; 327(7424):1151–5.
8. Ministério da Saúde. Secretaria de Atenção à Saúde Secretaria de Ciência, Tecnologia e Insumos Estratégicos. Protocolo Clínico e Diretrizes Terapêuticas - Doença Falciforme 2018.
9. Fainstein RSQ, Ramos MC, Mendonça D, Gesteira MF. Uso de hidroxiuréia no tratamento da doença falciforme. Rev Baiana Pediat. 2006;2(1):46–55.
10. Eisenstein E. Adolescência: definições, conceitos e critérios. Adolesc Saud. 2005;2(2):6–7.
11. Lobo C, Marra VN, Silva RMG. Crises dolorosas na doença falciforme. Rev Bras Hematol Hemoter. 2007;29(3):247–58.
12. Amaral JL, Almeida NA, Santos OS, Oliveira PP, Lanza FM. Socio-demographic, economic and health profile of adults with sickle-cell disease. Rev Rene. 2015;16(3):296–305.
13. Platt OS, Bamblia DJ, Rosse WF, Milner PF, Castro O, Steinberg MH, et al. Mortality in sickle cell disease – life expectancy and risk factors for early death. N Engl J Med. 1994;23(330):1639–44.
14. Cruz SV, Martelli DRB, Araújo MX, Leite BGL, Rodrigues LAM, Martelli JH. Avaliação da qualidade de vida em pacientes adultos com anemia falciforme no norte de Minas Gerais – Brasil. Rev Med Minas Gerais. 2016; 26(suppl. 5):S23–30.
15. Furtado NA, Motta J, Santos MDD. Estudo do perfil dos pacientes portadores de Síndromes Falciformes acompanhados no Serviço de Hematologia do Centro Estadual de Hemoterapia e Hematologia do Espírito Santo (HEMOES). Rev Bras Pesq Saúde. 2014;16(4):105–12.
16. Aleluia IP. Ocorrência de osteonecrose da cabeça femoral em pacientes com doença falciforme: um revisão sistemática. Trabalho de Conclusão de Curso (Medicina) – Universidade Federal da Bahia, Salvador, 2014.
17. Bennett OM, Namnyak SS. Bone and joint manifestations of sickle cell anaemia. J Bone Joint Surg Br. 1990;72(3):494–9.
18. Sachan AA, Lakhkar BN, Lakhkar BB, Sachan S. Is MRI necessary for skeletal evaluation in sickle cell disease. J Clin Diagn Res. 2015;9(6):TC08–12.
19. Balogun RA, Obalum DC, Giwa SO, Adekoya-Cole TO, Ogo CN, Enweluzo GO. Spectrum of musculo-skeletal disorders in sickle cell disease in Lagos, Nigeria. J Orthop Surg Res. 2010;5:2.
20. Akinyoola AL, Adediran IA, Asaleye CM. Avascular necrosis of the femoral head in sickle cell disease in Nigeria: a retrospective study. Niger Postgrad Med J. 2007;14(3):217–20.
21. Hernigou P, Habibi A, Bachir D, Galacteros F. The natural history of asymptomatic osteonecrosis of the femoral head in adults with sickle cell disease. J Bone Joint Surg Am. 2006;88(12):2565–72.
22. Iwegbu CG, Fleming AF. Avascular necrosis of the femoral head in sickle-cell disease. A series from the Guinea Savannah of Nigeria. J Bone Joint Surg Br. 1985;67(1):29–32.
23. Hughes M, Akram Q, Rees DC, Jones AKP. Haemoglobinopathies and the rheumatologist. Rheumatology (Oxford). 2016;55(12):2109–18.
24. Mont MA, Zywiel MG, Marker DR, McGrath MS. Delanois RE the natural history of untreated asymptomatic osteonecrosis of the femoral head: a systematic literature review. J Bone Joint Surg Am. 2010;92(12):2165–70.
25. Alonge TO, Shokunbi WA. The choice of arthroplasty for secondary osteoarthritis of the hip joint following avascular necrosis of the femoral head in sicklers. J Natl Med Assoc. 2004;96(5):678–81.
26. Rigano P, Franceschi L, Sainati L, Piga A, Piel FB, Capellini MD, Fidone C, Masera N, Palazzi G, Gianesin B, Forni GL. Italian Multicenter Study of Hydroxyurea in Sickle Cell Anemia Investigators. Real-life experience with hydroxyurea in sickle cell disease: a multicenter study in a cohort of patients with heterogeneous descent. Blood Cells Mol Dis. 2018;69:82–9.
27. Souza EQ, Sales AA, CVS S, Andrade SM, Lucio Neto MP, Oliveira EH. Uso da hidroxiuréia na anemia falciforme: uma revisão da literatura. Res, Soc Dev. 2020;9(2):102922058.

18

Osteoporotic fractures in rheumatoid arthritis patients in Argentina: A matched retrospective cohort study

Florencia S. Pierini*, Martin Brom, Marina Scolnik, Valeria Scaglioni, Javier E. Rosa and Enrique R. Soriano

Abstract

Background: To compare the incidence of osteoporotic fractures in patients with rheumatoid arthritis (RA) with matched controls from a university hospital.

Methods: Consecutive RA patients ($n = 100$) were matched (age and sex) with controls (1:2). The follow-up period began at the index date, defined as the date of diagnosis for RA patients and the date of the first medical claim at the Health Management Organization (HMO) for non-RA patients. Fracture incidence rates per 1000 persons-years (PY) for distinct types of fractures were calculated. Multivariate cox regression analysis was performed to identify factors associated with fractures.

Results: One hundred RA patients were followed for a total of 975.1 patients-years and 200 controls for 1485.7 patients-years. No difference was found in the overall fracture incidence rate per 1000 PY between RA and controls (19.5, 95% CI 12.7–28.6 vs 12.1, 95% CI 7.7–18.7, $p = 0.07$). In the Cox regression analysis, only age (HR 1.06, 95% CI 1.02–1.11, $p = 0.006$) and history of a prior fracture (HR 9.85, 95% CI 2.97–32.64, $p < 0.001$) were associated with fractures after the index date. The stratified analysis of the fractures by location showed that only the vertebral fractures were more frequent in RA patients compared with controls (12.9 per 1000 PY, 95% CI 8.9–25.8, vs. 3.4, 95% CI 1.4–8.1, respectively, $p = 0.01$).

Conclusion: Patients with RA didn't show an overall increased risk of osteoporotic fractures compared with matched controls, but vertebral fractures were more frequently observed in patients with RA.

Keywords: Rheumatoid arthritis, Incidence, Osteoporosis, Fragility fractures, Glucocorticoids

Introduction

Osteoporosis (OP) is a systemic skeletal disease characterized by decreased bone strength with a consequent increase in bone fragility and susceptibility to fracture due to low bone mass and microarchitecture alterations that generate a reduction of bone resistance to torsion and compression [1–3]. These fractures, known as fragility fractures, are bone cracks caused by a low-energy trauma (i.e. falling from a standing height) that should not be able to break a healthy bone [4].

* Correspondence: florpierini@gmail.com
Rheumatology Unit, Internal Medicine Department, Hospital Italiano de Buenos Aires, Perón 4190, 1181 Buenos Aires, Argentina

OP is a very prevalent condition that affects over 200 million people worldwide and causes an important economic and health burden. The principal risk factors for OP are sex and age, and it is estimated to affect 50% of women and 20% of men over 50 years [5]. The incidence of hip fractures in Argentina for women over 50 years is 276.5 per 100,000 person-years, and 114.7 every 100,000 person-years for men [4, 6–8]. The LAVOS study (Latin American Study of Vertebral Osteoporosis) showed an estimated vertebral fractures' prevalence of 16.2% [9]. Fragility fractures can be underdiagnosed because they are frequently non-symptomatic and consequently, not registered [6–8, 10, 11].

On the other hand, Rheumatoid Arthritis is the most frequent inflammatory arthritis in the adult population, affecting between 0.3 and 1% of the population in Argentina [12, 13]. It is an important risk factor for osteoporosis and osteoporotic fractures [4] since it affects bone structure in a multifactorial fashion, including chronic inflammation [14], immobility, use of corticosteroids (GC), vitamin D deficiency, and augmented fall risk [15]. Nevertheless, the relative weight of each of these factors is still unknown [16, 17]. Current data suggests that the pro-inflammatory cytokines (TNF-α, IL-1, IL-6, and IL-17) enhance the expression of RANKL (Receptor Activator of NF-kβ Ligand), leading to increased osteoclast differentiation, and thereafter producing bone resorption [14, 15, 18].

Several recently published studies show the impact of corticosteroids on bone mineral density (BMD) in patients with RA. Cheng T. et al. found that those patients with RA who received low doses of GC had a lower BMD at the spine (L1–4), a higher rate of fractures, and a significantly higher risk of fractures after 10 years compared to patients with RA who did not receive treatment with GC [19]. There is scarce literature in Latin America regarding the incidence of osteoporotic fractures in patients with RA. Moreover, the numerous advances in recent years for the treatment of RA may have changed the OP epidemiology in these patients. Our objective was to compare the incidence of fragility fractures in rheumatoid arthritis patients diagnosed after the year 2000 with matched controls from a University hospital-based health management organization (HMO) [13, 20–23].

Materials and methods

Data source and study population

We performed a retrospective cohort study on patients enrolled in a HMO in Buenos Aires City, Argentina. We included 100 consecutive incident RA patients diagnosed at our rheumatology unit between 01/01/2000 and 31/12/2015, that fulfilled ACR/EULAR 2010 criteria [24], and 200 controls (1:2) matched by age at diagnosis of RA and by sex.

We excluded all patients who suffered fragility fractures prior to the diagnosis of RA, or regarding controls, before the date of diagnosis of RA of their matched patient (Index Date). Patients who were affiliated to the HMO for under a year were also excluded to avoid possible prevalent cases that might have been affiliated to the HMO with the disease (RA or fractures).

The follow-up period began at the index date, defined as the date of RA diagnosis for cases and the date of the first medical claim at the HMO for the non-RA patients. Subjects were followed until they voluntarily left the HMO, death, or the end of study (05/01/2018).

We reviewed each patient's electronic medical records and recorded demographic information (sex and age), clinical data (comorbidities, weight, body mass index, current or past smoking, type and location of fracture), laboratory results (positivity for anti-citrullinated peptide antibody and/or rheumatoid factor, erythrosedimentation rate, ultrasensitive c reactive protein at the time of diagnosis), images (annual bone densitometry) and treatment data (chronic use of corticosteroid, use of another immunosuppressant, treatment for osteoporosis and osteopenia). We defined low-dose of GC as a 2.5–7.5 mg/day of prednisone or equivalent dose and prolonged corticosteroid use as equal or more than 3 months of use.

Fractures were evaluated by using X-rays, Computerized Tomography, and Nuclear Magnetic Resonance, many of which were ordered by other specialists for many other clinical reasons. All images that allowed to see the bones were carefully reviewed looking for fractures. Vertebral morphology of fractures was evaluated by Genant Classification [25].

The primary outcome was the incidence rate of all new fragility fractures after the index date, defined as bone cracks caused by a low-energy trauma [26]; and the secondary outcomes were incidence rates of each site fragility fractures (ribs, proximal extremity of the femur/hip, pelvis, vertebra, humerus, distal extremity of the radius and ulna). We excluded fractures produced by high impact trauma and fractures in sites that are not mentioned above.

Statistical analysis

Descriptive statistics were performed. Categorical variables were expressed as percentages with their corresponding 95% confidence intervals (95% CI). Continuous variables were expressed as means and medians, according to their distribution, with their corresponding standard deviations (SD) or interquartile ranges (IQR). Categorical variables were compared using a chi-square test or Fisher's test, and continuous variables using Student's t-test or Mann's Whitney test.

The incidence rates for all fractures and for each type of fragility fracture (vertebral, radius and femur) were calculated, both for patients with rheumatoid arthritis and controls, and the rate ratio between both groups was reported. The analysis was done at fracture level and not at patient level (each patient could have had more than one fracture after the index date).

We then performed a multivariate logistic regression analysis, evaluating possible factors associated with fractures (RA diagnosis, treatment with biologic DMARDs, sex, age, prior fracture after the index date, prolonged corticosteroid use – equal or more than 3 months-, osteoporosis diagnosis, osteoporosis treatment).

Results

Patient's demographic and clinical characteristics

One hundred patients with RA and 200 age and sex-matched controls were included. RA patients were followed for a total of 975.1 patients-years (PY) and controls for 1485.7 patients-years. As shown in Tables 1, 78% were female in both groups and the mean age at index date was 62 years. The median duration of follow-up was 9.5 years (IQR 5.9–13.4) for the RA group and 7.4 years (IQR 2.4–12.3) for the control group.

Regarding the RA patients, 97.9% (95% CI 92.0–99.5) were seropositive for Rheumatoid Factor and/or Anti Citrullinated Peptide Antibodies (ACPA), 94% (95% CI 87.1–97.3) were treated with conventional Disease-Modifying Antirheumatic Drugs (DMARDs), and 20% (95% CI 13.2–29.1) with biologic DMARDs. Sixty-nine percent of the patients with RA (69.0%, CI 0.59–77.3) used GC at some time of their disease vs. 5 patients in the control group (2.5%, CI 1.0–5.9), being this difference statistically significant ($p < 0.001$). In the same line, there was a statistically significant difference between groups (p < 0.001) for the prolonged use of GC, showing that 63 RA patients were exposed to prolonged GC (63.0%, CI 53.1–71.9) (p < 0.001) vs. 4 controls (2.0%, CI 0.7–5.2).

At least one Bone Mineral Density test was performed during follow-up in 74 of the RA patients (74, 95% CI 64.4–81.7) and in 88 of controls (44, 95% CI 37.2–50.9), $p < 0.001$. Osteoporosis was diagnosed by BMD in 36.5% (95% CI 26.2–48.1) of RA patients and 27.3% (CI 18.9–37.6) of controls, $p = 0.21$, according to The International Society for Clinical Densitometry (ISCD) [27] and WHO criteria [28]. There was no statistically significant difference in the use of antiresortive treatment between patients with RA (24, 95% CI 16.6–33.4) and controls (15, 95% CI 10.7–20.7) ($p = 0.06$).

Fractures incidence rates

The 100 RA patients contributed with a total of 975.1 patients/years, and showed a global fracture incidence rate of 19.5/1000 PY (95% CI 12.7–28.6) with 25 fractures occurring in 16 patients. The control group contributed with a total of 1485.7 patients/years, and presented a fracture incidence rate of 12.1/1000 PY (95% CI 7.7–18.7), with 23 fractures in 15 patients. The between-group difference is non-significant ($p = 0.07$).

When analyzing each type of fracture, only the vertebral fractures were more frequently found in RA patients compared with controls (12.9 per 1000 PY, 95% CI 8.9–25.8, versus 3.4, 95% CI 1.4–8.1, $p = 0.01$, respectively) (Table 2). The remaining incidence rates for other site fractures were similar across groups (Table 2).

Cox regression analysis association between fracture and other factors

After adjusting for RA diagnosis, treatment with biologic DMARDs, sex, age, history of prior fracture after the index date, prolonged corticosteroid use, osteoporosis diagnosis and treatment for osteoporosis, we found that age (HR 1.06, 95% CI 1.02–1.11, $p = 0.006$) and a

Table 1 Patient characteristics

	RA patients (*n* = 100)	Controls (*n* = 200)	p
Age at index date, years, mean (SD)	62.1 (12.9)	62.4 (13.9)	0.87
Female, n (%, 95 CI)	78 (78, 68.7–85.1)	156 (78, 71.7–83.2)	1
Follow up, years, median (IQR)	9.5 (5.9–13.4)	7.4 (IQR 2.4–12.3)	**< 0.001**
Seropositive Rheumatoid Factor and/or ACPA, n (%, 95 CI)	97,7 (97,7, 92.0–99.5)		
Use DMARDs, n (%, 95 CI)	94 (94, 87.1–97.3)		
Use biologic DMARDs, n (%, 95 CI)	20 (20, 13.2–29.1)		
BMI < 20, n (%, 95 CI)	5 (5.3, 2.2–12.1)	1 (0.6, 0.1–4.3)	**0.02**
Ever Smoker, n (%, 95 CI)	33 (33, 24.4–42.9)	31 (15.6, 11.1–21.3)	**0.001**
Menopause age, years, median (IQR)	47.8 (40.7–51)	48.4 (44.6–51.4)	0.27
Age at first Bone Mineral Densitometry, years, median (IQR)	62.7 (54.4–74.8)	67.0 (58.9–75.5)	0.09
Osteopenia at first densitometry, n (%, 95 CI)	21 (28.4, 19.2–39.8)	31 (35.6, 26.2–46.3)	0.33
Osteoporosis at first densitometry, n (%, 95 CI)	23 (31.3, 21.5–42.6)	22 (25, 16.9–35.2)	0.39
Osteoporosis at any densitometry, n (%, 95 CI)	27 (36.5, 26.2–48.1)	24 (27.3, 18.9–37.6)	0.21
Anti-resorptives use ever, n (% 95 CI)	24 (24.0%, 16.6–33.4)	30 (15.0%, 10.7–20.7)	0.06
Corticosteroid use ever, n (%, 95 CI)	69 (69.0, 59.2–77.3)	5 (2.5, 1.0–5.9)	**< 0.001**
Prednisone use > = 20 mg/day ever, n (%, 95 CI)	5 (5.0, 2.1–11.5)	1 (0.5, 0.1–3.5)	**0.01**
Corticosteroid use > = 3 months, n (%, 95 CI)	63 (63.0, 53.1–71.9)	4 (2.0, 0.7–5.2)	**< 0.001**

Table 2 Incidence rates of distinct types of fractures

	RA patients ($n = 100$)			Controls ($n = 200$)			P value
	Number of fractures	Patient/ years	Incidence rate per 1000 persons/years (95% CI)	Number of fractures	Patient/ years	Incidence rate per 1000 persons/years (95% CI)	
All fractures	24	1230.76	19.5 (12.7–28.6)	23	1900.82	12.1 (7.7–18.7)	0.07
Vertebral fractures	9	697.67	12.9 (8.9–25.8)	5	1470.58	3.4 (1.4–8.1)	**0.01**
Radius fracture	5	675.67	7.4 (3.6–14.9)	4	851.06	4.7 (2.3–9.8)	0.21
Ulna fracture	1	1000	1.0 (0.1–7.1)	1	1428.57	0.7 (0.1–4.7)	0.39
Humerus fracture	1	1000	1.0 (0.1–7.1)	5	1219.51	4.1 (1.8–8.9)	0.09
Rib fracture	0	0	0	1	1428.57	0.7 (0.1–4.7)	0.30
Hip fracture	5	793.65	6.3 (2.8–13.4)	5	1470.58	3.4 (1.4–8.0)	0.16
Pelvis fracture	2	625	3.2 (0.9–9.4)	2	1428.57	1.4 (0.3–5.3)	0.19

previous fracture (after index date) (HR 9.85, 95% CI 2.97–32.64, $p < 0.001$) were the only variables independently associated with fragility fractures. Neither RA diagnosis (HR 0.86, 95% CI 0.24–3.07, $p = 0.81$) nor a prolonged use (> 3 months) of low dose corticosteroids (HR 1.57, 95% CI 0.39–6.23, $p = 0.52$) were associated with increased fracture risk.

When analyzing vertebral fractures separately in a multivariate cox regression analysis (adjusting for age, RA diagnosis, gender, and a prior fracture), the use of low dose corticosteroids for more than 3 months was not associated in these patients with an increased vertebral fracture risk (HR 3.43, 95% CI 0.74–15.82, $p = 0.11$).

Discussion

Osteoporosis risk in RA patients is influenced by both general background factors (such as female gender, body mass index, age) and RA specific factors (ACPAs positivity, disease activity, immobility, systemic inflammation, and treatments) [29]. Additionally, the GIOTTO study reported that RA patients received sub-optimal prevention of BMD loss [30].

Since sex, age, and having had a prior fragility fracture are well-known risk factors for fragility fractures [16, 31, 32], we matched RA patients with controls by sex and age, and excluded any patient who had fragility fractures prior to the index date.

Our study shows a similar incidence rate of fragility fractures in RA patients compared with a recent systematic review and meta-analyses 19.5 (95% CI 12.7–28.6) vs 15.31 (95% CI 10.43–22.47) per 1000 persons/years [33].

We did not find an overall increased incidence of fragility fractures in RA patients compared to the general population. We acknowledge that our data differs from most previous studies, which suggested a causal relationship between RA and fragility fractures [17, 19, 32–35]. A possible explanation for the discordance between our results and many of the previous studies in patients with RA is that we included patients diagnosed with RA after the year 2000, when several new and more effective treatment options – Biologic DMARDs – were developed, and when the "treat to target" strategy was incorporated to daily practice, leading to better control of RA activity and consequently, lowering the need for corticosteroids [36]. Although conventional DMARDs diminish the activity of pro-inflammatory cytokines, it is reported that biological DMARDs have a better protective effect on the bone [37] by suppressing inflammation [38], and hence, they might protect the bone from fractures. Only 20% of this cohort of RA patients were in treatment with biologic DMARDs, so we couldn't demonstrate a protective effect regarding fractures, perhaps due to the low number of cases.

In line with this, a recent meta-analysis suggested that there might be a change in fracture risk trends as a result of the change in therapeutic strategies in RA and earlier control of inflammation [33].

Vertebral fractures were the only type of fragility fractures that were more frequent in RA patients than in the general population in our study. On the multivariate logistic regression analysis, the only independently associated variables were age and history of previous fractures. Unfortunately, we could not analyze factors such as BMD in all patients and functional disability which could be associated with fractures. The possibility of finding differences between groups in the rate of osteoporosis might have been hampered by the statistically significant difference of BMD tests performed (77% vs. 44%, $p < 0.001$), explained by the increased awareness of the risk in RA patients and the fact that most of the controls did not have indication for screening of osteoporosis.

Remarkably, 35% of the patients with RA diagnosed with osteoporosis by BMD test and 45% of controls were not under antiresortive treatment. Although we cannot rule out that it might respond to the retrospective nature of this study and under-registration of the treatment, we believe that it might reflect real life up to some extent and the fact that patients diagnosed with OP often go undertreated until they have a fragility fracture.

Although steroids use is associated with loss of trabecular bone, the main component of vertebrae, we did not find an association between vertebral fractures and prolonged use of low-dose corticosteroids. We don't have a certain explanation for this, but we believe that although more than half of RA patients (63, 95% CI 53.1–71.9, Table 1) were on corticosteroids for more than 3 months, doses were in general low, and only 5% (95% CI 2.1–11.5, Table 1) of patients have ever received prednisone doses greater than 20 mg/d and low doses may not have had an impact on fractures risk.

Our finding on vertebral fractures is in opposition to the study by Kim D. et al. [17], where they found an increased risk on RA patients with longer duration and a higher dose of oral corticosteroids.

Despite radius is also mostly composed of trabecular bone, we did not find a higher incidence rate of fractures in patients with RA compared with controls.

Regarding the incidence of fragility fractures in controls, we found an incidence rate for hip fractures of 3.4 (95% CI 1.4–8.0) per 1000 persons/years. This result is similar to previous studies reported in Argentina, such as the study by A. Wittich et al. in Tucumán [6] with an incidence rate of 2.76 and 1.14 per 1000 persons/years for women and men respectively; the study by M. Morosano et al. in Rosario with 2.9 per 1000 persons/years [7]; and the study by A. Bagur et al. in La Plata with 3.79 and 1.01 per 1000 persons/year for women and men respectively [8]. Regarding the incidence rate of vertebral fractures in controls, our cohort shows an incidence of 3.4 per 1000 persons/years (95% CI 1.4–8.0), but we didn't find any another study in Argentina or Latin America to compare with. Recently, a worldwide study by Ballane, G. et al. [39], reported higher age-standardized incidence rates of vertebral fractures in South Korea (5,44 and 15,75 for men and women per 1000 persons/year), USA (7,07 and 10,83 for men and women per 1000 persons/year) and Hong Kong (2,02 y 7,64 for men and women per 1000 persons/year); and the lowest incidence for the UK (0,48 and 0,84 for women and men per 1000 persons/year). The incidence rate for vertebral fractures reported in our study was similar to Germany (0.87 and 2.05 for men and women per 1000 persons/year) and Italy (2.11 and 2.49 for men and women per 1000 persons/year), within the range of lower values.

This study has several limitations. Due to the retrospective nature of the study, we lacked information on some possible risk factors for osteoporosis, such as functional disability, malabsorption, vitamin D levels, supplementation with vitamin D or calcium, and RA disease activity. We were also unable to stratify patients according to FRAX and to properly register the RA disease activity and its relationship with fracture risk.

On the other hand, some strengths should be listed. First, our HMO offers comprehensive health and medical services to approximately 140,000 outpatients on two central hospitals and 24 peripheral centers, and is broadly representative of the population from Buenos Aires city [13]. Second, all included patients fulfill strict classification criteria, and were compared with 2 matched controls. Third, only patients with incident diagnosis of RA were included and only incident fractures were considered. Finally, we included all types of fragility fractures in the analysis. Since less than half of vertebral fractures are symptomatic, we performed a revision of all the dorsal and lumbar spine x-rays, eliminating the possibility of under-diagnosis of asymptomatic fractures.

Conclusions

In this cohort of RA patients with diagnosis after the year 2000, no overall increased risk of fractures was found in comparison with matched controls, but an increased incidence of vertebral fractures in these patients versus matched controls was found.

Acknowledgements

Not applicable.

Authors' contributions

FP, MB and VS performed the examination of the patients' data in medical records and were a major contribution in writing the manuscript. MS, JR and ERS analyzed and interpreted the patient data statistically. All authors read and approved the final manuscript.

Authors' information

Not applicable.

References

1. NIH Consensus Development Panel on Osteoporosis Prevention, Diagnosis, and Therapy. Osteoporosis Prevention, Diagnosis, and Therapy. JAMA. 2001; 285(6):785–795. https://doi.org/10.1001/jama.285.6.785.
2. Assessment of fracture risk and its application to screening for postmenopausal osteoporosis. Report of a WHO Study Group. World Health Organ Tech Rep Ser. 1994;843:1 129.
3. Siris ES, Chen Y-T, Abbott TA, Barrett-Connor E, Miller PD, Wehren LE, et al. Bone mineral density thresholds for pharmacological intervention to

prevent fractures. Arch Intern Med. 2004;164(10):1108–12. https://doi.org/10.1001/archinte.164.10.1108.
4. Mosquera MT, Maurel DL, Pavón S, Arregui A, Moreno C, Vázquez J. Incidencia y factores de riesgo de la fractura de fémur proximal por osteoporosis [Incidence and risk factors in fractures of the proximal femur due to osteoporosis]. Rev Panam Salud Publica. 1998;3(4):211–9. Spanish. https://doi.org/10.1590/s1020-49891998000400001.
5. Wright NC, Looker AC, Saag KG, Curtis JR, Delzell ES, Randall S, et al. The recent prevalence of osteoporosis and low bone mass in the United States based on bone mineral density at the femoral neck or lumbar spine. J Bone Miner Res. 2014;29(11):2520–6. https://doi.org/10.1002/jbmr.2269.
6. Wittich A, Bagur A, Mautalen C, Cristofari A, Escobar O, Carrizo G, et al. Epidemiology of hip fracture in Tucuman. Argentina. Osteoporos Int. 2010; 21(11):1803–7. https://doi.org/10.1007/s00198-009-1135-3.
7. Morosano M, Masoni A, Sánchez A. Incidence of hip fractures in the city of Rosario. Argentina Osteoporos Int. 2005;16(11):1339–44. https://doi.org/10.1007/s00198-005-1839-y.
8. Bagur A, Mautalen C, Rubin Z. Epidemiology of hip fractures in an urban population of Central Argentina. Osteoporos Int. 1994;4(6):332–5. https://doi.org/10.1007/BF01622193.
9. Clark P, Cons-Molina F, Deleze M, Ragi S, Haddock L, Zanchetta JR, et al. The prevalence of radiographic vertebral fractures in Latin American countries: the Latin American vertebral osteoporosis study (LAVOS). Osteoporos Int. 2009;20(2):275–82. https://doi.org/10.1007/s00198-008-0657-4.
10. Harvey N, Dennison E, bone CC-P on the metabolic, 2008 undefined. Epidemiology of osteoporotic fractures. books.google.com.
11. Cummings SR, Melton LJ. Epidemiology and outcomes of osteoporotic fractures. Lancet. 2002;359(9319):1761–7. https://doi.org/10.1016/S0140-6736(02)08657-9.
12. Scublinsky D, Venarotti H, Citera G, Messina OD, Scheines E, Rillo O, et al. The prevalence of rheumatoid arthritis in Argentina. JCR J Clin Rheumatol. 2010;16(7):317–21. https://doi.org/10.1097/RHU.0b013e3181f3bfdd.
13. Di WT, Vergara F, Bertiller E, de LA Gallardo M, Gandino I, Scolnik M, et al. Incidence and Prevalence of Rheumatoid Arthritis in a Health Management Organization in Argentina: A 15-year Study. J Rheumatol. 2016;43(7):1306–11 Available from: http://www.ncbi.nlm.nih.gov/pubmed/27084906. [cited 2020 Apr 16].
14. Goldring SR. Inflammatory signaling induced bone loss. Bone. 2015;80:143–9. https://doi.org/10.1016/j.bone.2015.05.024.
15. Heinlen L, Humphrey MB. Skeletal complications of rheumatoid arthritis. Osteoporos Int. 2017;28(10):2801–12. https://doi.org/10.1007/s00198-017-4170-5.
16. Van Staa TP, Laan RF, Barton IP, Cohen S, Reid DM, Cooper C. Bone density threshold and other predictors of vertebral fracture in patients receiving oral glucocorticoid therapy. Arthritis Rheum. 2003;48(11):3224–9. https://doi.org/10.1002/art.11283.
17. Kim SY, Schneeweiss S, Liu J, Daniel GW, Chang C-L, Garneau K, et al. Risk of osteoporotic fracture in a large population-based cohort of patients with rheumatoid arthritis. Arthritis Res Ther. 2010;12(4):R154. https://doi.org/10.1186/ar3107.
18. Lane NE, Pressman AR, Star VL, Cummings SR, Nevitt MC. Rheumatoid arthritis and bone mineral density in elderly women. J Bone Miner Res. 2009;10(2):257–63. https://doi.org/10.1002/jbmr.5650100212.
19. Cheng T-T, Lai H-M, Yu S-F, Chiu W-C, Hsu C-Y, Chen J-F, et al. The impact of low-dose glucocorticoids on disease activity, bone mineral density, fragility fractures, and 10-year probability of fractures in patients with rheumatoid arthritis. J Investig Med. 2018;66(6):1004–7. https://doi.org/10.1136/jim-2018-000723.
20. Pierini FS, Scolnik M, Scaglioni V, Mollerach F, Soriano ER. Incidence and prevalence of granulomatosis with polyangiitis and microscopic polyangiitis in health management organization in Argentina: a 15-year study. Clin Rheumatol. 2019;38(7):1935–40. https://doi.org/10.1007/s10067-019-04463-y.
21. Rosa J, Garrot LF, Navarta DA, Saucedo C, Scolnik M, Bedran Z, et al. Incidence and prevalence of Polymyositis and Dermatomyositis in a health Management Organization in Buenos Aires. J Clin Rheumatol. 2013;19(6): 303–7. https://doi.org/10.1097/RHU.0b013e3182a21ba8.
22. Soriano ER, Rosa J, Velozo E, Schpilberg M, Imamura PM, Diaz J, et al. Incidence and prevalence of psoriatic arthritis in Buenos Aires, Argentina: a 6-year health management organization-based study. Rheumatology. 2011; 50(4):729–34. https://doi.org/10.1093/rheumatology/keq369.
23. Scolnik M, Marin J, Valeiras SM, Marchese MF, Talani AS, Avellaneda NL, et al. Incidence and prevalence of lupus in Buenos Aires, Argentina: a 11-year health management organisation-based study. Lupus Sci Med. 2014;1(1): e000021. https://doi.org/10.1136/lupus-2014-000021.
24. Aletaha D, Neogi T, Silman AJ, Funovits J, Felson DT, Bingham CO, et al. 2010 rheumatoid arthritis classification criteria: an American College of Rheumatology/European league against rheumatism collaborative initiative. Arthritis Rheum. 2010;62(9):2569–81. https://doi.org/10.1002/art.27584.
25. Genant HK, Wu CY, van Kuijk C, Nevitt MC. Vertebral fracture assessment using a semiquantitative technique. J Bone Miner Res. 1993;8(9):1137–48 Available from: https://pubmed.ncbi.nlm.nih.gov/8237484/. [cited 2021 Feb 9].
26. Fragility fractures | International Osteoporosis Foundation [Internet]. [cited 2021 Feb 10]. Available from: https://www.osteoporosis.foundation/health-professionals/fragility-fractures
27. Lewiecki EM, Gordon CM, Baim S, Leonard MB, Bishop NJ, Bianchi ML, et al. International Society for Clinical Densitometry 2007 adult and pediatric official positions. Bone. 2008;43(6):1115–21. https://doi.org/10.1016/j.bone.2008.08.106.
28. Kanis JA, Kanis JA. Assessment of fracture risk and its application to screening for postmenopausal osteoporosis: Synopsis of a WHO report. Osteoporos Int. 1994;4(6):368–81. https://doi.org/10.1007/BF01622200 [cited 2021 Feb 23].
29. Briot K, Geusens P, Em Bultink I, Lems WF, Roux C. Inflammatory diseases and bone fragility. Osteoporosis Int. 2017;28:3301–14.
30. Rossini M, Viapiana O, Vitiello M, Malavolta N, La Montagna G, Maddali Bongi S, et al. Prevalence and incidence of osteoporotic fractures in patients on long-term glucocorticoid treatment for rheumatic diseases: the glucocorticoid induced OsTeoporosis TOol (GIOTTO) study. Reumatismo. 2017;69(1):30. https://doi.org/10.4081/reumatismo.2017.922.
31. Akkawi I, Zmerly H. Osteoporosis: current concepts. Joints. 2018;6:122–7.
32. Kim D, Cho S-K, Park B, Jang EJ, Bae S-C, Sung Y-K. Glucocorticoids are associated with an increased risk for vertebral fracture in patients with rheumatoid arthritis. J Rheumatol. 2018 May;45(5):612–20. https://doi.org/10.3899/jrheum.170054.
33. Jin S, Hsieh E, Peng L, Yu C, Wang Y, Wu C, et al. Incidence of fractures among patients with rheumatoid arthritis: a systematic review and meta-analysis. Osteoporos Int. 2018;29(6):1263–75. https://doi.org/10.1007/s00198-018-4473-1
34. Van Staa TP, Geusens P, Bijlsma JWJ, Leufkens HGM, Cooper C. Clinical assessment of the long-term risk of fracture in patients with rheumatoid arthritis. Arthritis Rheum. 2006;54(10):3104–12. https://doi.org/10.1002/art.22117.
35. Xue A-L, Wu S-Y, Jiang L, Feng A-M, Guo H-F, Zhao P. Bone fracture risk in patients with rheumatoid arthritis. Medicine (Baltimore). 2017;96(36):e6983. https://doi.org/10.1097/MD.0000000000006983.
36. Grigor C, Capell H, Stirling A, McMahon AD, Lock P, Vallance R, et al. Effect of a treatment strategy of tight control for rheumatoid arthritis (the TICORA study): a single-blind randomised controlled trial. Lancet. 2004;364(9430): 263–9. https://doi.org/10.1016/S0140-6736(04)16676-2.
37. Killinger Z, Gajdarova L, Kuzma M, Krajcovicova A, Brazdilova K, Jackuliak P, et al. Biologic treatment in comparison to methotrexate has positive effect on trabecular bone score in rheumatoid arthritis patients: 1-year follow-up. Acta Clin Belg. 2019;74(2):121–5. https://doi.org/10.1080/17843286.2018.1512189. Epub 2018 Aug 23.
38. Zerbini CAF, Clark P, Mendez-Sanchez L, Pereira RMR, Messina OD, Uña CR, et al. Biologic therapies and bone loss in rheumatoid arthritis. Osteoporos Int. 2017;28(2):429–46. https://doi.org/10.1007/s00198-016-3769-2.
39. Ballane G, Cauley JA, Luckey MM, El-Hajj FG. Worldwide prevalence and incidence of osteoporotic vertebral fractures. Osteoporos Int. 2017;28(5): 1531–42. https://doi.org/10.1007/s00198-017-3909-3.

Translation, cultural adaptation and reproducibility of a Portuguese version of the Functional Index for Hand Osteoarthritis (FIHOA)

Francisco Vileimar Andrade de Azevedo[1], Hermano Alexandre Lima Rocha[2,3], Anamaria Jones[4], Jamil Natour[4] and Francisco Airton Castro da Rocha[1,5*]

Abstract

Background: The Functional Index for Hand Osteoarthritis (FIHOA) is a simple, reliable, and reproducible specific instrument to evaluate hand OA that can be applied both in clinical practice and research protocols. In order to be used in Brazil, FIHOA has to be translated into Portuguese, culturally adapted and have the reliability of the translated FIHOA version tested, which is the purpose of this study.

Methods: The FIHOA was translated into Brazilian Portuguese and administered to 68 patients with hand OA recruited between May 2019 and February 2020. The test-retest was applied to 32 patients and the reliability was assessed using Spearman's correlation coefficient and intraclass correlation coefficient (ICC). The internal consistency reliability was evaluated using Cronbach's alpha. External construction validity was assessed using the Spearman's correlation test between FIHOA and pain, assessed with a Visual Analogue Scale (VAS), the Cochin Hand Functional Scale (CHFS) and Health Assessment Questionnaire (HAQ).

Results: The 30 participants that initially answered the translated version of the FiHOA did not report difficulties in understanding or interpreting the translated version. The test-retest reliability for the total score was strong ($r = 0.86$; ICC = 0.89). Mean differences (1.37 ± 0.68) using Bland Altman's analysis did not significantly differ from zero and no systematic bias was observed. Cronbach's alpha was also high (0.89) suggesting a strong internal coherence in the test items. There were also correlations between FIHOA and the CHFS ($r = 0.88$), HAQ ($r = 0.64$) and pain in the hands both at rest ($r = 0.55$) and in motion ($r = 0.44$).

Conclusion: The translation of the FIHOA into Brazilian Portuguese proved a valid instrument for measuring the functional capacity of patients with hand OA who understand Brazilian Portuguese.

Keywords: FIHOA, Hand, Osteoarthritis, Patient health questionnaires, Validation studies

* Correspondence: arocha@ufc.br
[1]Department of Internal Medicine - Faculdade de Medicina, Universidade Federal do Ceará, Fortaleza, CE, Brazil
[5]Instituto de Biomedicina – Laboratório de Investigação em Osteoartropatias, Rua Cel. Nunes de Melo, 1315 - 1°. Andar, Rodolfo Teófilo, Fortaleza, CE 60430-270, Brazil

Background

Osteoarthritis (OA) is the most prevalent chronic arthropathy, involving particularly the hands, knee, cervical and lumbar spine and the hip [1, 2]. This is also true in Brazil, as it was recently reported, indicating a high OA prevalence [3]. Hand OA usually evolves with worsening symptoms with advanced age, being more prevalent in women. It is most commonly bilateral with symmetrical joint involvement [1, 4]. In addition to the pain component there is usually impairment of grip and pinch function particularly in those with a severe form [2, 4]. Initiatives published by the Outcome Measures in Rheumatology Clinical Trials (OMERACT) and Osteoarthritis Research Society International (OARSI) recommend the application of function measures to evaluate hand OA [5, 6]. The Functional Index for Hand Osteoarthritis (FIHOA) is a free-of-charge, simple, reliable, and reproducible specific instrument to evaluate hand OA that can be applied both in clinical practice and research protocols [7, 8]. It has been originally published in an English version and various translations into other languages have been provided [9–12]. In order to be used in another language, a questionnaire has to be translated, culturally adapted and validated [13]. Our aim was to translate, culturally adapt and test the reliability of a Portuguese version of the FIHOA.

Methodology

Translation and cultural adaptation

The translation process was performed according to the guidelines for validation and cross-cultural adaptation, as described previously [13]. The original version of FIHOA was translated into Portuguese by two independent native Portuguese-speaking persons. Minor differences were observed between the versions of the texts of the 02 translators. The discrepancies between the translations were discussed with the translators and a consensus Portuguese translation was made. The consensus Portuguese version was then translated back into English by two bilingual native English speakers that were unaware of the original version. This consensus version was compared with the original questionnaire in order to assess semantic equivalence between the two versions and thus confirm a final translated version of the questionnaire. Following, the final version of the translated text was analyzed by three independent rheumatologists and a physiotherapist, also native Portuguese speakers, reaching a final cross-culturally adapted Portuguese consensus translation (Table 1).

Patients

A total of 68 consecutive patients attending the outpatient clinic of the Rheumatology Service of the Hospital das Clínicas of the Faculdade de Medicina of the Universidade Federal do Ceará were recruited between May 2019 and February 2020. The protocol was approved by the Local Ethics Committee (CAAE:07360819930015045; May 20, 2019) and all participants signed an informed consent prior to inclusion. Patients had to be native Portuguese speakers, within 40 to 75 years-old age range and meet the classification criteria for Hand OA according to the American College of Rheumatology [14]. Exclusion criteria included skin lesions restricting range of motion, crystal-related arthropathies (gout, calcium pyrophosphate

Table 1 Portuguese version of the Functional Index for Hand Osteoarthritis

	Original version of FIHOA	Portuguese version of FIHOA
Question 1	Are you able to turn a key in a lock?	Você consegue girar uma chave em uma fechadura?
Question 2	Are you able to cut meat with a knife?	Você consegue cortar a carne com uma faca?
Question 3	Are you able to cut cloth or paper with a pair of scissors?	Você consegue cortar tecido ou papel com uma tesoura?
Question 4	Are you able to lift a full bottle with the hand?	Você consegue levantar uma garrafa cheia com a mão?
Question 5	Are you able to clench your fist?	Você consegue fechar a sua mão totalmente?
Question 6	Are you able to tie a knot?	Você consegue dar um nó?
Question 7A Question 7B	For women - Are you able to sew? For men - Are you able to use a screwdriver?	Para mulheres – Você consegue costurar? Para homens – Você consegue usar uma chave de fenda?
Question 8	Are you able to fasten buttons?	Você consegue abotoar uma roupa?
Question 9	Are you able to write for a long period of time (10 min)?	Você consegue escrever por um longo período de tempo? (10 min)
Question 10	Would you accept a handshake without reluctance?	Você aceitaria um aperto de mão sem medo?
Scoring system		
0	Possible without difficulty	Possível sem dificuldade
1	Possible with slight difficulty	Possível com pouca dificuldade
2	Possible with importante difficulty	Possível com muita dificuldade
3	Impossible	Impossível

disease), other immune-mediated diseases (rheumatoid arthritis, spondyloarthropathies, Sjögren's syndrome, systemic lupus erythematosus), hemochromatosis, history of upper limb trauma in the past 20 years, previous hand surgery, presence of a neurological disease or other musculoskeletal disease affecting the function of the upper limb.

Initially, 30 participants with hand OA answered the translated version of the questionnaire in order to assess the complete understanding of all items and whether the questions included the expected concepts without redundancy. Questions that could not be understood by more than 20% of the responders were analyzed, revised and resubmitted to another 30 group of patients. This procedure would be repeated until all questions were understood by over 80% of the patients in order to assure cultural adaptation. None of the participants reported difficulty in understanding and interpreting the questions involved in the final Portuguese version of FIHOA and the expert committee decided that no resubmission of the questionnaire to another group of participants and no further adjustments were necessary.

Subsequently, another group of patients was recruited to answer the questionnaire three times (test-retest phase). At first, participants were interviewed twice by different evaluators to check for inter-observer reliability. The second interview was conducted between 7 and 15 days after the first visit to assess intra-observer reliability. All questionnaires were answered under the supervision of an interviewer.

Functional Index for Hand Osteoarthritis score and other measures

FIHOA

The FIHOA contains 10 questions with one sex specific question included. The responses are scaled on a four-point Likert scale (0 = possible without difficulty, 1 = possible with slight difficulty, 2 = possible with important difficulty, 3 = impossible), to avoid any centralization of the answers. The range of scores is 0 to 30 [6].

Visual Analogue Scale for Hand Pain

Pain was assessed using a Visual Analogue Scale (VAS, 0–100 mm) for pain at rest and movement considering overall pain in the index hand during the last week.

Cochin Hand Functional Scale (CHFS)

The CHFS is an instrument for assessing functional disability of the hands that was initially developed in France to be used in patients with rheumatoid arthritis. It consists of a questionnaire of 18 questions (range 0–90) about activities of daily living that has been applied in other diseases involving the hand, including OA, and has been translated and validated into Brazilian Portuguese [15].

Health Assessment Questionnaire (HAQ)

The HAQ is a validated scale to assess functional daily living activities that can be used with arthritis patients and has been translated into Brazilian Portuguese (range 0–60) [16].

Statistical analysis

All data were analyzed using the Statistical Package for Social Science (SPSS) version 23 and the R program (version 3). A minimum sample size was defined as 50, based on a 5:1 criterion considering at least 5 respondents for each question, as described previously [17]. In this case, a minimum of 50 respondents for the 10 questions FIHOA questionnaire. Demographic and clinical characteristics were described using the mean and standard deviation for continuous variables and percentages for categorical variables. The main variable analyzed was the total score of the sum of the instrument's items. The Wilcoxon test was used to compare FIHOA scores between test and retest.

Test-retest reliability

The analysis of the intraclass correlation coefficient (ICC), Spearman's rank correlation coefficient and the Bland-Altman graph were used to assess inter-observer and intra-observer reproducibility. A level of ICC $\geq$ 0.7 was considered strong at the scale level. Intraclass correlation coefficients (ICCs) considering a 95% confidence interval (95% CI) were calculated for each isolated item as well as for total scores using a two-way random model. Spearman's coefficient of 0.1–0.3, 0.31–0.5 and > 0.5 were considered weak, moderate and strong correlation, respectively.

Internal consistency

Cronbach's alpha test was performed to assess the internal consistency of FIHOA. This instrument was used to measure the global correlation between items within the scale and levels > 0.7 were considered an adequate performance [16]. We calculated the total item correlations adjusted for the specific item. A correlation of at least 0.4 was considered adequate to validate the internal consistency of the scale.

Internal construct and external validity

Internal construction validity was assessed with analysis factor according to the standard "eigenvalue > 1" rule (the Kaiser criterion). Spearman's correlation test was used to verify the validity of external construction. External validity was assessed with the correlation of FIHOA with VAS of pain and the CHFS and HAQ instruments.

Results

Clinical and demographic characteristics

The Portuguese version of FIHOA was applied to 68 patients. The average time to answer the questionnaire was around 3 min. The clinical and demographic characteristics are shown in Table 2. Initially, 30 participants with hand OA answered the translated version of the questionnaire in order to assess the complete understanding of all items and none of the participants reported difficulty in understanding and interpreting the questions involved in the final Portuguese version of FIHOA. Following, the test-retest phase was performed with 38 participants. In this phase, six participants didn't complete the 1st FIHOA assessment (5 did not answer item 7 and 1 did not answer question 7 and question 4) and were excluded from the analysis (Table 2).

Test - retest reliability

The Portuguese version of FIHOA was applied on two occasions with an interval of 7 or 15 days. No statistically significant difference between the evaluations was observed (Wilcoxon test: $p = 0.32$). The average score of each item and the total score of the FIHOA test-retest are reported in Table 3 showing no differences between the two evaluations. The average of the total score of the FIHOA was 9.9 ± 7.2 in the first assessment and 8.6 ± 6.5 in the second evaluation. The Spearman value for the total score was 0.86 and there was a variation for each item ranging from 0.4 to 0.8. The ICC of 0.89 for the total score was considered strong and the ICC for each single item was considered good to strong (0.6–0.9) and ICC for interobserver, which was 0.92, was also strong. Mean differences (1.37 ± 0.68) using Bland Altman's analysis did not significantly differ from zero and no systematic bias was observed, as illustrated in Fig. 1.

Internal consistency

A high (0.89) Cronbach's alpha was achieved, meaning a strong internal consistency between the test item. These values were also high even after deleting an item, ranging from 0.91 to 0.93, further confirming the internal consistency of the translated version of the test. The individual items of the Brazilian version of FIHOA showed a moderate correlation adjusted to the total of the items. All correlations were statistically significant ($p < 0.01$), as shown in Table 4.

Validity of internal construction

Factor analysis was performed to assess the internal structural validity of the Brazilian version of FIHOA. The Kaiser-Meyer-Olkin was 0.821, which suggests that the sample size was adequate. Bartlett's sphericity test produced a high $\chi 2$ of 185.0 ($P < 0.01$), which indicates that the factorial model was appropriate. The selection of two components represented 67.8% of the overall variation. The two factors represented 54.3 and 13.4%, of the total variation, respectively.

All 10 FIHOA items were positively correlated with factor 1 (representing 54.3% of the variance). Therefore, factor 1 may reflect the general capacity to perform activities composing the FIHOA. The correlation model became clearer with the varimax rotation, establishing a two-dimensional model for the Brazilian version of FIHOA.

The rotation suggested that the first factor captured items such as activities that require coordination of the fingers and activities related to holding objects for a long period of time by pinching fingers. This factor also captured activities that need to hold objects in the hand applying a higher level of force. The first factor consists of the following six items: item 4 ("Are you able to lift a full bottle with the hand?"); item 6 ("Are you able to tie a knot?"); item 3 ("Are you able to cut cloth or paper with

Table 2 Demographic and clinical characteristics of patients that answered the Portuguese version of the FIHOA questionnaire

Variable	Cultural adaptation (30)	Test-retest (32)	Total (62)
Age (y)	51.7 ± 9.8	61.8 ± 10.1	56.9 ± 11.2
Female(%)	93	97	95
Duration of symptoms onset(m)	33.3 ± 44.1	131 ± 115	83.7 ± 100.8
Time of diagnosis(m)	17.2 ± 39.3	74.3 ± 101.6	46.7 ± 83
Right hand dominant (%)	97	100	98
FIHOA	4.6 ± 7.1	9.9 ± 7.2	7.4 ± 7.6
VAS 1		37.8 ± 28	
VAS2		68.7 ± 25	
CHFS		20.9 ± 15.9	
HAQ		12.6 ± 8.37	

A total of 62 patients answered a Portuguese version of the FIHOA questionnaire. Values represent n (%) of mean ± SD, as indicated. CHFS, Cochin Hand Functional Scale; HAQ, Health Assessment Questionnaire; y, years; m, months; SD, standard deviation; VAS (0–100 mm), visual analogue scale at rest (1) or following movement (2)

Table 3 Test-retest of reliability of the Brazilian version of the FIHOA questionnaire

FIHOA test -retest	Test	Retest	Spearman's rho	ICC
Item 1 – item 1 retest	0.53 ± 0.71	0.5 ± 0.62	0.66	0.81
Item 2 – item 2 retest	0.97 ± 0.88	0.87 ± 0.88	0.63	0.81
Item 3 – item 3 retest	0.97 ± 0.88	0.83 ± 0.82	0.73	0.84
Item 4 – item 4 retest	1.06 ± 0.90	0.97 ± 0.87	0.51	0.62
Item 5 – item 5 retest	1.09 ± 1.07	1.10 ± 1.08	0.76	0.90
Item 6 – item 6 retest	0.63 ± 0.74	0.63 ± 0.84	0.40	0.60
Item 7 – item 7 retest	0.97 ± 0.98	0.57 ± 0.67	0.65	0.80
Item 8 – item 8 retest	0.75 ± 0.83	0.57 ± 0.67	0.67	0.81
Item 9 – item 9 retest	1.56 ± 1.12	1.37 ± 1.11	0.80	0.87
Item 10 – item 10 retest	1.44 ± 1.12	1.2 ± 1.11	0.72	0.83
FIHOA Total Score	9.9 ± 7.2	8.6 ± 6.5	0.86	0.89

Values are given as mean ± standard deviation

a pair of scissors?"); item 8 ("Are you able to fasten buttons?"); item 9 ("Are you able to write for a long period of time?") and item 2 ("Are you able to cut meat with a knife?").

The second factor explains 13.4% of the total variance and is made up of item 5 ("Are you able to clench your fist?"), 1 (Are you able to turn a key in a lock?), 7 ("Are you able to sew?" Or "Are you able to use a screwdriver?") and 10 (would you accept a handshake without reluctance?"). These activities seem to be particularly related to the ability to perform rotation, flexion and extension of the wrist and hand grip movement. Item 7 had a strong correlation with both factors (factor 1 (519) and factor 2 (698)), meaning that the activity evaluated in item 7 is also related to the ability of coordinated finger movements. Factor 2 was opposed from item 5 to item 8, suggesting that individuals who were able to close their hands more easily had a lot of difficulty in performing the task of fastening buttons.

Validity of external construction

We calculated Spearman's rho values between the total score of the Brazilian version of FIHOA, VAS of hand pain at rest and in motion, CHFS and HAQ. There was a strong direct correlation between FIHOA and CHFS (Spearman's rho = 0.89, $P < 0.01$) and moderate correlation for FIHOA and HAQ (Spearman's rho = 0.64, $P < 0.01$). There was also a moderate correlation with VAS values for pain in the hands at rest (Spearman's rho = 0.55, $P < 0.01$) and a moderate correlation with VAS values for pain in the hands when in motion (Spearman's rho = 0.44, $P < 0.01$).

The Bland and Altman graph concerning the analysis of the FIHOA x HAQ tools showed that the mean differences were distributed close to zero and within 2 SD. Almost all observations were within the upper and lower limits identified by the SD, with only 03 values differing from the mean in more than three SD. The Bland and Altman analysis of the FIHOA x CHFS tools showed that the mean differences were close to 10, between 02 SD. Almost all observations were within the upper and lower limits identified by the SD, and none differed from the mean by more than three SD. No systematic trend of differences was observed in both analyzes.

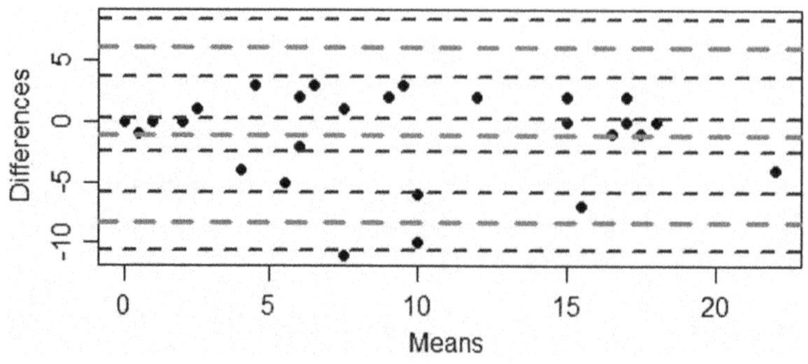

Fig. 1 Bland-Altman Plot of the Portuguese version of total FIHOA score for test and retest with 95% CI

Table 4 Internal consistency of the Brazilian version of FIHOA

Item	Score	Scale mean if item is deleted	Scale variance if item is deleted	Ajusted total item correlation	Cronbach's alpha if item is deleted
Item 1	0.53 ± 0.71	9.44	46.06	0.726	0.918
Item 2	0.97 ± 0.88	9.00	42.97	0.839	0.911
Item 3	0.97 ± 0.88	9.00	43.61	0.778	0.914
Item 4	1.06 ± 0.90	8.91	43.77	0.748	0.915
Item 5	1.09 ± 1.07	8.88	46.05	0.434	0.934
Item 6	0.63 ± 0.74	9.34	45.85	0.711	0.918
Item 7	0.97 ± 0.98	9.00	42.45	0.783	0.913
Item 8	0.75 ± 0.83	9.22	44.95	0.707	0.918
Item 9	1.56 ± 1.12	8.41	40.51	0.821	0.911
Item 10	1.44 ± 1.12	8.53	41.93	0.710	0.918

Values are given as mean ± standard deviation

Discussion

This study provides the Portuguese version of the FIHOA questionnaire with cultural adaptation to Brazilian patients, demonstrating a good reliability, validity, and internal consistency in patients with hand OA. Cultural adaptation was not a major issue given the similarity of the meaning of each FIHOA items which can be considered very similar in any culture. Although we did not aim to compare total scores among our patients, our mean of 7.4, which could be considered revealing a moderate functional impairment, are lower than values reported in similar studies carried out in Belgium (10.9), Iran (9.9) and Norway (9.3) [10, 18, 19]. On the other hand, one may consider that our patients presented greater impairment when comparing to scores obtained in studies performing translation of FIHOA in Italy (6.5), Japan (5.5), Morocco (5.0) and Korea (4.4) [11, 12, 20, 21].

We performed an assessment of the level of hand pain at rest and movement, which had not been done in previous FIHOA validation studies. The average level of pain at rest by VAS of the patients in this study was 38.7 mm, similar to the average pain in the population assessed in other studies such as in Belgium (42.9), Italy (35), Norway (41.7) and Korea (35.2) [9, 11, 12, 19]. The average level of global pain in moving hands (67.8) showed an important increase when compared to the level of pain at rest in our study and the other validation studies [9–12, 19, 21]. Although we initially thought that the level of pain in moving hands could be better correlated with the total score of a functional assessment instrument such as FIHOA, the results showed that there was a better correlation with the mean VAS score of pain in the hands at rest (0.55) compared to the VAS score of pain in the hands in motion (0.44) although the latter still has a moderate level of correlation. Actually, patients report that type of movement and intensity of the force applied influence the level of pain. Studies with a larger number of patients using VAS assessment at rest and movement can be carried out in the future to clarify the correlation of these two characteristics with the FIHOA score.

A good reliability was obtained given the good consistency of answers in the test-retest analysis which may be due to the clarity and simplicity of the questions in the original FIHOA questionnaire, making it possible to be easily translated. This aspect reinforces the validity of applying FIHOA in our patients.

The strong internal consistency of this Portuguese version of FIHOA is illustrated by a high Cronbach's alpha result. Cronbach's alpha showed a slight increase if any of the items were deleted and remained at a high value, indicating that the items are suitable for use. The correlation for adjusted item-total is> 0.4 for all items, confirming that there is a strong of association between individual items and the remainder of the scale.

Similar to most studies, the Factor of Analysis of this Portuguese version of FIHOA shows that it is not a one-dimensional tool, as reported by Dreiser et al. [7]. Indeed, similar to results obtained when translating into Persian, we found 2 factors, whereas similar studies performed in Italy and Korea found a greater number of factors [10–12]. Remarkably, the Norwegian version of FIHOA was the only one reporting only one dimension [19]. Our results were also able to discriminate the two components, functions of the hands such as: 1) coordination of the fingers and clamping objects at length and 2) rotation, flexion and extension of the wrist and hand grip movement. Other aspects, such as the level of pain in the hands, may have influenced the response pattern of component 2, as most patients with a higher level of disability in item 10 had a higher level of pain measured with the VAS.

The validity of external consistency was also considered good when compared to other instruments that assess functionality such as HAQ and CHFS. Even in comparison with instruments that assess pain level (VAS of pain in hands at rest and in movement), the analysis showed a good level of external correlation.

This study has some limitations, including the relatively low number of patients. We also had only 3 male patients (5%), which preclude a reliable analysis of item 7b, judged to be specific to that gender. It is worth mentioning that hand OA is very predominant in females and most previous similar FIHOA translational studies also had a similar low prevalence of male participants [9, 11, 12, 19, 22, 23]. There was a mean 10-year difference between the groups that participated in the pre-test and test-retest phases. The selection was at random and we believe this difference was irrelevant since the understanding of the phrasing was similar between both groups.

The evaluation of hand functionality through gender-specific questions can have its added value quite questionable in societies where a high and growing number of individuals of both genders have been performing similar tasks in their daily lives. It is assumed that there is a greater influence of a socio-cultural aspect than a functional difference between the two specific questions for each gender. Further studies are needed to investigate whether this gender-specific issue can be eliminated or replaced. Neither did we assess the number and location of the affected joints, nor the presence of Heberden and Bouchard nodes and deformities caused by OA, which may influence dexterity and functional capacity of the fingers. Indeed, the number of nodes in the hands and involvement of the base of the thumb and wrists may be associated with a higher level of pain and functional limitation [19, 24–26]. Six patients didn't complete the 1st FIHOA assessment, leaving some blank items in the questionnaire and were excluded from the analysis. The answers were similar and they justified that they hadn't performed that task in many years or had never done it (06 patients didn't know how to sew) and one patient also didn't know how to answer question 4 and justified that this item didn't specify the weight of the bottle that he would try to lift.

Conclusion

The Brazilian Portuguese version of the FIHOA questionnaire proved to be a fast, easy-to-handle, reliable valid instrument for measuring the functional capacity of patients with hand OA in native Portuguese speaking patients.

Abbreviations

CHFS: Cochin Hand Functional Scale; FIHOA: Functional Index for Hand Osteoarthritis; HAQ: Health Assessment Questionnaire; ICC: Intraclass correlation coefficient; OA: Osteoarthritis; OARSI: Osteoarthritis Research Society International; OMERACT: Outcome Measures in Rheumatology Clinical Trials; VAS: Visual Analogue Scale

Acknowledgements

We acknowledge the support we received from Dr. Emmanuel Maheu (Saint Antoine Hospital, Department of Rheumatology, Paris, France) that provided authorization for the translation and advice on the methods for our validation study. We acknowledge partial support of this work from the Conselho Nacional de Desenvolvimento Científico e Tecnológico (CNPQ), Brasil – Grant 308429/2018-4.

Authors' contributions

FVAA, JN, and FACR conceived the article. Data acquisition, analysis and/or interpretation: FVAA, AJ, HALR, JN, FACR. Draft and revision of the work: FVAA, AJ, HALR, JN, FACR. All authors approved the final version of the manuscript. All authors are accountable for all aspects of the work particularly regarding integrity of the data and collection of material.

Author details

[1]Department of Internal Medicine - Faculdade de Medicina, Universidade Federal do Ceará, Fortaleza, CE, Brazil. [2]Department of Global Health and Population, Harvard T. H. Chan School of Public Health, Boston, MA, USA. [3]Department of Community Health, Federal University of Ceará, Fortaleza, CE, Brazil. [4]Division of Rheumatology – Escola Paulista de Medicina, Universidade Federal de São Paulo, São Paulo, SP, Brazil. [5]Instituto de Biomedicina – Laboratório de Investigação em Osteoartropatias, Rua Cel. Nunes de Melo, 1315 - 1°. Andar, Rodolfo Teófilo, Fortaleza, CE 60430-270, Brazil.

References

1. Zhang Y, Jordan JM. Epidemiology of osteoarthritis. Clin Geriatr Med. 2010; 26(3):355–69. https://doi.org/10.1016/j.cger.2010.03.001.
2. Bijsterbosch J, Watt I, Meulenbelt I, Rosendaal FR, Huizinga TWJ, Kloppenburg M. Clinical and radiographic disease course of hand osteoarthritis and determinants of outcome after 6 years. Ann Rheum Dis. 2011;70(1):68–73. https://doi.org/10.1136/ard.2010.133017.
3. Coimbra IB, Plapler PG, Campos GC. Generating evidence and understanding the treatment of osteoarthritis in Brazil: a study through Delphi methodology. Clinics. 2019;74:e722. https://doi.org/10.6061/clinics/2019/e722.
4. Zhang W, Doherty M, Leeb BF, Alekseeva L, Arden NK, Bijlsma JW, et al. EULAR evidence-based recommendations for the diagnosis of hand osteoarthritis: report of a task force of ESCISIT. Ann Rheum Dis. 2009;68(1):8–17. https://doi.org/10.1136/ard.2007.084772.
5. Maheu E, Altman RD, Bloch DA, Doherty M, Hochberg M, Mannoni A, et al. Design and conduct of clinical trials in patients with osteoarthritis of the hand: recommendations from a task force of the Osteoarthritis Research Society International. Osteoarthr Cartil. 2006;14(4):303–22. https://doi.org/10.1016/j.joca.2006.02.010.
6. Pham T, van der Heijde D, Altman RD, Anderson JJ, Bellamy N, Hochberg M, et al. OMERACT-OARSI initiative: Osteoarthritis Research Society International set of responder criteria for osteoarthritis clinical trials revisited. Osteoarthr Cartil. 2004;12(5):389–99. https://doi.org/10.1016/j.joca.2004.02.001.
7. Dreiser RL, Maheu E, Guillou GB, et al. Validation of an algofunctional index for osteoarthritis of the hand. Rev Rhum Engl. 1995;62(6 suppl 1):43s–53s.
8. Kloppenburg M, Maheu E, Kraus VB, Cicuttini F, Doherty M, Dreiser RL, et al. Clinical trials recommendations: design and conduct of clinical trials for hand osteoarthritis. Osteoarthr Cartil. 2015;23(5):772–86. https://doi.org/10.1016/j.joca.2015.03.007.
9. Wittoek R, Cruyssen BV, Maheu E, et al. Cross-cultural adaptation of the Dutch version of the Functional Index for Hand Osteoarthritis (FIHOA) and a study on its construct validity. Osteoarthr Cartil. 2009;17(5):607–12. https://doi.org/10.1016/j.joca.2008.10.006.
10. Yoosefinejad AK, Motealleh A, Babakhani M. Evaluation of validity and reliability of the Persian version of the functional index of hand

osteoarthritis. Rheumatol Int. 2017;37(5):719–25. https://doi.org/10.1007/s00296-016-3645-6.

11. Gandini F, Giannitti C, Fattore G, Giordano N, Galeazzi M, Fioravanti A. Validation of an Italian version of the Functional Index for Hand Osteoarthritis (FIHOA). Mod Rheumatol. 2012;22(5):758–65. https://doi.org/10.1007/s10165-011-0579-4.
12. Ahn GY, Cho S-K, Cha SJ, Nam E, Lee JE, Dreiser RL, et al. Cross-cultural adaptation and validation of the Korean version of the Functional Index for Hand Osteoarthritis (FIHOA). Int J Rheum Dis. 2018;00(12):1–9. https://doi.org/10.1111/1756-185X.13412.
13. Beaton DE, Bombardier C, Guillemin F, Ferraz MB. Guidelines for the process of cross-cultural adaptation of self-report measures. Spine. 2000;25(24):3186–91. https://doi.org/10.1097/00007632-200012150-00014.
14. Altman R, Alarcón G, Appelrouth D, et al. The American College of Rheumatology criteria for the classification and reporting of osteoarthritis of the hand. Arthritis Rheum. 1990;33(11):1601–10. https://doi.org/10.1002/art.1780331101.
15. Chiari A, Sardim CCS, Natour J. Translation, cultural adaptation and reproducibility of the Cochin Hand Functional Scale questionnaire for Brazil. Clin Sci. 2011;66(5):731–6. https://doi.org/10.1590/S1807-59322011000500004.
16. Ferraz MB, Oliveira LM, Araujo PMP, Atra E, Tugwell P. Cross cultural reability of the physical ability dimension of the health assessment questionnaire. J Rheumatol. 1990;17(6):813–7.
17. Tsang S, Royse CF, Terkawi AS. Guidelines for developing, translating, and validating a questionnaire in perioperative and pain medicine. Saudi J Anaesth. 2017;11(Suppl 1):S80–9. https://doi.org/10.4103/sja.SJA_203_17.
18. Gliem JA, Gliem RR. Calculating, interpreting, and reporting cronbach's alpha reliability coefficient for likert-type scales. Midwest research to practice conference in adult, continuing, and community education; 2004. p. 82–8. http://hdl.handle.net/1805/344. Acessed 20 Apr 2020
19. Moe RH, Garratt A, Slatkowsky-Christensen B, Maheu E, Mowinckel P, Kvien TK, et al. Concurrent evaluation of data quality, reliability and validity of the Australian/Canadian osteoarthritis hand index and the Functional Index for Hand Osteoarthritis. Rheumatology (Oxford). 2010;49(12):2327–36. https://doi.org/10.1093/rheumatology/keq219.
20. Nakagawa Y, Kurimoto S, Maheu E, Matsui Y, Kanno Y, Menuki K, et al. Cross-cultural translation, adaptation and validation of a Japanese version of the Functional Index for Hand Osteoarthritis (JFIHOA). BMC Musculoskelet Disord. 2020;21(1):173. https://doi.org/10.1186/s12891-020-03193-6.
21. Taik FZ, Tahiri L, Rkain H, Aachari I, Maheu E, Allali F. Cross-cultural adaptation and validation of the Arabic version of the Functional Index for Hand Osteoarthritis. BMC Musculoskelet Disord. 2020;21(1):390. https://doi.org/10.1186/s12891-020-03418-8.
22. Chaisson CE, Zhang Y, McAlindon TE, Hannan MT, Aliabadi P, Naimark A, et al. Radiographic hand osteoarthritis: incidence, patterns, and influence of pre-existing disease in a population-based sample. J Rheumatol. 1997;24(7):1337–43.
23. Srikanth VK, Fryer JL, Zhai G, Winzenberg TM, Hosmer D, Jones G. A meta-analysis of sex differences prevalence, incidence and severity of osteoarthritis. Osteoarthr Cartil. 2005;13(9):769–81. https://doi.org/10.1016/j.joca.2005.04.014.
24. Marshall M, Van der Windt D, Nicholls E, et al. Radiographic hand osteoarthritis: patterns and associations with hand pain and function in a community dwelling sample. Osteoarthr Cartil. 2009;17(11):1440–7. https://doi.org/10.1016/j.joca.2009.05.009.
25. Bijsterbosch J, Visser W, Kroon HM, Stamm T, Meulenbelt I, Huizinga TWJ, et al. Thumb base involvement in symptomatic hand osteoarthritis is associated with more pain and funcional disability. Ann Rheum Dis. 2010;69(3):585–7. https://doi.org/10.1136/ard.2009.104562.
26. Kitisomprayoonkul W, Promsopa K. Chaiwanichsiri D (2010) do Heberden and Bouchard nodes affect finger dexterity in elderly? Rheumatol Int. 2010;30(4):543–5. https://doi.org/10.1007/s00296-009-1196-9.

20

The importance of lower extremity involvement type on exercise performances, function and quality of life in peripheral predominant forms of juvenile idiopathic arthritis

Sevtap Acer Kasman[1,2*], Özgür Zeliha Karaahmet[1], Ajda Bal Hastürk[1], Özge Başaran[3], Banu Çelikel Acar[3], Halise Hande Gezer[1] and Aytül Çakcı[1]

Abstract

Background: Juvenile idiopathic arthritis (JIA) can cause reduced exercise capacity, deterioration in functional activities, and poor health-related quality of life. This study aims to objectively reveal lower extremity involvement in the peripheral predominant forms of juvenile idiopathic arthritis through qualitative evaluations and to determine the effects of these involvements on exercise, function, and quality of life.

Methods: Thirty-two patients with a history of peripheral arthritis and aged between 7 and 16 years participated in the study. Demographics, JIA subtype, disease duration, arthritis and deformities of the lower extremity, disease activity score, 6-min walk test (6MWT), cycling exercise test (CYC-E), childhood health assessment questionnaire (CHAQ), and pediatric quality of life inventory (PedsQoL) scores were recorded. In case of clinical suspicion of arthritis, an ultrasonographic examination was performed for a definitive diagnosis. Regression analyses were performed to explore the most associated lower extremity involvement and patient characteristics for each of the dependent variables including 6MWT, CYC-E, CHAQ, and PedsQoL.

Results: Of the total number of patients, with a mean age of 12.91 (SD 2.37) years, 28.1% had knee arthritis, 15.6% foot arthritis, 12.5% hip arthritis, and 37.5% lower extremity deformity. The parameters that were most associated with CHAQ and PedsQoL were hip and knee arthritis, whereas CYC-E was found to be most associated with knee arthritis and height, and 6MWT was found to be most associated with hip arthritis, knee arthritis, and demographic characteristics.

* Correspondence: sevtap-acer@hotmail.com
[1]Department of Physical Medicine and Rehabilitation, University of Health Sciences Ankara Dışkapı Yıldırım Beyazıt Trainig and Research Hospital, Ankara, Turkey
[2]Present affiliation: Department of Rheumatology, University of Health Sciences Kartal Dr. Lütfi Kırdar Training and Research Hospital, Istanbul, Turkey

Conclusion: This study emphasizes the importance of hip and knee arthritis, which are among the determinants of walking endurance, function, and quality of life; and knee arthritis, which is among the determinants of cycling performance in JIA with lower extremity involvement.

Keywords: Juvenile idiopathic arthritis, Lower extremity, Deformity, Exercise, Function, Quality of life, Arthritis, Cycling, 6MWT

Background

Juvenile idiopathic arthritis (JIA) is the most common pediatric rheumatologic disease. Subluxation, fusion, and permanent joint deformities occur with damage to the joint surfaces and their adjacent structures. In addition to joint involvement, muscle strength, atrophy, weak endurance, gait disturbances, decreased exercise capacity, and decreased function and quality of life can be seen [1–4]. The hip, knee, and ankle are the most frequently affected lower extremity joints in JIA, with a prevalence rate of 30–50% [5]. It is also known that the most common joints requiring surgical intervention in adult JIA are the hip, knee, and ankle [6].

Children with JIA have poor function and exercise scores than healthy children [3, 4, 7–11]. When investigating the factors affecting these results, quantitative assessment methods, such as the number of swollen joints and tender joints, are generally used. Ultimately, it is recommended to reduce the number of tender/swollen joints (or decrease the disease activity scale scores) [12, 13]. However, the joint which mostly affects daily activities and quality of life in childhood, including exercise, is still a matter of curiosity.

Foot/ankle and hips can be affected in JIA, but these symptoms are more difficult to diagnose than knee arthritis. The impact of their subclinical involvement of them on daily life may sometimes be neglected [14]. Further, treatments may not necessarily cause complete remission of active arthritis in these joints [5]. Physical examination can easily diagnose knee arthritis; however, conditions such as arthritis, bursitis, or tenosynovitis of the ankle and hip are more difficult than knee to distinguish by physical examination [5, 15, 16]. In recent years, the introduction of ultrasonography (USG) in clinical use has enabled clinicians to easily differentiate these conditions. USG can demonstrate ongoing active disease in locations that are difficult to examine in JIA. It is reported to be more sensitive and reliable than physical examination and correlates better with disease activity indices as well as the progression of structural damage [17, 18]. Hence, a more objective examination is required in cases where physical examination is insufficient for evaluating the results affected by joint involvement.

The involvement and deformities of the lower extremity and the need for orthosis in JIA begin to appear in childhood; however, there is insufficient data in the literature regarding the comprehensive assessment of deformities [5]. To our knowledge, there is one validated damage scale, Juvenile Arthritis Damage Index - Articular (JADI-A), which includes assessment of the contracture of the hip, knee, ankle, and metatarsal joints and valgus knee deformity [19]. Nevertheless, it is unclear whether deformities are risk factors (independent from arthritis) for the poor exercise results.

In light of the aforementioned data, there is no study conducted with both qualitative, comprehensive, and objective evaluation methods that have revealed lower extremity impairments affecting exercise and daily life outcomes in JIA. We believe that investigating the qualitative effect (based on the location) rather than the number of joints swollen, objectively diagnosing arthritis with the use of USG, and including deformity in the analysis can increase the scope and provide more reliable results.

This study aims to objectively reveal lower extremity involvement in peripheral predominant forms of juvenile idiopathic arthritis through qualitative evaluations and to determine the effects of these involvements on two different exercise performances, function, and quality of life.

Methods

Patients

We included patients aged between 7 and 16 years and diagnosed with JIA according to the International League of Associations for Rheumatology criteria in Ankara Dışkapı Yıldırım Beyazıt Training and Research Hospital [20]. The diagnosis of JIA was made by a pediatric rheumatologist. Patients with axial involvement, systemic JIA (to minimize the systemic effects of disease), active infections, and patients who were newly diagnosed were excluded. Informed consent was obtained from the participants and their parents. Demographic characteristics, disease duration, disease subtypes, medications, Disease Activity Score28 (DAS-28) results, and the data below were recorded.

DAS28 was calculated with ESR (mm/h), tender and swollen joint count among 28 joints, and the patient's global assessment of disease activity on a visual analog scale. It predominantly evaluates the activity of the upper extremities.

Arthritis

Physical examination of the knee, hip, ankle, and foot joints was performed by the same physician. Patients with apparent arthritis were noted. Patients with suspicious arthritis (at least one of the following symptoms such as pain, tenderness, redness, warmth, or loss of function) were subjected to USG examination performed by an experienced specialist who was unaware of the clinical findings. For this purpose, General Electric Logiq 5 (frequency: 7–13 MHz) ultrasound device, linear probe, and gray scale were used. Definite arthritis on physical examination or at least grade 1 synovial fluid and/or grade 1 synovial hypertrophy on USG were considered arthritis positive [20].

Deformity

The patients' physical examination and goniometric measurements were performed by a physical medicine and rehabilitation specialist. The deformity status was determined according to the JADI-A [19] in which joint contracture and other deformities were only be scored when they are not due to active arthritis and present for at least six months. In addition, we distinguished the patients according to the lower extremity deformity (LED) presence. Since there was no standardization for the deformity assessment, we considered LED positive if a patient had any of the followings: hip internal rotation < 10 degrees, hip ankylosis/prosthesis, knee valgus > 15 degrees, knee flexion contracture, knee prosthesis, fixed valgus of the ankle, ankle ankylosis/arthrodesis/prosthesis, visible deformity of the metatarsophalangeals due to arthritis, or arthroplasty of the forefoot (measurements are from JADI-A) [19].

Primary outcome measurements (in order of application)

1. Function. The childhood health assessment questionnaire (CHAQ) was used for the assessment of functional ability. The ratings of the scale were determined by the physician with face-to-face encounters with the patients and their parents. For each item of CHAQ, the patient's difficulty level experienced while performing a relevant activity is questioned. The scoring was done using a four-point scale ranging from 0 (without any difficulty), 1 (with some difficulty), 2 (with much difficulty), 3 (unable to do). If assistance was required of a person or device, the scoring was increased to 2 if 0 or 1 points whereas ratings of 2 and 3 points remained unaffected. The CHAQ score was calculated as the sum of the scores of all the eight sections divided by 8, which is in the range 0–3. The Turkish validity and reliability study of this score has been performed [21].
2. Quality of life. The PedsQL 3.0 Arthritis Module (PedsQL-3A), which evaluates the QoL based on patient-reported outcomes, was used. There were 3 forms of the questionnaire, classified according to the following age groups: 5–7, 8–12, and 13–18 years. It consisted of 5 sub-items including pain/ache, activities of daily living, treatment, anxiety, and communication. The total score of Likert-type questions was between 0 and 100 and the best score was 100. It has been validated in Turkish [22]. The physician conducted the questionnaires face-to-face with patients.
3. Cycling exercise performance. The cycling exercises (CYC-E) were applied on the CareFusion Type MasterScreen-CPX device to simulate home cycling. Since there was not a standardized and validated cycling protocol for home exercise in JIA, a cycling protocol was created for this study [13, 23]. The protocol should be partially achievable for healthy and active children, with no floor and ceiling effect for children with JIA [23]. Therefore, pilot tests were performed on 11 JIA and 11 age-matched healthy children to decide on the protocol. The final cycling protocol was developed where the results of the healthy subjects exhibited a ceiling effect in a 20-min exercise without observing floor or ceiling effect in patients (no more than 15% of respondents having the lowest and highest possible response) and close to submaximal difficulty: After warming up at 90–100 rpm without any load for 3 min, the participants continued the test with a load equivalent to half of their weight at 90–100 rpm, then a 20-min exercise was performed with a 1-watt load increase every 3 min. Participants were informed about 3 h of fasting, maximal effort, degree of strain, and possible symptoms before cycling. Simultaneously, the heart rate was measured with a probe. The age-predicted maximum heart rate (HRmax) was calculated for each participant and the peak heart rate (HRpeak) reached during the test was measured [23, 24]. The exercise test was terminated prematurely if the patient stated that he could not continue the exercise for any reason or when indications for termination of the exercise test occurred [25]. Cycling exercise duration (CYC-ED) was recorded as an outcome.
4. Walking endurance. The 6-min walk test (6MWT) was used for this purpose. Unlike all other evaluations, the 6MWT was performed on the next day so that the cycling test would not affect the 6MWT results. It was conducted in a straight 8-m corridor. Patients were instructed to walk the longest possible distance within 6 min at their normal walking pace with turning points at both ends of the 8-m

distance. The patient was motivated at each turn. The distance covered at the end of the exercise was recorded. The 6MWT is a reliable method for evaluating exercise capacity in JIA [26, 27].

All exercise tests were performed during noontime and under the control of a physical medicine and rehabilitation specialist experienced in cardiac rehabilitation.

Statistics

Statistical analysis was done using the SPSS V.20. Descriptive statistics were presented as percentages for categorical variables, as mean (with SD) for normally distributed continuous data, and as median (with IQR) for non-normal distributed continuous data. To determine relationships with potential independent variables (age, gender, height, weight, BMI, disease duration, hip arthritis, knee arthritis, foot/ankle arthritis, JADI-A, and LED score) that may affect primary outcome measurements (CHAQ, PedsQL-3A, CYC-ED, 6MWT), Pearson test for normally distributed continuous quantitative data, Spearman test for non-normally distributed continuous quantitative data, Student T-test for normally distributed categorical variables, and Mann–Whitney U test for non-normally distributed categorical variables were performed. Backward multivariate linear regression analysis was used to determine the best predictors of CHAQ, PedsQl-3A, CYC-E, and 6MWT. In addition to hip, knee, and foot/ankle arthritis, the parameters that were found to be significant in the tests mentioned above were included in the models. $P < 0.05$ was considered significant.

Results

Thirty-two patients with a diagnosis of JIA (13 boys, 19 girls) were included in the study. 6MWT data of 2 patients (1 boy, 1 girl) were missing. There was no other missing data. Data regarding demographics, clinical, and exercise tests of the patients with a diagnosis of JIA are shown in Table 1. Bilateral knee arthritis was found in one patient and unilateral or no lower extremity arthritis in all other patients.

During CYC-E, the heart rate increased to an average of 83% (95% CI 0.80–0.87) of maximal heart rate and stabilized after 3–6 min. A significant correlation was found between the 6MWT and CYC-E results of the patients (Pearson's correlation coefficient 0.534, p: 0.002).

Associations between the dependent and independent variables are shown in Table 2. Several individual and disease-related characteristics were associated with various outcome measures.

For each primary outcome measure, foot/ankle, knee, and hip arthritis that were likely to clinically affect the outcomes were included in each regression model. In addition, the independent variables shown in italics in Table 2 were included in the relevant model, except JADI-A. The JADI-A was not included as it showed collinearity with the presence of lower limb deformity. The final models of the backward multivariate linear regression analysis for each primary outcome measure are shown in Table 3.

Table 1 Demographic and clinical characteristics of the patients

Characteristic	Mean (or Median) or Percentage
Gender, male rate	40%
Age, years	12.91 (SD 2.37)
BMI, kg/m^2	20.23 (SD 3.87)
JIA subtype	
Oligoarticular	75%
Polyarticular	16%
Undifferentiated	9%
Pharmacological treatment	
Follow-up without medication	19%
NSAID only	19%
DMARD (with or without NSAID)	62%
Disease duration, months	41.00 (SD 38.05)
DAS28	2.85 (SD 1.23)
Hip arthritis	12.5%
Knee arthritis	28.1%
Foot/ankle arthritis	15.6%
JADI-A	0 (IQR 1) (min 0, max 8)
LED positivity rate	37.5%
6MWT, m (n: 30)	427.76 (SD 107.47)
CYC-E test duration, min	10.46 (SD 4.22)
CHAQ	0.13 (IQR 0, 0.69)
PedsQL-3A	84.37 (SD 13.45)

NSAID non-steroid anti-inflammatory drug, *DMARD* biologic or conventional disease-modifying anti-rheumatic drug, *DAS28* disease activity score 28, *JADI-A* Juvenile Arthritis Damage Index – Articular, *LED* lower extremity deformity, *6MWT* 6-min walk test, *CYC-E* cycling exercise, *CHAQ* Childhood Health Assessment Questionnaire, *PedsQL-3A* PedsQL 3.0 Arthritis Module

Discussion

This study is the first to investigate the contribution of lower limb arthritis, particularly hip and knee arthritis, in poor outcomes in walking, cycling, function, and quality of life in children with JIA with peripheral arthritis. In JIA with lower extremity involvement, the most important determinants of walking endurance, function, and quality of life are hip and knee arthritis, whereas knee arthritis is crucial in cycling performance. The literature search showed us when investigating factors affecting poor outcomes in children with JIA, quantitative assessment methods, such as the number of swollen

Table 2 Associations between the dependent and independent variables

Independent variables	Dependent variables			
	CHAQ (n:32)	PedsQL-3A (n:32)	CYC-ED (n:32)	6DYT (n:30)
Age*, years	0.186	0.647	0.366	*0.044 (0.371)*
Gender†	0.563	0.803	0.340	0.126
Height*, cm	0.106	0.629	*0.033 (0.390)*	*0.019 (0.425)*
Weight*, kg	0.067	0.883	0.276	*0.033 (0.390)*
BMI*, kg/m^2	0.111	0.551	0.907	0.222
Disease duration*, months	0.635	0.782	0.720	0.379
Hip arthritis†	*0.002*	*0.003*	0.602	*0.044*
Knee arthritis†	*0.009*	0.059	*0.002*	*0.010*
Ankle/foot arthritis†	*0.033*	0.253	*0.001*	0.082
LED positive†	0.613	0.459	0.572	*0.022*
JADI-A*	0.204	0.224	0.895	*0.016 (−0.437)*

**p* value for Pearson or Spearman's correlation test, correlation coefficients were given in parentheses in case of significance
†*p* value for Student T or Mann Whitney U test
CHAQ Childhood Health Assessment Questionnaire, *PedsQL-3A* PedsQL 3.0 Arthritis Module, *CYC-ED* cycling exercise duration, *6MWT* 6-min walk test, *LED* lower extremity deformity, *JADI-A* Juvenile Arthritis Damage Index – Articular

Table 3 Predictors of CHAQ, PedsQL-3A, CYC-E, and 6MWT found in backward regression analysis*

Primary outcome	Independent variable (explaining variance)	Beta	95% CI for B		p
			Lower	Upper	
CHAQ[a]					
	Hip arthritis	0.755	0.755	1.377	< 0.001
	Knee arthritis	0.559	0.351	0.809	< 0.001
PedsQL-3A[b]					
	Hip arthritis	−0.741	−40.624	−19.783	< 0.001
	Knee arthritis	−0.405	−19.819	− 4.484	0.003
CYC-ED[c]					
	Knee arthritis	−0.408	−6.719	− 835	0.014
	Height	0.368	0.016	0.217	0.025
6MWT[d]					
	Hip arthritis	−0.628	− 272.608	− 118.109	< 0.001
	Knee arthritis	−0.524	− 176.551	−65.090	< 0.001
	Gender	−0.239	−104.092	−0.952	0.046
	Age	0.293	−0.972	28.040	0.066
	Weight	0.268	−0.350	4.270	0.093

*Final models for regression analysis
[a] 2nd model for CHAQ (Childhood Health Assessment Questionnaire); Model $p < 0.001$, R^2: 0.683, F: 31.213
[b] 2nd model for PedsQL-3A (PedsQL 3.0 Arthritis Module); Model $p < 0.001$, R^2: 0.572, F: 19.365
[c] 3rd model for CYC-ED (cycling exercise duration); Model p: 0.006, R^2: 0.299, F: 6.196
[d] 4th model for 6MWT (6-min walk test); Model $p < 0.001$, R^2: 0.701, F: 11.738

joints and tender joints, have often been used. It has been proposed to ultimately reduce the number of tender/swollen joints (or lower disease activity scale scores) [12, 13, 28]. On the other hand, the present study indicates that different joints affect the result differently with the qualitative assessment.

In this study, knee arthritis was observed at a rate of 28.1%, foot/ankle 15.6%, and hip 12.5% when clinical and subclinical arthritis were evaluated together. These rates correspond with the findings in the literature. In a study conducted in patients under one year of treatment, the prevalence of knee, ankle, foot, and hip synovitis was 8–20%, 6–12%, 5, and < 5%, respectively, and walking difficulty was observed at rates of 25–30% [29]. The joint involvement that would best explain this difficulty in walking seen in the majority of the patients is not specified, and the diagnosis of arthritis is based solely on physical examination. However, it is important to distinguish subclinical synovitis in children, especially in feet and hip joints, and not to omit them while investigating the causes associated with the result. Each patient should be specifically evaluated for these joints by clinical and, if necessary, subclinical examination [15, 16].

It is well known that children with JIA have a decreased functional competence and quality of life than healthy children [4]. In a previous large sample study, predictors of disability assessed by HAQ were female gender, symmetrical arthritis, hip joint involvement, long-term high ESR, and rheumatoid factor [11]. Regarding the quality of life, the effect of the number of swollen joints was highlighted in another study [30]. It is noteworthy that in the current study, a significant part of the variance in both functional loss and quality of life was explained by hip and knee arthritis.

The average of 6MWT in our study was at expected levels when compared with the previous study [31] and was lower than healthy Turkish children [32]. The findings of our study highlight that out of all the factors, hip arthritis may have the greatest impact on this low score of 6MWT. In addition to hip arthritis, knee arthritis, gender, age, and weight explain 70.1% of the variance in 6MWT. This result suggests that walking endurance can be widely affected by active hip and knee arthritis. However, 6MWT is a widely used method to assess cardiovascular exercise capacity, and it has also been included in home exercise programs given to children with JIA in clinical trials [27, 33–35]. Hence, we also investigated a different exercise performance that was less likely to be affected by the effect of active arthritis in assessing actual cardiovascular performance. Although respiratory and metabolic requirements differ during cycling and walking exercise [36], we hypothesized that the effect of arthritis on cycling performance would not be as great as that on walking endurance.

In our study, a protocol that can provide a cycling exercise result with a wide variance was applied. CYC-E correlated moderately with 6MWT and remained at the submaximal exercise level determined by heart rate measurement. Ultimately, as intended, an intense home exercise cycling performance was provided [23]. When we investigated the contribution of lower extremity involvement to cycling performance, it was seen that 29.9% of the variance was explained by the presence of knee arthritis and height. Although this data is similar to the effect of height determined in the study of Paap et al. [27], our study is unique in that it also includes the contributing joints. In conclusion, this study contributes to the literature by indicating that walking and cycling endurances are affected by different factors in these patients and hip arthritis has a greater influence on walking than cycling.

Although lower extremity deformity examined in this study is not found as an independent risk factor for poor outcome, it can be assumed that there is a questionable effect on walking endurance. On the other hand, it was not associated with CHAQ, unlike a previous study [37]. The failure to identify lower extremity deformities as an independent factor may be since it is indeed not so or may be because our sample did not include a great sample size. Future studies are required to investigate the effect of the presence of deformity on adverse outcomes with larger samples and established disease. Apart from arthritis and deformity, one of the conditions most likely to be associated with reduced physical activity in children with inflammatory diseases is pain [10]. However, the pain was not included in independent factors in this study, because it is a subjective complaint and our outcome variables could be influenced by any pain in children [38]. Hence, a definite diagnosis of arthritis has provided more reliable observations in understanding the contribution of lower extremity arthritis to the results. In addition to all, there is a need to design and validate tools assessing optimal LED (especially other deformities of the foot) and home exercise performances [5]. The pilot study that we conducted because of a lack of protocol that can be considered as a home program for cycling exercise in the literature, has ensured that this issue is relatively tolerated [23].

The results might have been different if the majority had been diagnosed with polyarticular or systemic JIA. The variances in the primer outcome measures might have probably not been explained that well. However, the main purpose of this study was to find out the value of lower extremity involvement type in itself. The results should not be generalized to all JIAs. Future research is needed to explain the variance of disability or QoL in the general JIA population.

Conclusions

This study highlights that hip and knee arthritis are the most important determinants of poor outcome in walking, function, and quality of life in children with JIA with peripheral arthritis alone; in addition, considering the cycling performance, the hip arthritis factor is relatively eliminated. Each patient should be evaluated especially in terms of these joints with clinical and, if necessary, subclinical examination.

Abbreviations

JIA: Juvenile idiopathic arthritis; 6MWT: 6-min walk test; CYC-E: Cycling exercise test; CHAQ: Childhood Health Assessment Questionnaire; PedsQoL: Pediatric Quality of Life Inventory Arthritis Module; USG: Ultrasonography; JADI-A: Juvenile Arthritis Damage Index Articular; DAS-28: Disease Activity Score 28; LED: Lower extremity deformity

Acknowledgements

Not applicable.

Authors' contributions

All authors contributed to the study conception and design. Material preparation and analysis were performed by SAK and AÇ. Data collection and diagnosis were made by ÖB and BÇA. Sonographic assessments were made by ABH. Exercise tests were made under the control of ÖZK and HHG. The first draft of the manuscript was written by SAK and all authors commented on previous versions of the manuscript. All authors read and approved the final manuscript.

Authors' information

SAK and HHG: Physicians specialized in Physical Medicine and Rehabilitation and Rheumatology. ÖZK: Associate Professor specialized in Physical Medicine and Rehabilitation. ABH: Professor specialized in Physical Medicine and Rehabilitation. ÖB: Physician specialized in Pediatric Rheumatology. BÇA: Professor specialized in Pediatric Rheumatology. AÇ: Physician specialized in Physical Medicine and Rehabilitation and the Chairperson.

Author details

[1]Department of Physical Medicine and Rehabilitation, University of Health Sciences Ankara Dışkapı Yıldırım Beyazıt Trainig and Research Hospital, Ankara, Turkey. [2]Present affiliation: Department of Rheumatology, University of Health Sciences Kartal Dr. Lütfi Kırdar Training and Research Hospital, Istanbul, Turkey. [3]Department of Pediatric Rheumatology, University of Health Sciences Ankara Child Health and Diseases Hematology Oncology Training and Research Hospital, Ankara, Turkey.

References

1. Oen K. Long-term outcomes and predictors of outcomes for patients with juvenile idiopathic arthritis. Best Pract Res Clin Rheumatol. 2002;16(3):347–60. https://doi.org/10.1053/berh.2002.0233.
2. Packham JC, Hall MA. Long-term follow-up of 246 adults with juvenile idiopathic arthritis: functional outcome. Rheumatology. 2002;41(12):1428–35. https://doi.org/10.1093/rheumatology/41.12.1428.
3. Van Brussel M, Lelieveld OTHM, Van Der Net J, et al. Aerobic and anaerobic exercise capacity in children with juvenile idiopathic arthritis. Arthritis Care Res. 2007;57(6):891–7. https://doi.org/10.1002/art.22893.
4. Takken T, Van Der Net J, Helders PJM. Relationship between functional ability and physical fitness in juvenile idiopathic arthritis patients. Scand J Rheumatol. 2003;32(3):174–8. https://doi.org/10.1080/03009740310002524.
5. Fellas A, Singh-Grewal D, Santos D, Coda A. Physical examination tools used to identify swollen and tender lower limb joints in juvenile idiopathic arthritis: a scoping review. Arthritis. 2018;2018:1–7. https://doi.org/10.1155/2018/3408162.
6. Malviya A, Johnson-Lynn S, Avery P, Deehan D, Foster H. Juvenile idiopathic arthritis in adulthood and orthopaedic intervention. Clin Rheumatol. 2009;28(12):1411–7. https://doi.org/10.1007/s10067-009-1266-0.
7. van Pelt PA, Takken T, van Brussel M, et al. Aerobic capacity and disease activity in children, adolescents and young adults with juvenile idiopathic arthritis (JIA). Pediatr Rheumatol Online J. 2012;10(1):25. https://doi.org/10.1186/1546-0096-10-25.
8. Takken T, Van Der Net J, Kuis W, Helders PJM. Physical activity and health related physical fitness in children with juvenile idiopathic arthritis. Ann Rheum Dis. 2003;62(9):885–9. https://doi.org/10.1136/ard.62.9.885.
9. Takken T, Hemel A, Van Der Net J, Helders PJM. Aerobic fitness in children with juvenile idiopathic arthritis: a systematic review. J Rheumatol. 2002;29(12):2643–7.
10. Bos GJ, Lelieveld OT, Armbrust W, et al. Physical activity in children with Juvenile Idiopathic Arthritis compared to controls. Pediatr Rheumatol Online J. 2016;14(1):42. https://doi.org/10.1186/s12969-016-0102-8.
11. Flatø B, Lien G, Smerdel A, et al. Prognostic factors in juvenile rheumatoid arthritis: a case-control study revealing early predictors and outcome after 14.9 years. J. Rheumatol. 2003;30(2):386–93.
12. Giannini EH, Ruperto N, Ravelli A, Lovell DJ, Felson DT, Martini A. Preliminary definition of improvement in juvenile arthritis. Arthritis Rheum. 1997;40(7):1202–9. https://doi.org/10.1002/1529-0131(199707)40:7<1202::AID-ART3>3.0.CO;2-R.
13. Cavallo S, Brosseau L, Toupin-April K, Wells GA, Smith CA, Pugh AG, et al. Ottawa panel evidence-based clinical practice guidelines for structured physical activity in the management of juvenile idiopathic arthritis. Arch Phys Med Rehabil. 2017;98(5):1018–41. https://doi.org/10.1016/j.apmr.2016.09.135.
14. Spraul G, Koenning G. A descriptive study of foot problems in children with juvenile rheumatoid arthritis (JRA). Arthritis Rheum. 1994;7(3):144–50. https://doi.org/10.1002/art.1790070308.
15. Magni-Manzoni S, Epis O, Ravelli A, Klersy C, Veisconti C, Lanni S, et al. Comparison of clinical versus ultrasound-determined synovitis in juvenile idiopathic arthritis. Arthritis Care Res. 2009;61(11):1497–504. https://doi.org/10.1002/art.24823.
16. Collado P, Jousse-Joulin S, Alcalde M, Naredo E, D'Agostino MA. Is ultrasound a validated imaging tool for the diagnosis and management of synovitis in juvenile idiopathic arthritis? A systematic literature review. Arthritis Care Res. 2012;64(7):1011–9. https://doi.org/10.1002/acr.21644.
17. Grassi W. Clinical evaluation versus ultrasonography: who is the winner? J Rheumatol. 2003;30(5):908–9.
18. Hendry GJ, Gardner-Medwin J, Steultjens MPM, Woodburn J, Sturrock RD, Turner DD. Frequent discordance between clinical and musculoskeletal ultrasound examinations of foot disease in juvenile idiopathic arthritis. Arthritis Care Res. 2012;64(3):441–7. https://doi.org/10.1002/acr.20655.
19. Viola S, Felici E, Magni-Manzoni S, Pistorio A, Buoncompagni A, Ruperto N, et al. Development and validation of a clinical index for assessment of long-term damage in juvenile idiopathic arthritis. Arthritis Rheum. 2005;52(7):2092–102. https://doi.org/10.1002/art.21119.
20. Szkudlarek M, Court-Payen M, Jacobsen S, Klarlund M, Thomsen HS, Østergaard M. Interobserver agreement in ultrasonography of the finger and toe joints in rheumatoid arthritis. Arthritis Rheum. 2003;48(4):955–62. https://doi.org/10.1002/art.10877.
21. Ruperto N, Ravelli A, Pistorio A, et al. Cross-cultural adaptation and psychometric evaluation of the Childhood Health Assessment Questionnaire (CHAQ) and the Child Health Questionnaire (CHQ) in 32 countries. Review of the general methodology. Clin. Exp. Rheumatol. 2001;19(4 SUPPL. 23):S1–9.
22. Tarakci E, Baydogan SN, Kasapcopur O, Dirican A. Cross-cultural adaptation, reliability, and validity of the Turkish version of PedsQL 3.0 arthritis module: a quality-of-life measure for patients with juvenile idiopathic arthritis in Turkey. Qual. Life Res. 2013;22(3):531–6. https://doi.org/10.1007/s11136-012-0180-0.
23. Noonan V, Dean E. Submaximal exercise testing: clinical application and interpretation. Phys Ther. 2000;80(8):782–807. https://doi.org/10.1093/ptj/80.8.782.
24. Machado FA, Denadai BS. Validity of maximum heart rate prediction equations for children and adolescents. Arq Bras Cardiol. 2011;97(2):136–40. https://doi.org/10.1590/S0066-782X2011005000078.
25. Washington RL, Bricker JT, Alpert BS, et al. Guidelines for exercise testing in the pediatric age group: From the Committee on Atherosclerosis and Hypertension in Children, Council on Cardiovascular Disease in the Young, the American Heart Association. Circulation. 1994;90(4 I):2166–79.
26. Pritchard L, Verschuren O, Roy M, Kaup C, Rumsey DG. Reproducibility of the Six-Minute Walk Test in Children and Youth with Juvenile Idiopathic Arthritis. Arthritis Care Res (Hoboken). 2020;10.1002/acr.24492. https://doi.org/10.1002/acr.24492.
27. Paap E, Van Der Net J, Helders PJM, Takken T. Physiologic response of the six-minute walk test in children with juvenile idiopathic arthritis. Arthritis Care Res. 2005;53(3):351–6. https://doi.org/10.1002/art.21175.
28. Giannini MJ, Protas EJ. Exercise response in children with and without juvenile rheumatoid arthritis: a case-comparison study. Phys Ther. 1992;72(5):365–72. https://doi.org/10.1093/ptj/72.5.365.
29. Hendry GJ, Shoop-Worrall SJ, Riskowski JL, et al. Prevalence and course of lower limb disease activity and walking disability over the first 5 years of juvenile idiopathic arthritis: results from the childhood arthritis prospective study. Rheumatol Adv Pract. 2018;2(2):rky039. https://doi.org/10.1093/rap/rky039.
30. Ezzahri M, Amine B, Rostom S, Badri D, Mawani N, Gueddari S, et al. Factors influencing the quality of life of Moroccan patients with juvenile idiopathic arthritis. Clin Rheumatol. 2014;33(11):1621–6. https://doi.org/10.1007/s10067-014-2489-2.
31. Lelieveld OTHM, Takken T, Van Der Net J, Van Weert E. Validity of the 6-minute walking test in juvenile idiopathic arthritis. Arthritis Care Res. 2005;53(2):304–7. https://doi.org/10.1002/art.21086.
32. Kanburoglu MK, Ozdemir FM, Ozkan S, Tunaoglu FS. Reference values of the 6-minute walk test in healthy Turkish children and adolescents between 11 and 18 years of age. Respir Care. 2014;59(9):1369–75. https://doi.org/10.4187/respcare.02891.
33. Tarakci E, Yeldan I, Nilay Baydogan S, Olgar S, Kasapcopur O. Efficacy of a land-based home exercise programme for patients with juvenile idiopathic arthritis: a randomized, controlled, single-blind study. J Rehabil Med. 2012;44(11):962–7. https://doi.org/10.2340/16501977-1051.
34. Sule SD, Fontaine KR. Slow speed resistance exercise training in children with polyarticular juvenile idiopathic arthritis. Open Access Rheumatol Res Rev. 2019;11:121–6.
35. Klepper S, Mano Khong TT, Klotz R, Gregorek AO, Chan YC, Sawade S. Effects of structured exercise training in children and adolescents with juvenile idiopathic arthritis. Pediatr Phys Ther. 2019;31(1):3–21. https://doi.org/10.1097/PEP.0000000000000555.
36. Palange P, Forte S, Onorati P, Manfredi F, Serra P, Carlone S. Ventilatory and metabolic adaptations to walking and cycling in patients with COPD. J Appl Physiol. 2000;88(5):1715–20. https://doi.org/10.1152/jappl.2000.88.5.1715.
37. Sarma PK, Misra R, Aggarwal A. Physical disability, articular, and extra-articular damage in patients with juvenile idiopathic arthritis. Clin Rheumatol. 2008;27(10):1261–5. https://doi.org/10.1007/s10067-008-0901-5.
38. Costa MDC, Natour J, Oliveira HAV, Terreri MT, Len CA. Gait in children and adolescents with idiopathic musculoskeletal pain. Adv. Rheumatol. (London, England). 2019;59(1):7.

21

The efficacy of low dose short-term prednisone therapy for remission induction in newly diagnosed rheumatoid arthritis patients

John M. Stacy[1†], Jacob R. Greenmyer[1†], James R. Beal[2], Abe E. Sahmoun[3] and Erdal Diri[4*]

Abstract

Background: The ACR/EULAR recommendations endorse the use of glucocorticoids (GCs) for rheumatoid arthritis (RA) patients' flares and as a bridge to a DMARD. However, the recommendation of low dose short-term monotherapy with (GCs) remains open to the discretion of the clinician. The aim of this study was to assess whether a short-term use of low dose prednisone monotherapy was effective in inducing remission in newly diagnosed RA patients.

Methods: A retrospective analysis of patients newly diagnosed with RA at a Community Health Center in North Dakota was performed based on the ACR/EULAR RA classification criteria. Demographic and clinical data were abstracted from patients' medical charts. Patients treated with ($\leq$ 10 mg/day) of prednisone up to 6 months were included. Response to prednisone was analyzed according to pre- and post-treatment DAS28-ESR score and EULAR response criteria.

Results: Data on 201 patients were analyzed. The mean prednisone dose was 8 mg/day (range: 5–10; SD = 1.2) and the mean treatment duration was 42.2 days (12–177; 16.9). Disease severity significantly improved from baseline to follow-up for: tender joint count (8.6 ± 4.8 vs. 1.5 ± 3.3; $P < 0.001$), swollen joint count (6.2 ± 5.0 vs. 1.4 ± 3.0; $P < 0.001$), and visual analog pain score (4.8 ± 2.6 vs. 2.1 ± 2.5; $P < 0.001$). DAS28-ESR disease severity significantly improved from baseline to follow-up: (5.1 ± 1.2 vs. 2.7 ± 1.3; $P < 0.001$). Per EULAR response criteria, 69.7% of patients showed good response to treatment and 20.4% showed moderate response. 54.2% of patients reached remission.

Conclusion: Short-term use of low dose prednisone monotherapy induced disease remission and improved clinical severity of RA in the majority of newly diagnosed patients.

Keywords: Rheumatoid arthritis, Prednisone, Efficacy, Low dose, Short-term, Remission, Disease severity

* Correspondence: erdal.diri@trinityhealth.org
†John M. Stacy and Jacob R. Greenmyer contributed equally to the creation of this manuscript.
[4]Division of Rheumatology, Trinity Medical Group, Minot, ND, USA

Background

Rheumatoid arthritis (RA) is a chronic, inflammatory synovial joint disorder characterized by symmetrical polyarticular arthritis [1]. The prevalence of RA has increased significantly, affecting 1.5 million adults in the U.S. [2].

RA is expensive not only for patients and payers through direct healthcare related costs, but also to society in the form of lost productivity secondary to the loss of functionality that comes with advanced disease [3, 4]. RA-associated morbidity is directly correlated with the amount of time patients spend in a state of severe disease activity [5]. Therefore, early intervention and optimal management is paramount to limiting long-term complications.

Glucocorticoids (GCs) were reported to be effective in treating RA as early as 1949 [6]. GCs have strong anti-inflammatory properties that act quickly, and are therefore effective in inducing early remission in newly diagnosed RA patients while bridging to a synthetic disease-modifying anti-rheumatic drug (DMARD) and in fighting flares [7, 8].

The 2016 EULAR recommends that GCs be tapered as rapidly as clinically feasible, preferably within 3 months. However, they leave the dosing regimen and route of administration up to the decision of the individual rheumatologist [9]. Similarly, the 2015 ACR guidelines also acknowledge the efficacy of less than 3 months of low dose GC bridging therapy, but their dosing and administration recommendations are to some extent unclear [10].

Early RA has previously been defined as duration of symptoms for < 12 months [11]. For early RA, the international guidelines recommend the use of GCs without indicating the best starting dosage and duration of use of GCs [9–13]. Despite these shortcomings, GCs prescription rates remain high ranging from 30 to 74% [14–16]. The use of GCs as monotherapy has been overlooked in recent years and the risks of GC exposure vary widely based on patient characteristics [17].

The purpose of this study was to assess whether short-term use of low dose prednisone monotherapy was effective in inducing remission in newly diagnosed RA patients.

Methods

Study design

A retrospective electronic medical records review was conducted of patients newly diagnosed with RA (ICD-9: 714) between January 1, 2005 and September 1, 2018 at a community medical center, North Dakota, USA. Diagnoses were made based on the ACR/EULAR 2010 RA classification criteria [18].

Criteria of eligibility

Inclusion criteria consisted of: newly diagnosed RA patients treated with ≤ 10 mg/day of prednisone and had received a maximum of 6-month therapy. Patients were considered newly diagnosed if they had a duration of symptoms of less than 12 months. The international recommendations agree that a dose < 10 mg/day GC is considered a low dose, and GC should be tapered in less than 3 months, or 7.5 mg/day GC prescribed for up to 6 months [19]. Exclusion criteria were: 1) patients ever treated with a DMARD or started on a DMARD during the treatment period; 2) patients already actively on GCs upon entry into study; and 3) insufficient information in the electronic medical records to calculate disease severity.

The following variables were recorded for each patient: age, gender, race, prednisone dose, treatment duration, additional anti-inflammatory medications, rheumatoid factor status, rheumatoid factor titer, anti-cyclic citrullinated peptide antibody status, erythrocyte sedimentation rate, C-reactive protein, hemoglobin, platelets, tender joint count, swollen joint count, visual analogue scale, and DAS-28 ESR score. Response to prednisone treatment was calculated using the DAS-28 ESR score prior to initiating treatment and 6 weeks after initiation.

We computed: 1) the difference in DAS28-ESR score before and after prednisone treatment; 2) the disease activity severity score before and after treatment; and 3) the change via EULAR response criteria.

Disease activity severity DAS28-ESR was classified as: remission (< 2.6), low/minimal (≥ 2.6 to < 3.2), moderate (≥ 3.2 to 5.1), and high/severe (> 5.1). EULAR response criteria were used to compare improvement in DAS28-ESR scores with achieved disease severity upon follow up, taking into account both improvement in DAS28-ESR score over the study period as well as the absolute value of the DAS28-ESR score at the end of the study [9, 10, 20].

Statistical analysis

SPSS 25.0 for Windows was used to analyze demographic and clinical characteristics of patients. Proportions and percentages were computed for each categorical variable. Paired t-tests were performed to determine which continuous variables were significantly different from one another. All p-values were two-sided, and p-value < 0.05 was considered significant.

Results

Six hundred seventy-five patients were screened and 201 patients fulfilled the criteria (supplemental). The mean age (standard deviation) was 55.1 ± 15.9 years, 65.7% were female and 91.5% were white (Table 1). The mean

Table 1 Characteristics of patients newly diagnosed with rheumatoid arthritis

Number of patients	N = 201
Age (years)	
Mean ± SD (Range)	55.1 ± 15.9 (18–91)
Gender, female n (%)	132 (66)
Time between symptom onset and diagnosis (days)	
Mean ± SD (Range)	200.4 ± 133.9 (3–365)
Treatment duration (days)	
Mean ± SD (Range)	42.2 ± 16.9 (12–177)
Race	
White n (%)	184 (92)
Other	17 (8)
Prednisone dose (mg/day)	
Mean ± SD (Range)	8.0 ± 1.2 (5–10)

SD Standard Deviation

prednisone dose was 8.0 ± 1.2 mg and the mean treatment duration was 42.2 ± 16.9 days.

Clinical measures of disease severity significantly improved with reductions in tender joint count from baseline 8.6 ± 4.8 vs. 1.5 ± 3.3 at follow-up ($P < 0.001$), swollen joint count, 6.2 ± 5.0 vs. 1.4 ± 3.0 ($P < 0.001$), and visual analog pain score, 4.8 ± 2.6 vs. 2.1 ± 2.5 ($P < 0.001$) (Table 2). Biomarkers of inflammation also showed significant improvement from baseline to follow-up with ESR decreasing from 33.7 ± 22.6 vs.19.9 ± 16.0 ($P < 0.001$) and a CRP from 2.5 ± 3.2 vs. 1.2 ± 1.3 ($P < 0.001$) (Table 2).

Overall, DAS28-ESR improved significantly from 5.1 ± 1.2 baseline vs. 2.7 ± 1.3 at follow up ($P < 0.001$). DAS28-ESR also significantly improved in both seropositive and seronegative patients from baseline to follow-up. In seropositive patients the mean DAS28-ESR changed from 5.2 ± 1.1 vs. 2.7 ± 1.3 ($P < 0.001$) and in seronegative patients the mean DAS28-ESR changed from 4.9 ± 1.2 vs. 2.6 ± 1.1 ($P < 0.001$) (Table 2).

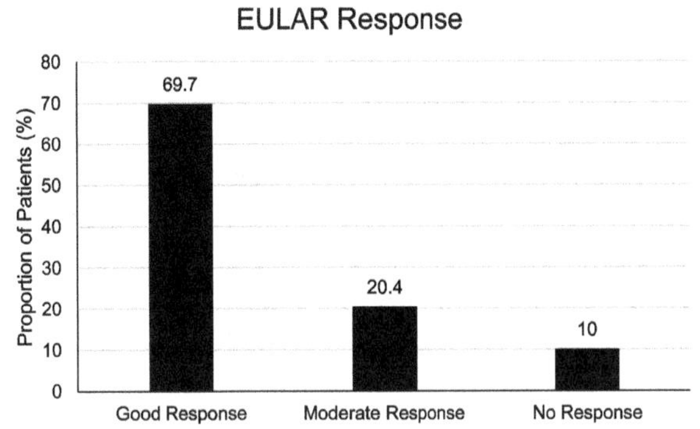

Fig. 1 Response rate based on EULAR criteria

Most patients showed marked improvement in disease severity at follow-up according to both DAS28-ESR severity classification and EULAR response criteria. According to the EULAR response criteria, the vast majority, 69.7% of the patients showed good response, with 20.4% showing moderate response and only 10% of the patients showing no response (Fig. 1). Prior to treatment, 95% of our patients exhibited either severe or moderate disease activity according to the DAS28-ESR classification (Fig. 2). Following treatment, 54.2% of patients had achieved remission, 16.9% exhibited low disease activity, with an additional 23.9% having moderate disease activity. Only 5% displayed severe disease state (Fig. 3).

Discussion

This study found that low dose, short-term prednisone monotherapy significantly improved the disease severity indexes. Furthermore, the majority of patients achieved remission while only 5% still showed signs of severe disease. Early exposure to (GCs) in RA patients has been associated with improved outcomes and reduced need for biologicals [21–23].

Table 2 Response rate of disease activity measurements

	Baseline	Follow-up	*P*-value
ESR, mean ± SD mm/hr	33.7 ± 22.6	19.9 ± 16.0	< 0.001
CRP, mean ± SD mg/L	2.5 ± 3.2	1.2 ± 1.3	< 0.001
Hemoglobin, mean ± SD g/dL	13.5 ± 1.56	13.9 ± 1.42	< 0.001
Platelets, mean ± SD 1000/mm^3	163.1 ± 174.4	154.4 ± 157.2	0.02
Tender joint count, mean ± SD	8.6 ± 4.8	1.5 ± 3.3	< 0.001
Swollen Joint Count, mean ± SD	6.2 ± 5.0	1.4 ± 3.0	< 0.001
Visual Analog Scale, mean ± SD	4.8 ± 2.6	2.1 ± 2.5	< 0.001
DAS28-ESR, mean ± SD	5.1 ± 1.2	2.7 ± 1.3	< 0.001
Seropositive, mean ± SD ($n = 134$)	5.2 ± 1.1	2.7 ± 1.3	< 0.001
Seronegative, mean ± SD ($n = 67$)	4.9 ± 1.2	2.6 ± 1.1	< 0.001

SD Standard deviation, *ESR* erythrocyte sedimentation rate, *CRP* C-reactive protein, *DAS28* disease activity score at 28 joints

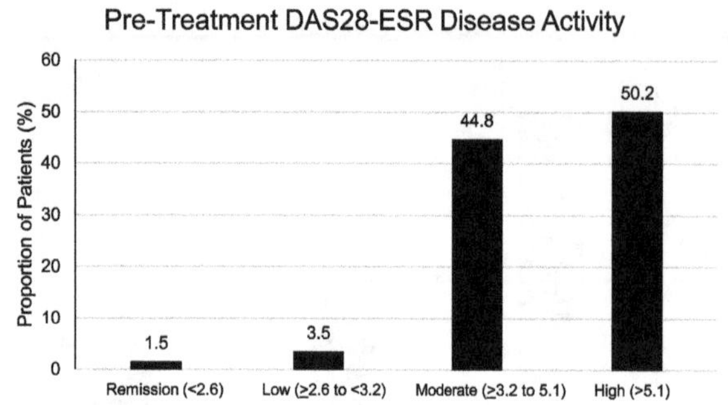

Fig. 2 DAS28-ESR severity prior to treatment

The BARFOT study found that 7.5 mg/d of prednisone resulted in 55.5% remission rate in newly diagnosed RA patients at 2 years [24]. A meta-analysis of 11 controlled trials also showed clinical improvement in disease after a month of treatment with low-dose GCs [8]. However, this analysis defined "low dose" as < 15 mg/day, and included patients on bridging therapy as well as those on GC monotherapy.

The 2015 ACR guidelines recommend GC should be considered for short-term, defined as < 3 months, in lowest possible dose in conjunction of a DMARD for early RA treatment (10). However. they did not defined the GC dose and left it to practitioner to decide. Therefore, particularly early RA patients are quite often overdosed with GC treatment with prednisone from 10 up to 60 mg daily that exposes RA patients to potentially multiple GC systemic toxicities. Our study suggests that low dose prednisone, < 10 mg daily, is adequate for remission induction in a short period of time, in most of early RA patients. Furthermore, we have an experience that low dose prednisone is not only effective in remission induction, but also in even 5 mg daily, can be as effective as a DMARD in maintenance of remission in a significant number of RA patients (data not shown).

While we did not document specific adverse events, several studies have assessed the safety profile related to low-dose prednisone [25–27]. A meta-analysis of six randomized trials (389 patients, average dose of prednisone equivalent: 5–10 mg/day for at least 2 years) revealed a good efficacy to toxicity ratio with a number needed to harm/number needed to treat of 0.25 [28]. The ESPOIR study found that low-dose (< 5 mg/d) prednisone therapy for 6 months was not associated with significant side effects [29]. The GLORIA trial is currently underway to evaluate the safety and effectiveness of low dose GC therapy (5 mg/day prednisone for 2 years) versus placebo in 800 elderly patients with RA and might soon provide valuable new evidence [30]. Waljee et al. [31] found that even short-term GC exposure was associated with venous thromboembolism, fractures and sepsis. In the Rabbit registry [32], the overall risk of death was increased in a manner independent of the activity of the disease for daily doses of GC greater than 5 mg/d (an increase of 40% in the risk for doses comprised between 5 and 10 mg/day). Glucocorticoid use in RA is associated with a dose-dependent increase in mortality rates, with a daily threshold dose of 8 mg, at which the number of deaths increased in a dose-dependent manner [33, 34]. Standardized guidelines on RA evaluation of adverse events are lacking.

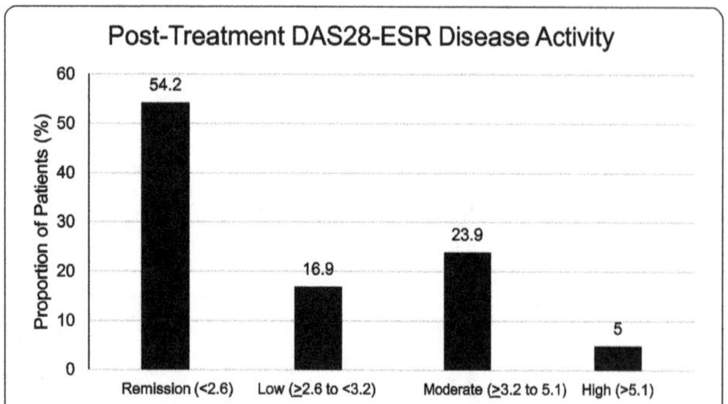

Fig. 3 DAS28-ESR severity after treatment

We acknowledge some limitations inherent to this study. First, these data are retrospectively obtained from electronic medical records of RA patients that carries potential multiple variables effecting results. Second, vast majority of analyzed patients are white not reflecting racial differences. Third, missing data related exclusion of patients may cause selection bias. Nonetheless, we believe the strength of our study is including quite homogeneous data, obtained from a single practice, that minimizes most of above concerns.

Conclusions

Our study showed that low dose and short-term GC monotherapy to be efficacious in inducing remission in newly diagnosed RA patients. These findings may assist clinicians in selecting the appropriate prednisone dosage and duration of use, as a first line monotherapy, for newly diagnosed RA patients. The side effects of GCs are clearly dose- dependent but are also affected by patient's risk factors, which should be considered when GCs are prescribed. More research needs to be done to perform side effects of induction with low dose GC monotherapy vs. alternative therapies and the long term consequences of both therapies for matched treatment groups.

Supplementary Information

Additional file 1: Supplemental 1. Electronic medical record search results and case inclusion.

Acknowledgements

Not applicable.

Authors' contributions

ED conceived the hypothesis, provided clinical guidance, and interpretation of the findings, JG and JS performed data collection and drafted the manuscript. JB participated in study design, conducted data analysis, and edited the final manuscript. AS participated in the study design, updated the literature review, and edited the final manuscript. The authors read and approved the final manuscript.

Author details

[1]University of North Dakota School of Medicine and Health Sciences, Grand Forks, ND, USA. [2]Department of Family and Community Medicine, University of North Dakota School of Medicine and Health Sciences, Grand Forks, ND, USA. [3]Department of Internal Medicine, University of North Dakota School of Medicine and Health Sciences, Forks, ND, USA. [4]Division of Rheumatology, Trinity Medical Group, Minot, ND, USA.

References

1. Aletaha D, Smolen JS. Diagnosis and Management of Rheumatoid Arthritis: a review. JAMA. 2018;320(13):1360–72. https://doi.org/10.1001/jama.2018.13103.
2. Kawatkar AA, Gabriel SE, Jacobsen SJ. Secular trends in the incidence and prevalence of rheumatoid arthritis within members of an integrated health care delivery system. Rheumatol Int. 2019;39(3):541–9. https://doi.org/10.1007/s00296-018-04235-y.
3. Kobelt G, Woronoff AS, Richard B, Peeters P, Sany J. Disease status, costs and quality of life of patients with rheumatoid arthritis in France: the ECO-PR study. Joint Bone Spine. 2008;75(4):408–15. https://doi.org/10.1016/j.jbspin.2007.07.015.
4. Van den Hoek J, Boshuizen HC, Roorda LD, Tijhuis GJ, Nurmohamed MT, van den Bos GA, et al. Mortality in patients with rheumatoid arthritis: a 15-year prospective cohort study. Rheumatol Int. 2017;37(4):487–93. https://doi.org/10.1007/s00296-016-3638-5.
5. Listing J, Kekow J, Manger B, Burmester GR, Pattloch D, Zink A, et al. Mortality in rheumatoid arthritis: the impact of disease activity, treatment with glucocorticoids, TNFα inhibitors and rituximab. Ann Rheum Dis. 2015; 74(2):415–21. https://doi.org/10.1136/annrheumdis-2013-204021.
6. Hench PS, Kendall EC, Slocumb CH, Polley HF. The effect of a hormone of the adrenal cortex (17-hydroxy-11-dehydrocorticosterone: compound E) and of pituitary adrenocortical hormone in arthritis: preliminary report. Ann Rheum Dis. 1949;8(2):97–104. https://doi.org/10.1136/ard.8.2.97.
7. Palmowski Y, Buttgereit T, Dejaco C, Bijlsma JW, Matteson EL, Voshaar M, et al. "Official View" on glucocorticoids in rheumatoid arthritis: a systematic review of international guidelines and consensus statements. Arthritis Care Res. 2017;69:1134–41.
8. Gøtzsche PC, Johansen HK. Short-term low-dose corticosteroids vs placebo and nonsteroidal anti-inflammatory drugs in rheumatoid arthritis. Cochrane Database Syst Rev. 2005(1):CD000189.
9. Smolen JS, Landewé R, Bijlsma J, Burmester G, Chatzidionysiou K, Dougados M, et al. EULAR recommendations for the management of rheumatoid arthritis with synthetic and biological disease-modifying anti-rheumatic drugs: 2016 update. Ann Rheum Dis. 2017;76(6):960–77. https://doi.org/10.1136/annrheumdis-2016-210715.
10. Singh JA, Saag KG, Bridges SL Jr, Akl EA, Bannuru RR, Sullivan MC, et al. American College of Rheumatology guideline for the treatment of rheumatoid arthritis. Arthritis Rheum. 2016;68:1–26.
11. Heidari B. Rheumatoid arthritis: early diagnosis and treatment Outcoms. Caspian J Intern Med. 2011;2(1):161–70.
12. GUIPCAR Group. Update of the clinical practice guideline for the management of rheumatoid arthritis in Spain. 2011.
13. Lau CS, Chia F, Harrison A, Hsieh TY, Jain R, Jung SM, et al. APLAR rheumatoid arthritis treatment recommendations. Int J Rheum Dis. 2015; 18(7):685–713. https://doi.org/10.1111/1756-185X.12754.
14. Black RJ, Joseph RM, Brown B, Movahedi M, Lunt M, Dixon WG. Half of UK patients with rheumatoid arthritis are prescribed oral glucocorticoid therapy in primary care: a retrospective drug utilization study. Arthritis Res Ther. 2015;17(1):375. https://doi.org/10.1186/s13075-015-0895-8.
15. Yamanaka H, Askling J, Berglind N, Franzen S, Frisell T, Garwood C, et al. Infection rates in patients from five rheumatoid arthritis (RA) registries: contextualizing an RA clinical trial programme. RMD Open. 2017;3(2): e000498. https://doi.org/10.1136/rmdopen-2017-000498.
16. Caplan L, Wolfe F, Russell AS, Michaud K. Corticosteroid use in rheumatoid arthritis: prevalence, predictors, correlates, and outcomes. J Rheumatol. 2007;34(4):696–705.
17. Strehl C, Bijlsma JW, de Wit M, Boers M, Caeyers N, Cutolo M, et al. Defining conditions where long-term glucocorticoid treatment has an acceptably low level of harm to facilitate implementation of existing recommendations: view points from an EULAR task force. Ann Rheum Dis. 2016;75(6):952–7. https://doi.org/10.1136/annrheumdis-2015-208916.
18. Kay J, Upchurch KS. ACR/EULAR 2010 rheumatoid arthritis classification criteria. Rheumatology. 2012;51(suppl. 6):vi5–9.
19. Gaujoux-Viala C, Gossec L. When and for how long should glucocorticoids be used in rheumatoid arthritis? International guidelines and recommendations. Ann N Y Acad Sci. 2014;1318(1):32–40. https://doi.org/10.1111/nyas.12452.
20. Fransen J, Van Riel PL. The disease activity score and the EULAR response criteria. Clin Exp Rheumatol. 2005;23:S93.
21. Safy M, Jacobs JWG, Ijff ND, Bijlsma JWJ, van Laar JM, de Hair MJH, et al. Long-term outcome is better when a methotrexate-based treatment strategy is combined with 10 mg prednisone daily: follow-up after the second Computer-Assisted Management in Early Rheumatoid Arthritis trial. Ann Rheum Dis. 2017;76:1432–5.
22. Jacobs JW, Van Everdingen AA, Verstappen SM, Bijlsma JW. Follow up radiographic data on patients with rheumatoid arthritis who participated in a two-year trial of prednisone therapy or placebo. Arthritis Rheum. 2006; 54(5):1422–8. https://doi.org/10.1002/art.21809.
23. Van Tuyl LH, Boers M, Lems WF, Landewé RB, Han H, Van der Linden S, et al. Survival, comorbidities and joint damage 11 years after the COBRA combination therapy trial in early rheumatoid arthritis. Ann Rheum Dis. 2010;69(5):807–12. https://doi.org/10.1136/ard.2009.108027.
24. Galicia-Hernandez G, Parra-Salcedo F, Ugarte-Martinez P, Contreras-Yanez I, Ponce-de-Leon A, Pascual-Ramos V. Sustained moderate-to-high disease activity and higher Charlson score are predictors of incidental serious infection events in RA patients treated with conventional disease-modifying anti-rheumatic drugs: a cohort study in the treat-to-target era. Clin Exp Rheumatol 2016;34:261–69.
25. Svensson B, Boonen A, Albertsson K, Van Der Heijde D, Keller C, Hafstrom I. Low-dose prednisolone in addition to the initial disease-modifying antirheumatic drug in patients with early active rheumatoid arthritis reduces joint destruction and increases the remission rate: a two-year randomized trial. Arthritis Rheum. 2005;52(11):3360–70. https://doi.org/10.1002/art.21298.
26. Van der Goes MC, Jacobs JW, Boers M, Andrews T, Blom-Bakkers MA, Buttgereit F, et al. Monitoring adverse events of low-dose glucocorticoid therapy: EULAR recommendations for clinical trials and daily practice. Ann Rheum Dis. 2010;69(11):1913–9. https://doi.org/10.1136/ard.2009.124958.
27. Da Silva JA, Jacobs JW, Bijlsma JW. Revisiting the toxicity of low-dose glucocorticoids: risks and fears. Ann N Y Acad Sci. 2006;1069(1):275–88. https://doi.org/10.1196/annals.1351.026.
28. Montecucco C, Todoerti M, Sakellariou G, Scirè CA, Caporali R. Low-dose oral prednisone improves clinical and ultrasonographic remission rates in early rheumatoid arthritis: results of a 12-month open-label randomized study. Arthritis Res Ther. 2012;14(3):R112. https://doi.org/10.1186/ar3838.
29. Roubille C, Rincheval N, Dougados M, Flipo RM, Daures JP, Combe B. Seven-year tolerability profile of glucocorticoids use in early rheumatoid arthritis: data from the ESPOIR cohort. Ann Rheum Dis. 2017;76(11):1797–802. https://doi.org/10.1136/annrheumdis-2016-210135.
30. Ravindran V, Rachapalli S, Choy EH. Safety of medium- to long-term glucocorticoid therapy in rheumatoid arthritis: a meta-analysis. Rheumatology. 2009;48(7):807–11. https://doi.org/10.1093/rheumatology/kep096.
31. Hartman L, Rasch LA, Klausch T, Bijlsma HW, Christensen R, Smulders YM, et al. Harm, benefit and costs associated with low-dose glucocorticoids added to the treatment strategies for rheumatoid arthritis in elderly patients (GLORIA trial): study protocol for a randomized controlled trial. Trials. 2018; 19(1):67. https://doi.org/10.1186/s13063-017-2396-3.
32. Waljee AK, Rogers MAM, Lin P, Singal AG, Stein JD, Marks RM, et al. Short-term use of oral corticosteroids and related harms among adults in the United States: population based cohort study. BMJ. 2017;357:j1415.

33. Listing J, Kekow J, Manger B, Burmester GR, Pattloch D, Zink A, et al. Mortality in rheumatoid arthritis: the impact of disease activity, treatment with glucocorticoids, TNFa inhibitors and rituximab. Ann Rheum Dis. 2015; 74(2):415–21. https://doi.org/10.1136/annrheumdis-2013-204021

34. del Rincón I, Battafarano DF, Restrepo JF, Erikson JM, Escalante A. Glucocorticoid dose thresholds associated with all-cause and cardiovascular mortality in rheumatoid arthritis. Arthritis Rheum. 2014;66(2):264–72. https://doi.org/10.1002/art.38210.

22

Long non-coding RNA KCNQ1OT1 promotes cell viability and migration as well as inhibiting degradation of CHON-001 cells by regulating miR-126-5p/TRPS1 axis

Binfeng Wang and Xiangwei Liu*

Abstract

Background: Osteoarthritis (OA) is defined as a degenerative disease. Pivotal roles of long non-coding RNA (lncRNAs) in OA are widely elucidated. Herein, we intend to explore the function and molecular mechanism of lncRNA KCNQ1OT1 in CHON-001 cells.

Methods: Relative expression of KCNQ1OT1, miR-126-5p and TRPS1 was determined by quantitative real-time polymerase chain reaction (qRT-PCR). Cell viability was examined by MTT assay. The migratory ability of chondrocytes was assessed by transwell assay. Western blot was used to determine relative protein expression of collagen II, MMP13 and TRPS1. Dual-luciferase reporter (DLR) assay was applied to test the target of lncRNA KCNQ1OT1 or miR-126-5p.

Results: Relative expression of KCNQ1OT1 and TRPS1 was reduced, whereas miR-126-5p was augmented in cartilage tissues of post-traumatic OA patients compared to those of subjects without post-traumatic OA. Increased KCNQ1OT1 or decreased miR-126-5p enhanced cell viability and migration, and repressed extracellular matrix (ECM) degradation in CHON-001 cells. MiR-126-5p was the downstream target of KCNQ1OT1, and it could directly target TRPS1. There was an inverse correlation between KCNQ1OT1 and miR-126-5p or between miR-126-5p and TRPS1. Meantime, there was a positive correlation between KCNQ1OT1 and TRPS1. The promoting impacts of KCNQ1OT1 on cell viability and migration as well as the suppressive impact of KCNQ1OT1 on ECM degradation were partially abolished by miR-126-5p overexpression or TRPS1 knockdown in CHON-001 cells.

Conclusions: Overexpression of KCNQ1OT1 attenuates the development of OA by sponging miR-126-5p to target TRPS1. Our findings may provide a possible therapeutic strategy for human OA in clinic.

Keywords: Post-traumatic osteoarthritis, KCNQ1 overlapping transcript 1, miR-126-5p, Tricho-rhino-phalangeal syndrome type I

* Correspondence: liuxiangwei338@163.com
Orthopaedic Ward 2 (Trauma Surgery), Chifeng Municipal Hospital, No.1, Zhaowuda Road, Chifeng City 024000, Inner Mongolia, China

Introduction

Osteoarthritis (OA) is a degenerative bone and joint disease, which is featured by destruction of joint matrix and the decrease of articular chondrocytes [1, 2]. Its clinical symptoms include swelling, stiffness and arthralgia [3]. As previously reported, OA can be caused by diverse factors, such as genetic predisposition, failure of nutrient supply, abnormal mechanical loading and trauma [1]. Currently, drug treatment, stem cell treatment, electromagnetic therapy and acupuncture therapy have been clinically applied for OA therapy [4–7]. However, the treatment effect is unsatisfactory. Thence, it is imperative to explore more effective targets for OA management.

Recent years, the crucial roles of long non-coding RNAs (lncRNAs) in OA have been gradually recognized [8–10]. For instance, MALAT1 and MFI2-AS1 are deeply involved in chondrocytes proliferation and extracellular matrix (ECM) degradation in OA [8, 9]. Similarly, TUG1 can facilitate ECM degradation of chondrocytes in OA [10]. Notably, lncRNA KCNQ1 overlapping transcript 1 (KCNQ1OT1), located in the KCNQ1 locus at 11p15.5 [11], has been reported to play important role in the proliferation and differentiation of chondrocytes in fracture or osteolysis [12, 13]. However, the role and mechanism of lncRNA KCNQ1OT1 in OA are not elucidated.

It is well known that lncRNAs participate in post-transcriptional regulation by binding to microRNAs (miRNAs) [14]. Ample evidence has revealed that miRNAs are critical regulators in the pathogenesis of OA [15], such as miR-335-5p [16] and miR-140 [17]. More importantly, miR-126 is also uncovered to possess a regulatory role in OA [18, 19]. For example, inhibition of miR-126 promotes the viability and migration of chondrocytes in a cell model of OA [18]. The viability of chondrocytes is enhanced by down-regulation of miR-126 [19]. In addition, miR-126 is revealed to be a target of lncRNA DNM3OS to regulate OA progression [19]. Nonetheless, the regulatory effect of lncRNA KCNQ1OT1 on miR-126-5p in OA has not been explored.

Tricho-rhino-phalangeal syndrome type I (TRPS1) is known as an oncogene to promote cell proliferation and metastasis in several types of human cancers, such as breast cancer [20], osteosarcoma [21], and colon cancer [22]. In recent years, the promoting role of TRPS1 in chondrocytes differentiation and proliferation has attracted increasing attention [23, 24]. Wuelling et al. found that loss of TRPS1 represses the differentiation of chondrocytes via Wnt5a [23]. Suemoto et al. demonstrated that overexpression of TRPS1 facilitates chondrocytes proliferation by reduction the level of Stat3 [24]. However, studies of TRPS1 effects on OA are limited.

Here, the roles of lncRNA KCNQ1OT1 and miR-126-5p were examined in CHON-001 cells. To further explore the regulatory mechanism of lncRNA KCNQ1OT1, the regulatory relation among KCNQ1OT1, miR-126-5p and TRPS1 was tested in CHON-001 cells. This investigation provided a new theoretical reference for OA treatment.

Materials and methods

Patients

The OA cartilage tissues were obtained from knees of post-traumatic OA (PTOA) patients (14 males and 9 females, an average age of 56.58 years) who underwent total knee arthroplasty. Normal cartilage tissues were collected from subjects without PTOA (8 males and 8 females, an average age of 51.66 years) who underwent the amputation. All samples were collected from our hospital between March 2017 and December 2019. The tissues samples were used to detect the expression levels of KCNQ1OT1, miR-126-5p, and TRPS1, as well as the correlations among them. The current study was approved by the ethics committees of our hospital, and all participants had signed written informed consents.

Cell culture

A human chondrocyte cell line (CHON-001) was bought from American Type Culture Collection (ATCC; Manassas, Virginia, USA). CHON-001 cells were grown in Dulbecco's Modified Eagle's Medium (DMEM; Gibco, Waltham, MA, USA) supplemented with 0.1 mg/mL G-418 (Gibco) and 10% fetal bovine serum (FBS; Gibco), and maintained in an incubator with a temperature of 37 °C and 5% CO_2.

Cell transfection

The pcDNA3.1-negative control (NC), pcDNA3.1-KCNQ1OT1 (containing full-length of KCNQ1OT1), short hairpin (sh)-NC, sh-KCNQ1OT1, mimics NC, miR-126-5p mimics, inhibitor NC, miR-126-5p inhibitor, sh-TRPS1 were bought from RiboBio (Guangzhou, China). Then these oligonucleotides and plasmids were transfected into CHON-001 cells through Lipofectamine3000 (Invitrogen, Carlsbad, CA, USA) for 48 h. Afterwards, the transfected CHON-001 cells were used to perform the functional experiments of KCNQ1OT1/miR-126-5p/TRPS1 axis in vitro.

Quantitative Real-Time Polymerase Chain Reaction (qRT-PCR)

Total RNA from cartilage tissues and CHON-001 cells was extracted using TRIzol® reagent (Invitrogen), and RNA concentration was detected by NanoDropND-1000 spectrophotometer. After that, extracted RNA was converted to complementary DNA (cDNA) via a PrimeScript™ RT reagent kit (Takara, Beijing, China). The cDNA was used for performing qRT-PCR according to instructions of a SYBR Green PCR kit (Takara). The reaction procedures were shown as follows: 95 °C for 20 s, 35 cycles of 95 °C for 10 s, 60 °C for 30 s and 72 °C for 10 s. All primers (Table 1) were bought from Sangon Biotech (Shanghai, China). Finally, relative expression of KCNQ1OT1, miR-126-5p and TRPS1 was calculated via the $2^{-\Delta\Delta Ct}$ method. U6 and GADPH were used as internal references.

3-(4, 5-Dimethyl-2-Thiazolyl)-2, 5-Diphenyl-2-H-tetrazolium bromide (MTT) assay

CHON-001 cells (6×10^3/well) were seeded in 96-well plates, and then reacted with MTT (10 µL). After 4 h of reaction, and dimethyl sulfoxide (150 µL) were added into each well for dissolving formazan crystals. Cell viability was assessed by measuring the optical density (OD) at 450 nm using a microplate reader (BMG LABTECH, Durham, NC, USA).

Dual Luciferase Reporter (DLR) assay

The 3′-UTR sequence of KCNQ1OT1 or TRPS1 containing miR-126-5p binding sites was cloned into a pGL3 Basic Vector (Promega, Madison, WI) to construct KCNQ1OT1 wt or TRPS1 wt. KCNQ1OT1 mut or TRPS1 mut was obtained by mutating binding sites of miR-126-5p and then introduced into the pGL3 Basic Vector (Promega). Then CHON-001 cells were transfected with above plasmids along with mimics NC/miR-126-5p mimics. Following 48 h of transfection, Firefly and Renilla luciferase activity was examined through a dual-luciferase reporter assay system (Biotek, Winooski, VT, USA). Relative luciferase activity was defined as the ratio of Firefly luciferase activity and Renilla luciferase activity.

Western blot

Total proteins were isolated from CHON-001 cells using RIPA lysis (Beyotime, Shanghai, China), and the concentration of proteins was measured through a bicinchoninic acid kit (Pierce, Waltham, MA, USA). Next, protein samples were separated by sodium dodecyl sulphate-polyacrylamide gel electrophoresis (SDS-PAGE) gel, followed by transferring onto polyvinylidene difluoride (PVDF) membranes (Millipore, Billerica, MA, USA). After being blocked with 5% skim milk, the membranes were incubated with the following primary antibodies overnight at 4 °C: anti-TRPS1 (1:1000, ab227867, Abcam), anti-collagen II (1:2000, ab188570, Abcam), anti-MMP13 (1:1000, ab51072, Abcam) and anti-α-tubulin (1:2000, ab52866, Abcam). After the membranes were washed with tris buffered saline Tween (TBST), the membranes were nurtured with the secondary antibody (1:10,000, ab205718, Abcam) at 37 °C for 2 h. Finally, the immune-reactivity was visualized using electrochemiluminescence (Thermo Fisher Scientific, Shanghai, China), and relative protein expression of MMP13, TRPS1 and collagen II over α-tubulin was quantified via Gel-pro Analyzer software (Media Cybernetics, Maryland, USA).

Transwell assay

For determining the migratory ability of CHON-001 cells, transwell assay was carried out with the 24-well transwell chamber (8-µm pore size; Corning, Cambridge, USA). CHON-001 cells (6×10^5 cells) in FBS-free medium were plated into the upper layer of the transwell chamber. Subsequently, the lower chamber was filled with 600 µL DMEM including 10% FBS. After incubation for 24 h, migratory cells on the lower chamber were fixed in 4% paraformaldehyde for 15 min and stained with 0.5% crystal violet for 10 min. The numbers of migratory cells were counted under a Leica microscope (Leica Microsystems, Wetzlar, Germany). The percentage of migration was calculated as the following formula: (the numbers of migratory cells in the treat group)/ (the numbers of migratory cells in the control group) × 100%.

Statistical analysis

Data were analyzed by the SPSS 22.0 software (IBM, Armonk, NY, USA). All results were displayed as the mean ± standard deviation. One-way ANOVA was utilized for multiple comparisons, followed by Tukey's post hoc test. Student's t-test was applied to compare differences between two groups. A value of $P < 0.05$ was regarded as statistically significant.

Results

LncRNA KCNQ1OT1 promotes cell viability and migration, and represses ECM degradation in CHON-001 cells

In order to probe the function of lncRNA KCNQ1OT1 in OA, the expression of KCNQ1OT1 was firstly

Table 1 Primers for qRT-PCR

Gene	Forward	Reverse
KCNQ1OT1	5′-CTTTGCAGCAACCTCCTTGT-3′	5′-TGGGGTGAGGGATCTGAA-3′
MiR-126-5p	5′-GCGCGCATTATTACTTTTGG-3′	5′-TGGTGTCGTGGAGTCG – 3′
TRPS1	5′-CAAATCTCAGGCCTGAGTGA – 3′	5′-GTGAAGAGCTGATATCCTGCAG-3′
U6	5′-CTCGCTTCGGCAGCACA-3′	5′-AACGCTTCACGAATTTGCGT-3′
GAPDH	5′-CAAAGGTGGATCAGATTCAAG-3′	5′-GGTGAGCATTATCACCCAGAA-3′

determined in PTOA patients. We found that KCNQ1OT1 expression was lower in the PTOA group than that in the control group ($P < 0.001$, Fig. 1A). Subsequently, lncRNA KCNQ1OT1 was overexpressed or silenced in CHON-001 cells. As expected, KCNQ1OT1 expression was evidently diminished by addition of sh-KCNQ1OT1, and distinctly boosted by addition of pcDNA3.1-KCNQ1OT1 in CHON-001 cells (all $P < 0.001$, Fig. 1B). Then functional experiments were performed. Results from MTT and transwell assays displayed that the viability ($P < 0.001$, Fig. 1C) and migratory ability of CHON-001 cells ($P < 0.01$, Fig. 1D) were enhanced when KCNQ1OT1 was overexpressed, whereas silencing of KCNQ1OT1 resulted in opposite results. Moreover, data from western blot indicated that up-regulation of KCNQ1OT1 elevated relative protein expression of the ECM protein (collagen II) ($P < 0.01$, Fig. 1E), whereas reduced relative protein expression of the cartilage-degrading enzyme (MMP13) in CHON-001 cells ($P < 0.001$, Fig. 1E), thereby repressing the ECM

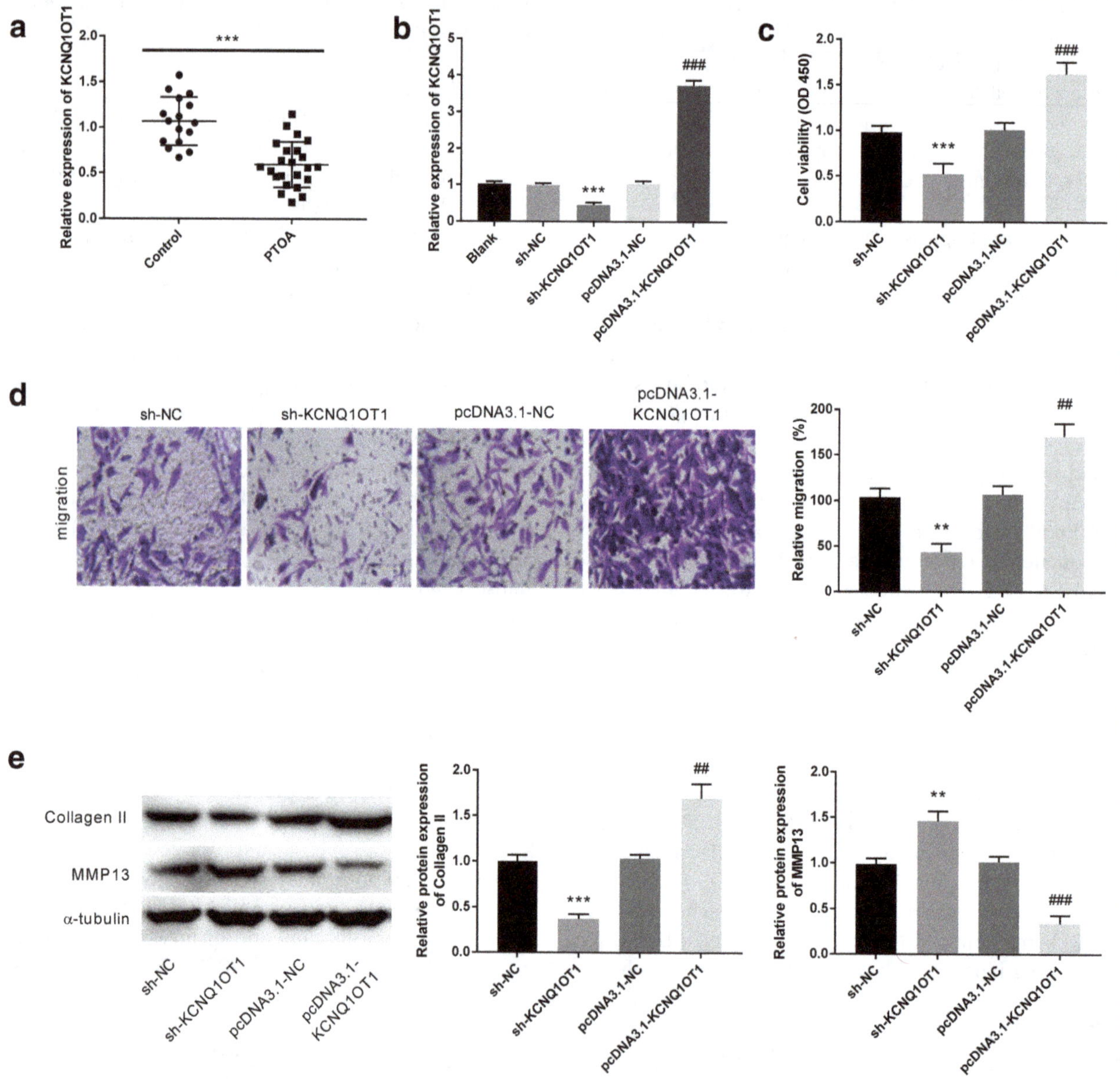

Fig. 1 LncRNA KCNQ1OT1 promotes cell viability and migration, and suppresses ECM degradation in CHON-001 cells. **a** Relative expression of KCNQ1OT1 was detected by qRT-PCR in cartilage tissues of PTOA patients and normal cartilage tissues. $^{***}P < 0.001$, vs. Control. **b** Relative expression of KCNQ1OT1 was determined by qRT-PCR in CHON-001 cells. $^{***}P < 0.001$, vs. sh-NC. $^{\#\#\#}P < 0.001$, vs. pcDNA3.1-NC. **c** The cell viability was determined by MTT assay in CHON-001 cells. $^{***}P < 0.001$, vs. sh-NC. $^{\#\#\#}P < 0.001$, vs. pcDNA3.1-NC. **d** Relative migration was assessed by transwell assay in CHON-001 cells. $^{**}P < 0.01$, vs. sh-NC. $^{\#\#}P < 0.01$, vs. pcDNA3.1-NC. **e** Relative protein expression of collagen II and MMP13 was determined by western blot in CHON-001 cells. $^{**}P < 0.01$, $^{***}P < 0.001$, vs. sh-NC. $^{\#\#}P < 0.01$, $^{\#\#\#}P < 0.001$, vs. pcDNA3.1-NC

degradation of CHON-001 cells. In contrast to KCNQ1OT1 up-regulation, KCNQ1OT1 down-regulation made opposite effects on the protein expression of collagen II and MMP13 in CHON-001 cells.

LncRNA KCNQ1OT1 can directly bind to miR-126-5p

For exploring the downstream mechanism by which KCNQ1OT1 affected CHON-001 cells, we searched for targeting miRNAs of KCNQ1OT1 by starbase. Interestingly, we observed some complementary bases between miR-126-5p and KCNQ1OT1 (Fig. 2A). Meantime, DLR assay was used to verify the interaction of miR-126-5p and KCNQ1OT1. As shown in Fig. 2B, addition of miR-126-5p mimics markedly decreased relative luciferase activity of KCNQ1OT1 wt compared to addition of mimics NC ($P < 0.01$), while it failed to affect relative luciferase activity of KCNQ1OT1 mut in CHON-001 cells, confirming the direct binding between miR-126-5p and KCNQ1OT1 (Fig. 2B). Moreover, we discovered that relative expression of miR-126-5p was greatly boosted by knockdown of KCNQ1OT1 but reduced by overexpression of KCNQ1OT1 in CHON-001 cells (all $P < 0.001$, Fig. 2C). MiR-126-5p expression was higher in the PTOA group relative to that in the control group ($P < 0.001$, Fig. 2D). There was an inverse correlation between KCNQ1OT1 expression and miR-126-5p expression in cartilage tissues of PTOA patients ($P = 0.0171$, $R^2 = 0.2422$, Fig. 2E).

Decreased expression of miR-126-5p enhances the viability and migratory ability but represses ECM degradation in CHON-001 cells

Afterwards, to examine whether miR-126-5p made impacts on CHON-001 cells, CHON-001 cells were transfected with miR-126-5p mimics, miR-126-5p inhibitor and corresponding controls. As manifested in Fig. 3A, miR-126-5p mimics caused notable up-regulation of miR-126-5p, and miR-126-5p inhibitor led to distinct down-regulation of miR-126-5p in CHON-001 cells (all $P < 0.001$). Functionally, it was found that the cell viability ($P < 0.001$, Fig. 3B) and migratory ability ($P < 0.01$, Fig. 3C) were enhanced by miR-126-5p inhibitor, and reduced by miR-126-5p mimics in CHON-001 cells. Relative protein expression of collagen II was decreased by miR-126-5p mimics but elevated by miR-126-5p inhibitor in CHON-001 cells (all $P < 0.001$,

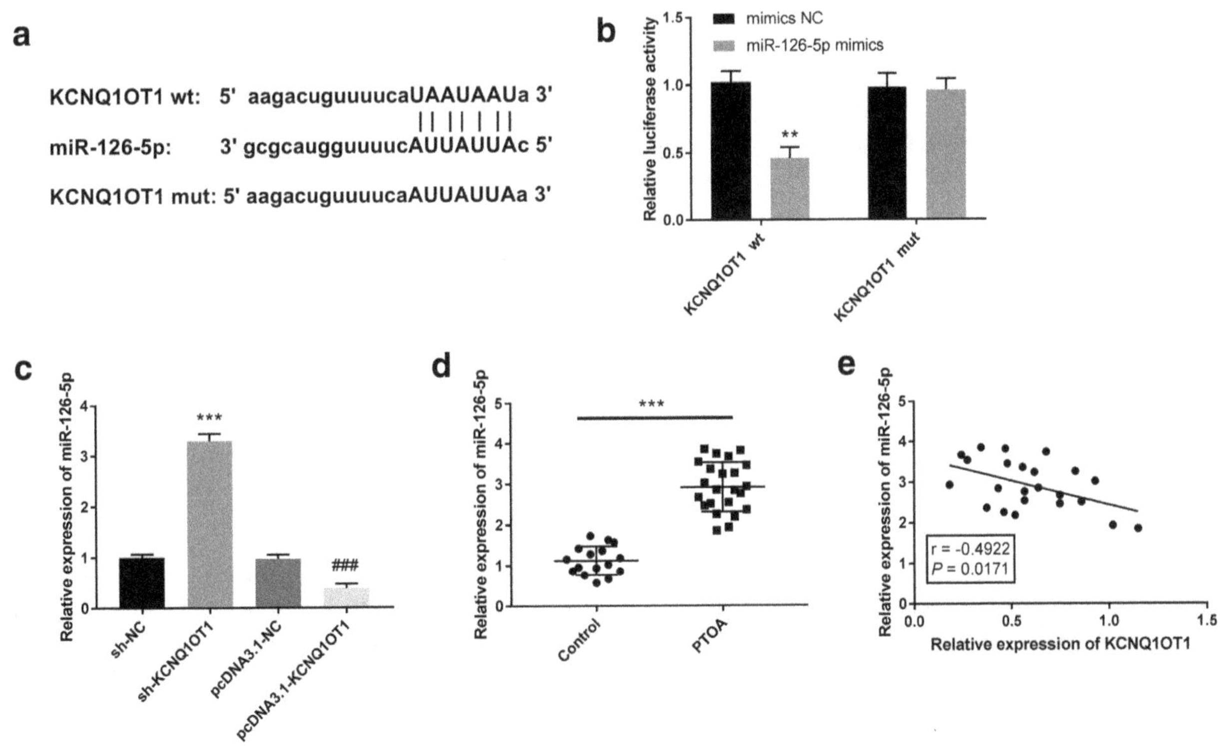

Fig. 2 LncRNA KCNQ1OT1 can directly bind to miR-126-5p. **a** The binding sequences between KCNQ1OT1 and miR-126-5p were predicted by starbase. **b** The interaction between KCNQ1OT1 and miR-126-5p in CHON-001 cells was verified by dual-luciferase reporter (DLR) assay. $^{**}P < 0.01$, vs. mimics NC. **c** Relative expression of miR-126-5p was detected by qRT-PCR in CHON-001 cells. $^{***}P < 0.001$, vs. sh-NC. $^{\#\#\#}P < 0.001$, vs. pcDNA3.1-NC. **d** Relative expression of miR-126-5p was detected by qRT-PCR in cartilage tissues of PTOA patients and normal cartilage tissues. $^{***}P < 0.001$, vs. Control. **e** The correlation between KCNQ1OT1 and miR-126-5p was analyzed by Pearson's correlation analysis in cartilage tissues of PTOA patients. $P = 0.0171$. $R^2 = 0.2422$

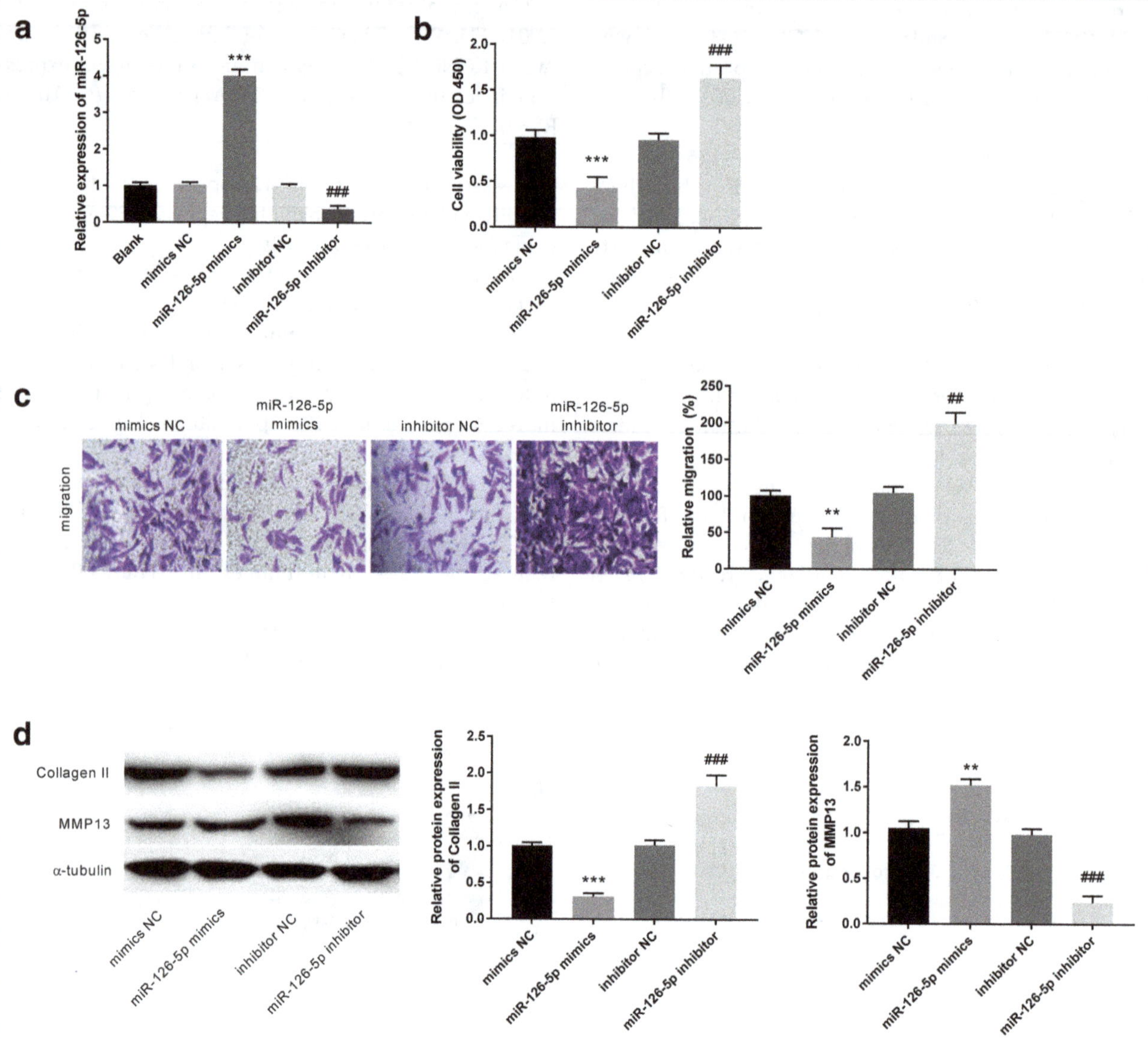

Fig. 3 Decreased expression of miR-126-5p enhances the viability and migratory ability of chondrocytes, and represses ECM degradation in CHON-001 cells. **a** Relative expression of miR-126-5p was determined by qRT-PCR in CHON-001 cells. ***$P < 0.001$, vs. mimics NC. ###$P < 0.001$, vs. inhibitor NC. **b** The cell viability was determined by MTT assay in CHON-001 cells. ***$P < 0.001$, vs. mimics NC. ###$P < 0.001$, vs. inhibitor NC. **c** Relative migration was assessed by transwell assay in CHON-001 cells. **$P < 0.01$, vs. mimics NC. ##$P < 0.01$, vs. inhibitor NC. **d** Relative protein expression of collagen II and MMP13 was determined by western blot in CHON-001 cells. **$P < 0.01$, ***$P < 0.001$, vs. mimics NC. ###$P < 0.001$, vs. inhibitor NC

Fig. 3D). Meantime, relative protein expression of MMP13 was boosted by miR-126-5p mimics ($P < 0.01$) but reduced by miR-126-5p inhibitor ($P < 0.001$) in CHON-001 cells (Fig. 3D).

TRPS1 was targeted by miR-126-5p

After that, target genes of miR-126-5p were predicted with starbase. It was uncovered that TRPS1 possessed binding regions of miR-126-5p (Fig. 4A). Meanwhile, the result of DLR displayed that relative luciferase activity of CHON-001 cells was evidently reduced after co-transfection of miR-126-5p mimics and TRPS1 wt ($P < 0.01$), while showed no significant change after co-transfection of miR-126-5p mimics and TRPS1 mut (Fig. 4B). Besides, we found that the protein expression of TRPS1 was decreased by miR-126-5p up-regulation and increased by miR-126-5p down-regulation in CHON-001 cells (all $P < 0.001$, Fig. 4C). The mRNA expression of TRPS1 was declined in the PTOA group compared to the control group ($P < 0.001$, Fig. 4D). TRPS1 was inversely correlated with miR-126-5p ($P = 0.0037$, $R^2 = 0.336$, Fig. 4E) and positively correlated with KCNQ1OT1 ($P < 0.0001$, $R^2 = 0.6136$, Fig. 4F) in cartilage tissues of PTOA patients.

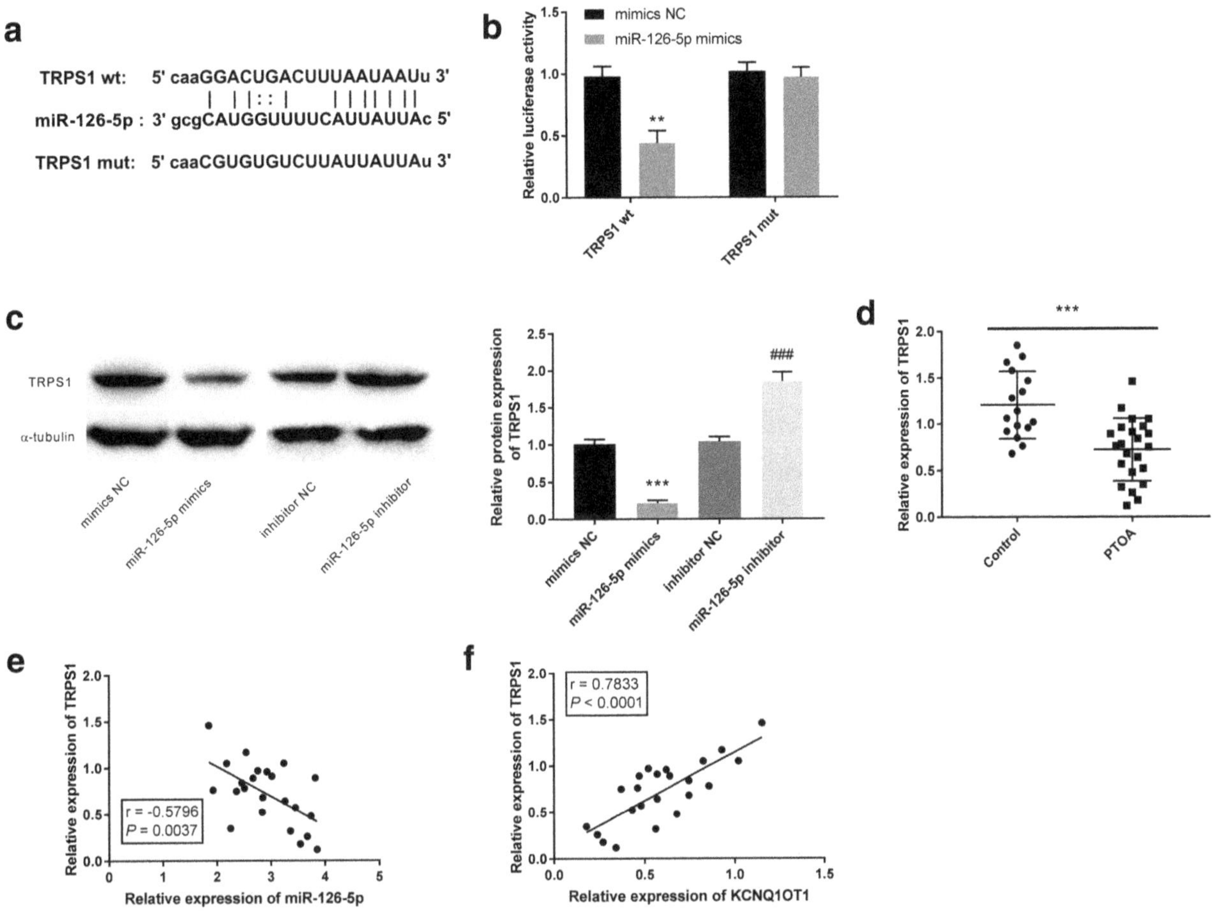

Fig. 4 TRPS1 was targeted by miR-126-5p. **a** The binding sequences between TRPS1 and miR-126-5p were predicted by starbase. **b** The interaction between TRPS1 and miR-126-5p in CHON-001 cells was verified by dual-luciferase reporter (DLR) assay. $^{**}P < 0.01$, vs. mimics NC. **c** Relative protein expression of TRPS1 was detected by western blot in CHON-001 cells. $^{***}P < 0.001$, vs. mimics NC. $^{###}P < 0.001$, vs. inhibitor NC. **d** Relative expression of TRPS1 was detected by qRT-PCR in cartilage tissues of PTOA patients and normal cartilage tissues. $^{***}P < 0.001$, vs. Control. **e** The correlation between TRPS1 and miR-126-5p was analyzed by Pearson's correlation analysis in cartilage tissues of PTOA patients. $P = 0.0037$. $R^2 = 0.336$. **f** The correlation between KCNQ1OT1 and TRPS1 was analyzed by Pearson's correlation analysis in cartilage tissues of PTOA patients. $P < 0.0001$. $R^2 = 0.6136$

LncRNA KCNQ1OT1 enhances the viability and migration but suppresses degradation of CHON-001 cells via sponging miR-126-5p to target TRPS1

Finally, we explored the interrelation among KCNQ1OT1, miR-126-5p and TRPS1 in CHON-001 cells. Firstly, TRPS1 knockdown was achieved by sh-TRPS1 transfection. As expected, the mRNA expression of TRPS1 was remarkably reduced by sh-TRPS1 transfection in CHON-001 cells ($P < 0.01$, Fig. 5A). Then, the regulatory relation of KCNQ1OT1, miR-126-5p and TRPS1 was tested. We found that TRPS1 expression was elevated by pcDNA3.1-KCNQ1OT1, and the elevation effect of pcDNA3.1-KCNQ1OT1 on TRPS1 expression was reversed by miR-126-5p mimics in CHON-001 cells (all $P < 0.001$, Fig. 5B). Next, rescue assays were implemented. It was proved that KCNQ1OT1 overexpression strengthened the viability and migratory ability of CHON-001 cells (all $P < 0.001$, Fig. 5C-D), and these enhanced effects were partially attenuated by miR-126-5p overexpression or TRPS1 knockdown in CHON-001 cells (all $P < 0.01$, Fig. 5C-D). Additionally, KCNQ1OT1 overexpression elevated the protein expression of collagen II but reduced the protein expression of MMP13 in CHON-001 cells (all $P < 0.001$, Fig. 5E), which was reversed by miR-126-5p overexpression or TRPS1 knockdown (all $P < 0.01$, Fig. 5E).

Discussion

OA is the most common joint disease with high morbidity in the middle-aged and elderly population [25, 26]. Numerous lncRNAs have been confirmed to be downregulated in OA [27–29], such as lncRNA ATB [27], lncRNA PACER [28], and lncRNA ANCR [29]. In line with the previous studies, a decreased expression of

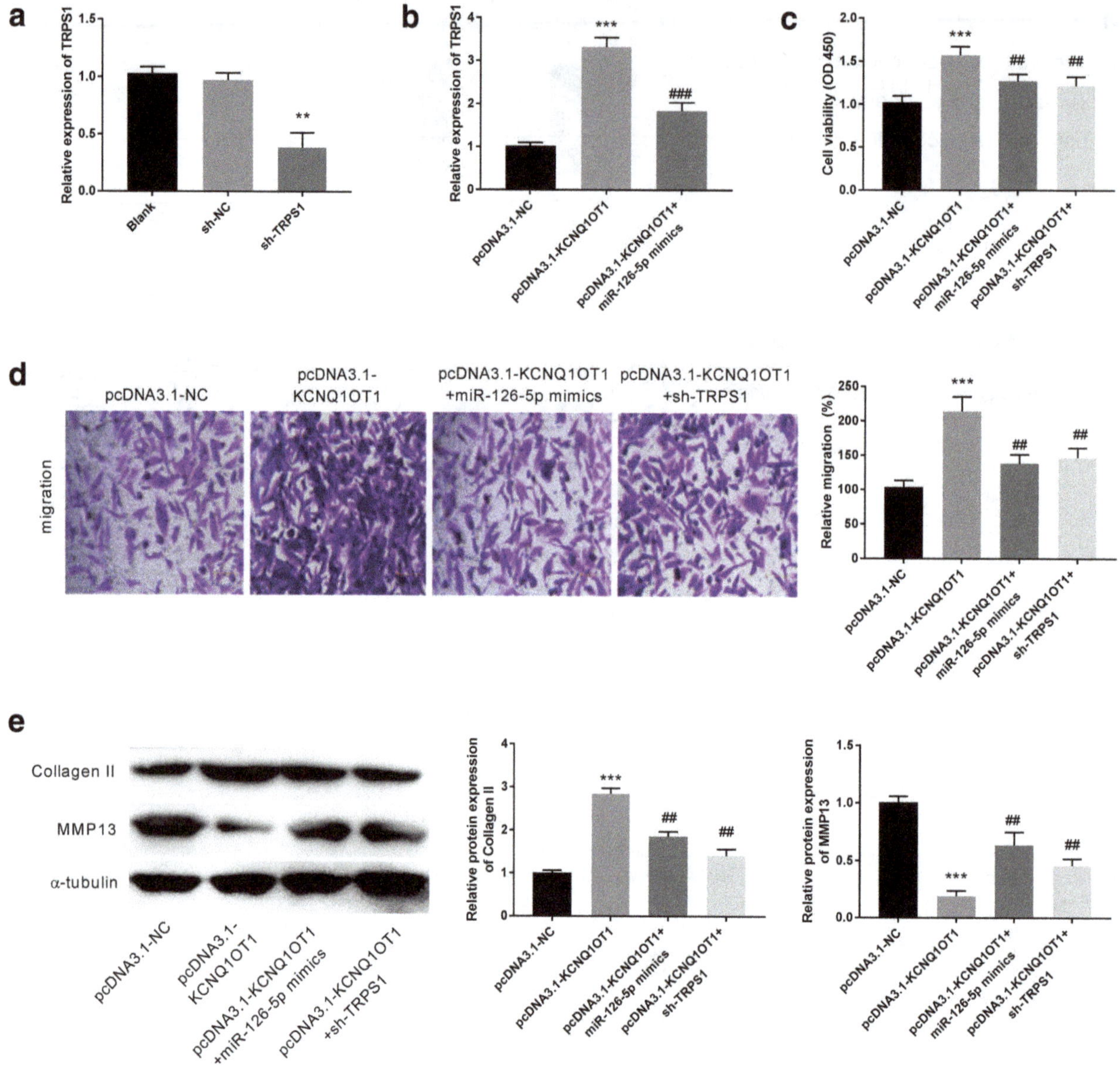

Fig. 5 LncRNA KCNQ1OT1 enhances the cell viability and migration but suppresses ECM degradation via sponging miR-126-5p to target TRPS1 in CHON-001 cells. **a** Relative expression of TRPS1 in CHON-001 cells was detected by qRT-PCR after transfection of sh-NC and sh-TRPS1. $^{**}P < 0.01$, vs. sh-NC. **b** Relative expression of TRPS1 was determined by qRT-PCR in CHON-001 cells. $^{***}P < 0.001$, vs. pcDNA3.1-NC. $^{\#\#\#}P < 0.001$, vs. pcDNA3.1-KCNQ1OT1. **c** The cell viability was determined by MTT assay in CHON-001 cells. $^{***}P < 0.001$, vs. pcDNA3.1-NC. $^{\#\#}P < 0.01$, vs. pcDNA3.1-KCNQ1OT1. **d** Relative migration was assessed by transwell assay in CHON-001 cells. $^{***}P < 0.001$, vs. pcDNA3.1-NC. $^{\#\#}P < 0.01$, vs. pcDNA3.1-KCNQ1OT1. **e** Relative protein expression of collagen II and MMP13 was determined by western blot in CHON-001 cells. $^{***}P < 0.001$, vs. pcDNA3.1-NC. $^{\#\#}P < 0.01$, vs. pcDNA3.1-KCNQ1OT1

lncRNA KCNQ1OT1 was also observed in cartilage tissues of PTOA patients compared to that of subjects without PTOA. The results implied that lncRNA KCNQ1OT1 may participate in the progression of OA. Given that loss of chondrocytes is the main cause of OA [30], numerous reports have focused on the impacts of lncRNAs on chondrocytes [8, 9, 31]. For instance, knockdown of lncRNA-p21 strengths cell viability and repress apoptosis in OA chondrocytes [31]. LncRNA MALAT1 promotes cell proliferation and inhibit ECM degradation in IL-1β-induced chondrocytes [8]. Silencing of lncRNA MFI2-AS1 elevates chondrocytes viability but represses ECM degradation [9]. In this study, we discovered that KCNQ1OT1 overexpression promoted the viability and migration as well as inhibition of ECM degradation in CHON-001 cells. Similarly, a recent study conducted by Gu et al. has indicated that KCNQ1OT1 facilitates the proliferation and suppress apoptosis of articular chondrocytes, thus accelerating fracture healing [12]. Therefore, we speculated that KCNQ1OT1 may be a favourable factor to prevent the development of OA due to its important role in promoting the viability and migration of chondrocytes.

Emerging evidence has shown that miR-162 is implicated in OA [32]. Yu et al. have indicated that miR-126 is highly expressed in OA tissues, whereas decreased miR-126 strengthens chondrocyte viability and migration [18]. Interestingly, Ai et al. also found an increased miR-126 in CHON-001 cells, and the cell proliferation can be promoted by suppression of miR-126 [19]. Similarly, we revealed that miR-126-5p was up-regulated in cartilage tissues of PTOA patients, suggesting that miR-126-5p may be involved in the development of OA. Then, our functional experiments on miR-126-5p demonstrated that inhibition of miR-126-5p enhanced the viability and migratory ability of CHON-001 cells, and repressed ECM degradation in CHON-001 cells. Based on these results, we speculated that miR-126-5p may be a pathogenic miRNA existed in OA progression. On the other hand, miR-126-5p is revealed to act as the downstream targets of varied lncRNAs, such as lncRNA CRNDE [33], lncRNA HOTAIR [34], and lncRNA TMPO-AS1 [35]. Here, miR-126-5p was also identified as the target of and negatively regulated by lncRNA KCNQ1OT1. Therefore, we speculated that KCNQ1OT1 may promote the viability and migration of CHON-001 cells by targeting miR-126-5p. The rescue experiments confirmed that miR-126-5p mimics reversed the promoting effects of KCNQ1OT1 on cell viability and migration as well as the suppressive effect of KCNQ1OT1 on ECM degradation in CHON-001 cells. These results verified our speculation.

Numerous studies have uncovered the vital role of TRPS1 in cellular processes of chondrocytes [24, 36]. Gai et al. have stated that TRPS1 can regulate the proliferation and apoptosis of chondrocytes [36]. Suemoto et al. have unveiled that overexpression of TRPS1 facilitates chondrocytes proliferation by reduction the level of Stat3 [24]. In the present study, we found that TRPS1 expression was reduced in cartilage tissues, suggesting that TRPS1 may exhibited an anti-osteoarthritis OA progression. It is noticed that TRPS1, an atypical member of the GATA transcriptional factor family, is initially identified as a transcriptional repressor [37]. Indeed, it was previously uncovered to be targeted by varied miRNAs, including miR-26b-5p [38], and miR-221 [39]. Additionally, convincing evidence has demonstrated that complex interactions between miRNAs and their target genes are essential in regulating of homeostatic pathways in OA [40]. Inspired by this perception, bioinformatics analysis was implemented to predict target genes of miR-126-5p. We found that TRPS1 was a direct target gene of miR-126-5p. Meanwhile, we observed the negative correlation between TRPS1 and miR-126-5p in cartilage tissues of PTOA patients. Taken together, we speculated that decreased miR-126-5p enhanced the viability and migratory ability as well as repressing ECM degradation by targeting TRPS1 in CHON-001 cells. More importantly, we discovered that TRPS1 was positively correlated with KCNQ1OT1 in cartilage tissues of PTOA patients. The promoting effects of KCNQ1OT1 on cell viability and migration as well as the inhibitory effect of KCNQ1OT1 on ECM degradation were reversed by TRPS1 knockdown in CHON-001 cells. Therefore, we believed that lncRNA KCNQ1OT1 could repress OA progression via mediating miR-126-5p/TRPS1 axis in vitro. In addition, there may be some other important genes or pathways related to this axis in several types of human diseases, such as TRPS1-SOX9 in hereditary hypertrichoses or chondrocytes differentiation [41], KCNQ1OT1-PI3K/AKT pathway in cardiomyocytes injury [42] or colorectal cancer [43], miR-126-5p-PI3K/AKT pathway in ovarian cancer [44], cervical cancer [45], and gastric cancer [46]. We speculated that these important genes or pathways may be also involved in regulation of OA pathogenesis via interaction of KCNQ1OT1/miR-126-5p/TRPS1 axis. This is a research direction in our future studies.

Furthermore, there are also some other limitations in this study: i) lncRNA KCNQ1OT1 may be related with paternal allele, and the differences on KCNQ1OT1 expression in female and male OA patients are needed to be studied; ii), CHON-001 cells combined with cytokine stimulation and osmotic pressure to establish a vitro model for OA or use of the isolated chondrocytes from OA patients may be more rigorous and significant; iii) this study is focused on a cellular level, and in vivo experiments should be performed.

Conclusions

In summary, lncRNA KCNQ1OT1 was decreased in the PTOA group compared to the control group. LncRNA KCNQ1OT1 acted as a sponge of miR-126-5p, and TRPS1 was the downstream target of miR-126-5p. Overall, lncRNA KCNQ1OT1 repressed OA progression via binding to miR-126-5p and indirectly regulating TRPS1 in vitro. Hence, our study provided insights into the development of a novel target for treating OA.

Abbreviations

OA: Osteoarthritis; LncRNAs: Long non-coding RNA; QRT-PCR: Quantitative real-time polymerase chain reaction; DLR: Dual-luciferase reporter; ECM: Extracellular matrix; KCNQ1OT1: LncRNA KCNQ1 overlapping transcript 1; MiRNAs: microRNAs; TRPS1: Tricho-rhino-phalangeal syndrome type I; PVDF: Polyvinylidene difluoride; TBST: Tris buffered saline Tween

Acknowledgements

Not applicable.

Authors' contributions

All authors made substantial contributions to conception and design, acquisition of data, or analysis and interpretation of data; took part in drafting the article or revising it critically for important intellectual content; gave final approval of the version to be published; and agree to be accountable for all aspects of the work.

References

1. Pereira D, Ramos E, Branco J. Osteoarthritis. Acta Medica Port. 2015;28(1):99 106. https://doi.org/10.20344/amp.5477.
2. Liu C, Wang B, Xiao L, Li Y, Xu L, Zhao Z, et al. Protective effects of the pericellular matrix of chondrocyte on articular cartilage against the development of osteoarthritis. Histol Histopathol. 2018;33(8):757–64. https://doi.org/10.14670/HH-11-967.
3. Suri P, Morgenroth DC, Hunter DJ. Epidemiology of osteoarthritis and associated comorbidities. PM R. 2012;4(5 Suppl):S10–9. https://doi.org/10.1016/j.pmrj.2012.01.007.
4. Wollheim FA. Current pharmacological treatment of osteoarthritis. Drugs. 1996;52(Suppl 3):27–38. https://doi.org/10.2165/00003495-199600523-00006
5. Richmond J, Hunter D, Irrgang J, Jones MH, Snyder-Mackler L, van Durme D, et al. American Academy of Orthopaedic surgeons clinical practice guideline on the treatment of osteoarthritis (OA) of the knee. J Bone Joint Surg Am. 2010;92(4):990–3. https://doi.org/10.2106/JBJS.I.00982.
6. Brosseau L, Wells G, Marchand S, Gaboury I, Stokes B, Morin M, et al. Randomized controlled trial on low level laser therapy (LLLT) in the treatment of osteoarthritis (OA) of the hand. Lasers Surg Med. 2005;36(3): 210–9. https://doi.org/10.1002/lsm.20137.
7. Hermann W, Lambova S, Muller-Ladner U. Current treatment options for osteoarthritis. Curr Rheumatol Rev. 2018;14(2):108–16. https://doi.org/10.2174/1573397113666170829155149.
8. Zhang Y, Wang F, Chen G, He R, Yang L. LncRNA MALAT1 promotes osteoarthritis by modulating miR-150-5p/AKT3 axis. Cell Biosci. 2019;9(1):54._ https://doi.org/10.1186/s13578-019-0302-2.
9. Luo X, Wang J, Wei X, Wang S, Wang A. Knockdown of lncRNA MFI2-AS1 inhibits lipopolysaccharide-induced osteoarthritis progression by miR-130a-3p/TCF4. Life Sci. 2020;240:117019. https://doi.org/10.1016/j.lfs.2019.117019
10. Tang LP, Ding JB, Liu ZH, Zhou GJ. LncRNA TUG1 promotes osteoarthritis-induced degradation of chondrocyte extracellular matrix via miR-195/MMP-13 axis. Eur Rev Med Pharmacol Sci. 2018;22(24):8574–81. https://doi.org/10.26355/eurrev_201812_16620.
11. Kanduri C. Kcnq1ot1: a chromatin regulatory RNA. Semin Cell Dev Biol. 2011; 22(4):343–50. https://doi.org/10.1016/j.semcdb.2011.02.020.
12. Gu H, Li Z, Lv XF, Zhao AB, Zhu MY, Zhang Y. LncRNA KCNQ1OT1 delayed fracture healing through the Wnt/beta-catenin pathway. Eur Rev Med Pharmacol Sci. 2019;23(11):4575–83. https://doi.org/10.26355/eurrev_201906_18034.
13. Gao X, Ge J, Li W, Zhou W, Xu L. LncRNA KCNQ1OT1 promotes osteogenic differentiation to relieve osteolysis via Wnt/beta-catenin activation. Cell Biosci. 2018;8(1):19. https://doi.org/10.1186/s13578-018-0216-4.
14. Paraskevopoulou MD, Hatzigeorgiou AG. Analyzing MiRNA-LncRNA interactions. Methods Mol Biol. 2016;1402:271–86. https://doi.org/10.1007/978-1-4939-3378-5_21.
15. Swingler TE, Niu L, Smith P, et al. The function of microRNAs in cartilage and osteoarthritis. Clin Exp Rheumatol. 2019;37(Suppl 120(5)):40–7.
16. Zhong G, Long H, Ma S, et al. miRNA-335-5p relieves chondrocyte inflammation by activating autophagy in osteoarthritis. Life Sci. 2019;226: 164–72. https://doi.org/10.1016/j.lfs.2019.03.071.
17. Si HB, Zeng Y, Liu SY, Zhou ZK, Chen YN, Cheng JQ, et al. Intra-articular injection of microRNA-140 (miRNA-140) alleviates osteoarthritis (OA) progression by modulating extracellular matrix (ECM) homeostasis in rats. Osteoarthr Cartil. 2017;25(10):1698–707. https://doi.org/10.1016/j.joca.2017.06.002.
18. Yu CD, Miao WH, Zhang YY, Zou MJ, Yan XF. Inhibition of miR-126 protects chondrocytes from IL-1beta induced inflammation via upregulation of Bcl-2. Bone Joint Res. 2018;7(6):414–21. https://doi.org/10.1302/2046-3758.76.BJR-2017-0138.R1.
19. Ai D, Yu F. LncRNA DNM3OS promotes proliferation and inhibits apoptosis through modulating IGF1 expression by sponging MiR-126 in CHON-001 cells. Diagn Pathol. 2019;14(1):106. https://doi.org/10.1186/s13000-019-0877-2.
20. Wang H, Huang Y, Yang Y. LncRNA PVT1 regulates TRPS1 expression in breast Cancer by sponging miR-543. Cancer Manag Res. 2020;12:7993–8004. https://doi.org/10.2147/CMAR.S263383.
21. Zhang J, Ma X, Zhou R, Zhou Y. TRPS1 and YAP1 regulate cell proliferation and drug resistance of osteosarcoma via competitively binding to the target of circTADA2A - miR-129-5p. Onco Targets Ther. 2020;13:12397–407. https://doi.org/10.2147/OTT.S276953.
22. Hong J, Sun J, Huang T. Increased expression of TRPS1 affects tumor progression and correlates with patients' prognosis of colon cancer. Biomed Res Int. 2013;2013:454085.
23. Wuelling M, Schneider S, Schrother VA, et al. Wnt5a is a transcriptional target of Gli3 and Trps1 at the onset of chondrocyte hypertrophy. Dev Biol. 2020;457(1):104–18. https://doi.org/10.1016/j.ydbio.2019.09.012.
24. Suemoto H, Muragaki Y, Nishioka K, Sato M, Ooshima A, Itoh S, et al. Trps1 regulates proliferation and apoptosis of chondrocytes through Stat3 signaling. Dev Biol. 2007;312(2):572–81. https://doi.org/10.1016/j.ydbio.2007.10.001.
25. Mandl LA. Osteoarthritis year in review 2018: clinical. Osteoarthr Cartil. 2019; 27(3):359–64. https://doi.org/10.1016/j.joca.2018.11.001.
26. Guan VX, Mobasheri A, Probst YC. A systematic review of osteoarthritis prevention and management with dietary phytochemicals from foods. Maturitas. 2019;122:35–43. https://doi.org/10.1016/j.maturitas.2019.01.005.
27. Dang X, Lian L, Wu D. The diagnostic value and pathogenetic role of lncRNA-ATB in patients with osteoarthritis. Cell Mol Biol Lett. 2018;23(1):55. https://doi.org/10.1186/s11658-018-0118-9.
28. Jiang M, Liu J, Luo T, et al. LncRNA PACER is down-regulated in osteoarthritis and regulates chondrocyte apoptosis and lncRNA HOTAIR expression. Biosci Rep. 2019;39(6):BSR20190404. https://doi.org/10.1042/BSR20190404.
29. Li Q, Zhang Z, Guo S, Tang G, Lu W, Qi X. LncRNA ANCR is positively correlated with transforming growth factor-beta1 in patients with osteoarthritis. J Cell Biochem. 2019;120(9):14226–32. https://doi.org/10.1002/jcb.28881.
30. Hosseinzadeh A, Kamrava SK, Joghataei MT, Darabi R, Shakeri-Zadeh A, Shahriari M, et al. Apoptosis signaling pathways in osteoarthritis and possible protective role of melatonin. J Pineal Res. 2016;61(4):411–25. https://doi.org/10.1111/jpi.12362.
31. Tang L, Ding J, Zhou G, Liu Z. LncRNAp21 promotes chondrocyte apoptosis in osteoarthritis by acting as a sponge for miR451. Mol Med Rep. 2018;18(6): 5295–301. https://doi.org/10.3892/mmr.2018.9506.
32. Fang Y, Shen C, Zhang H, et al. Effect of MiR-126 on cartilage regeneration in osteoarthritis rabbits through MAPK signaling pathway. Minerva Med. 2019.
33. Liu C, Hou J, Shan F, Wang L, Lu H, Ren T. Long non-coding RNA CRNDE promotes colorectal carcinoma cell progression and paclitaxel resistance by regulating miR-126-5p/ATAD2 Axis. Onco Targets Ther. 2020;13:4931–42. https://doi.org/10.2147/OTT.S237580.
34. Liu L, Cui S, Wan T, Li X, Tian W, Zhang R, et al. Long non-coding RNA HOTAIR acts as a competing endogenous RNA to promote glioma

progression by sponging miR-126-5p. J Cell Physiol. 2018;233(9):6822–31. https://doi.org/10.1002/jcp.26432.

35. Hu Y, Zhang Y, Ding M, et al. LncRNA TMPO-AS1/miR-126-5p/BRCC3 axis accelerates gastric cancer progression and angiogenesis via activating PI3K/Akt/mTOR pathway. J Gastroenterol Hepatol. 2020. Online ahead of print.
36. Gai Z, Gui T, Muragaki Y. The function of TRPS1 in the development and differentiation of bone, kidney, and hair follicles. Histol Histopathol. 2011; 26(7):915–21. https://doi.org/10.14670/HH-26.915.
37. Momeni P, Glockner G, Schmidt O, et al. Mutations in a new gene, encoding a zinc-finger protein, cause tricho-rhino-phalangeal syndrome type I. Nat Genet. 2000;24(1):71–4. https://doi.org/10.1038/71717.
38. Wilke CM, Hess J, Klymenko SV, Chumak W, Zakhartseva LM, Bakhanova EV, et al. Expression of miRNA-26b-5p and its target TRPS1 is associated with radiation exposure in post-Chernobyl breast cancer. Int J Cancer. 2018; 142(3):573–83. https://doi.org/10.1002/ijc.31072.
39. Penolazzi L, Lambertini E, Scussel Bergamin L, et al. Reciprocal Regulation of TRPS1 and miR-221 in Intervertebral Disc Cells. Cells. 2019;8(10):1170. https://doi.org/10.3390/cells8101170.
40. Oliviero A, Della Porta G, Peretti GM, Maffulli N. MicroRNA in osteoarthritis: physiopathology, diagnosis and therapeutic challenge. Br Med Bull. 2019; 130(1):137–47. https://doi.org/10.1093/bmb/ldz015.
41. Tan Z, Niu B, Tsang KY, Melhado IG, Ohba S, He X, et al. Synergistic co-regulation and competition by a SOX9-GLI-FOXA phasic transcriptional network coordinate chondrocyte differentiation transitions. PLoS Genet. 2018;14(4):e1007346. https://doi.org/10.1371/journal.pgen.1007346.
42. Pan F, Xu X, Zhan Z, et al. 6-Gingerol protects cardiomyocytes against hypoxia-induced injury by regulating the KCNQ1OT1/miR-340-5p/ PI3K/AKT pathway. Panminerva Med. 2020. Online ahead of print.
43. Duan Q, Cai L, Zheng K, Cui C, Huang R, Zheng Z, et al. lncRNA KCNQ1OT1 knockdown inhibits colorectal cancer cell proliferation, migration and invasiveness via the PI3K/AKT pathway. Oncol Lett. 2020;20(1):601–10. https://doi.org/10.3892/ol.2020.11619.
44. Bi X, Lv X, Liu D, et al. METTL3-mediated maturation of miR-126-5p promotes ovarian cancer progression via PTEN-mediated PI3K/Akt/mTOR pathway. Cancer Gene Ther. 2020;28(3-4):335–49.
45. Shi WJ, Liu H, Ge YF, Wu D, Tan YJ, Shen YC, et al. LINC00673 exerts oncogenic function in cervical cancer by negatively regulating miR-126-5p expression and activates PTEN/PI3K/AKT signaling pathway. Cytokine. 2020; 136:155286. https://doi.org/10.1016/j.cyto.2020.155286.
46. Hu Y, Zhang Y, Ding M, et al. Long noncoding RNA TMPO-AS1/miR-126-5p/ BRCC3 axis accelerates gastric cancer progression and angiogenesis via activating PI3K/Akt/mTOR pathway. J Gastroenterol Hepatol. 2020. Online ahead of print.

23

What is the diagnostic value of dual-energy computed tomography in patients with clinical diagnosis of gout?

Jung Sun Lee[*] and Wook Jang Seo

Abstract

Objectives: To investigate the frequency of monosodium urate (MSU) crystal deposits on dual-energy computed tomography (DECT) in patients with clinical diagnosis of gout and the factors associated MSU crystal positivity.

Methods: This study was conducted in patients with clinical diagnosis of gout who underwent DECT. Clinical features were compared between patients with positive and those with negative DECT results. A logistic regression analysis was performed to determine the factors associated with MSU crystal positivity on DECT.

Results: A total of 148 patients with clinical diagnosis of gout were included, and MSU crystal deposition on DECT was observed in 64 patients (43.3%). The patients with positive DECT results were more likely to have renal insufficiency, longer disease duration, and higher serum urate level than those with negative. In the multivariable analysis, first gout attack (odds ratio 0.462; 95% confidence interval 0.229–0.931, $p = 0.031$) was associated with a less likely MSU crystal deposit-positive DECT result. In the subgroup analysis of patients with first attack, serum urate level > 8 mg/dL was associated with DECT positivity.

Conclusion: Of the patients with clinical diagnosis of gout, those with renal insufficiency, longer disease duration, and high serum urate level were more likely to be positive of gout on DECT. First gout attack was associated with less likely to be positive for MSU crystal on DECT. Thus, performing DECT scan in the selected patients who had characteristics that highly probability of DECT positivity could increase positive predictive value.

Keywords: Monosodium urate, Gout, Dual-energy computed tomography, Diagnostic imaging

Introduction

Gout is caused by the deposition of monosodium urate (MSU) crystals in the joints, cartilage, and soft tissues. It is the most common inflammatory arthritis in the West, and its prevalence is constantly increasing in Korea [1]. An important test in diagnosing gout is to check for MSU crystals under polarizing microscopy through joint fluid aspiration in the affected joint [2]. However, in the case of the first metatarsal joint, puncture is not easy thus it may be difficult to confirm the presence of MSU crystals under polarizing microscopy. Furthermore, an experienced inspector is required to detect MSU crystals under polarizing microscopy [3].

When the presence of MSU crystal deposits cannot be confirmed by synovial fluid examination, imaging could be used as a diagnostic tool in patients with suspected gout. Plain radiographs showed punched-out erosions with overhanging or sclerotic margins and tophi as ill-defined mass lesions in chronic gout [4]. However, findings from plain radiographs are often normal, and the sensitivity of plain radiography for gout diagnosis is only 30% [5]. Recently, the use of ultrasonography in the diagnosis of gout has been increasing. The presence of MSU crystal deposits is suggested by the double-contour sign, tophus, and snowstorm appearance [6]. In addition, cortical bone erosion characterized by punched-out

* Correspondence: jungsunlee0820@gmail.com
Division of Rheumatology, Department of Internal Medicine, Seoul Veterans Hospital, 53 Jinhwangdo-ro 61-gil Gangdong-gu, Seoul 05368, South Korea

lesions can be detected on ultrasonography [7]. However, ultrasonography highly depends on operator experience and patient factors, including obesity or the involved joint. Conventional computed tomography and magnetic resonance imaging can demonstrate erosion or tophi in gout, but these findings are not specific to gout [8].

Dual-energy computed tomography (DECT), which has been widely used in recent years, is a computerized tomography test that does not use a contrast agent. It is a noninvasive test that can identify soft tissues and MSU crystals using tissue-specific image attenuation. Its known sensitivity and specificity are 78–89% and 93–100%, respectively [9–11]. Patients with short disease duration, with first gout attack, and taking uric acid-lowering drugs are known to most likely have false-negative test results for gout. In addition, in gout patients without tophi, the sensitivity of DECT is lower than in patients with tophi [12–15]. Thus, a negative result is difficult to interpret in patients with suspected gout.

Research is limited on whether clinical manifestations differ between positive and negative MSU crystals on DECT in patients with clinical diagnosis of gout, and on factors associated with the positive DECT results. Therefore, in this study, we aimed to examine the clinical characteristics of patients with positive MSU crystals on DECT in comparison with patients with negative MSU crystals and the factors associated with DECT positivity.

Materials and methods

Study population

In this retrospective cohort study, we reviewed the electronic medical records of patients who underwent DECT because of episode of inflammatory arthritis or tendinitis possibly caused by gout but could not undergo synovial fluid aspiration at Seoul Veterans Hospital, Seoul, South Korea, between January 2013 and March 2020. Clinical diagnosis of gout was on the basis of the 1977 or 2015 gout classification criteria [16, 17]. First, in accordance with the 2015 ACR/EULAR classification criteria, patients with a score of ≥8 excluding DECT results were included as clinical diagnosis of gout cases. Among the patients with scores < 8, those who met at least 6 or more of the 12 items of the 1977 ACR criteria were classified as having clinical diagnosis of gout. Patients taking urate-lowering agents (including allopurinol, febuxostat, or benzbromarone) were excluded from the analysis. From the medical records, the following data were collected: (1) demographic information, including age and sex; (2) data on accompanying medical conditions such as hypertension, diabetes mellitus, renal insufficiency (defined as an estimated glomerular filtration rate of < 60 mL/min/1.73 m^2 obtained using the Chronic Kidney Disease Epidemiology Collaboration equation), cardiovascular disease, and alcohol intake; (3) affected joint, number of attacks, and disease duration; and (4) laboratory data, including serum urate levels and glomerular filtration rate.

This study was approved by the institutional review board of the Seoul Veterans Hospital, Seoul, Korea (IRB No. BOHUN 2020-07-012-001). The requirement for informed consent was waived owing to the retrospective nature of the study.

DECT imaging scans

All of the patients underwent DECT of the painful joint under the clinical suspicion of gout attack. A dual-source DECT scanner (Somaton Definition Flash, Siemens Healthcare) with 80/Sn140 kV and 250 mAs for one tube and the other automatically adjusted to maintain a 2:1 ratio. All the datasets were reconstructed using a bone algorithm to 0.75-mm slices with a 0.5-mm increment. Post-processing was performed using a commercial software program ("gout," Syngo CT Workplace, Siemens Medical System). The MSU crystals were shown in green (Fig. 1a and b).

Erosion was defined as cortical disruption in any two planes (Fig. 1c and d). A musculoskeletal radiologist evaluated the DECT images and recorded the locations of the urate depositions.

Statistical analyses

The chi-square and Fisher exact tests were used for comparisons of categorical data between the 2 groups according to DECT results. Continuous values were expressed median (interquartile range) using the Mann-Whitney U test for comparing 2 groups of patients according to DECT results. A logistic regression analysis with a backward elimination procedure was performed to identify the factors associated with DECT positivity. Variables with P values < 0.2 in the univariate analysis were selected for the multivariable analysis. The SPSS 20.0 software (SPSS Inc., Chicago, IL, USA) was used for all the statistical analyses.

Results

Comparison of the MSU crystal deposit-positive and MSU crystal deposit-negative DECT groups

A total of 148 patients with clinical diagnosis of gout who underwent DECT were included. Among 148 included patients, 132 met the 2015 ACR/EULAR classification criteria excluding DECT results and 16 met the 1977 ACR criteria. Sixty-four patients had a first gout attack. Table 1 shows the baseline clinical characteristics and laboratory data of the included patients. Among the 148 patients, 64 had positive and 84 had negative DECT results for MSU crystal deposits. The mean age and sex distribution were similar between the 2 groups. No significant difference in the presence of comorbidities,

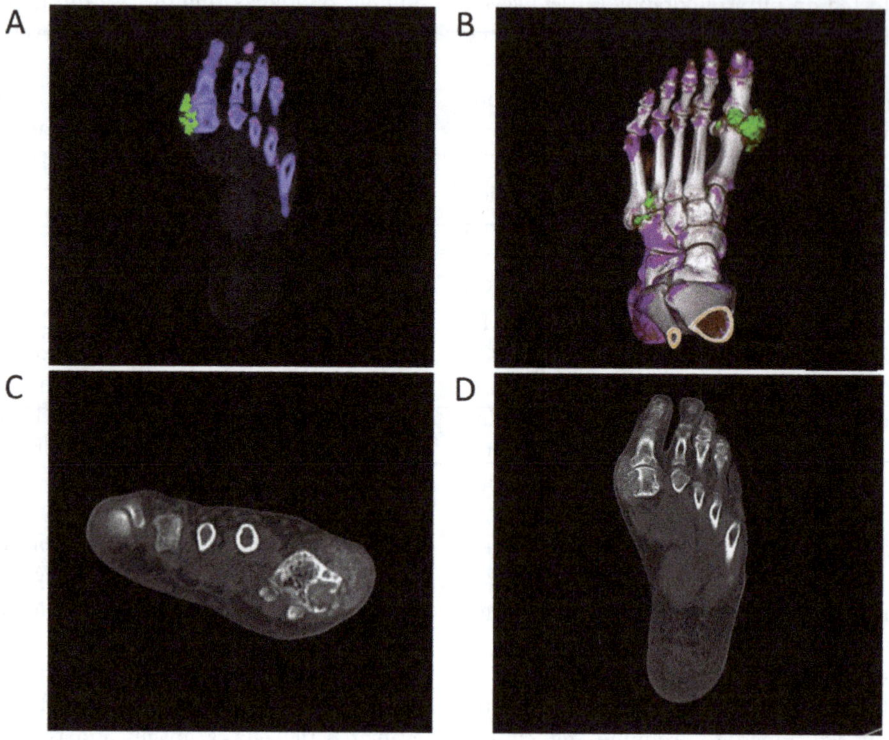

Fig. 1 Dual-energy computed tomography (DECT) images. A) Color mapping showing uric acid deposits (green) in the periarticular tissues of the first MTP joint. B) Three-dimensional DECT image with color mapping showing tophi (green) in the first MTP joint. C, D) Two-dimensional CT image showing high-attenuation tophi associated with erosions in the first MTP joint

including hypertension, diabetes mellitus, and cardiovascular disease, were found between the 2 groups. However, the patients with MSU crystal deposit- positive DECT results were more likely to have renal insufficiency (29/64, 45.3% vs. 20/84, 23.8%; $P = 0.006$) and longer gout disease durations (38.5 months [3.3–120 months] vs. 5 months [1.3–33.3 months]; $P < 0.001$). Furthermore, among the patients with the MSU crystal deposit-positive DECT results, the proportion of those who had a first attack was lower (21/64, 32.8% vs. 43/84, 51.2%; $P = 0.025$) than that among the patients with MSU crystal deposit-negative DECT results. The serum urate level was higher in the patients with positive than in those with negative DECT results for MSU crystal deposits. Among 16 patients who did not meet the 2015 gout classification criteria, 5 showed positive DECT result and met the 2015 ACR/EULAR classification criteria. Of 64 patients with positive DECT results, 60 started receiving urate-lowering agents after undergoing DECT.

Factors associated with DECT positivity

Table 2 shows the factors associated with DECT positivity. In the univariate analysis, age (odds ratio [OR] 1.043, 95% confidence interval [CI] 1.008–1.078, $p = 0.016$), renal insufficiency (OR 2.651, 95% CI 1.313–5.356, $p = 0.007$), first gout attack (OR 0.446, 95% CI 0.237–0.914, $p = 0.026$), and serum urate level > 8 mg/dL were significantly associated with DECT positivity. In the multivariable analysis, first attack (OR 0.462, 95% CI 0.229–0.931, $p = 0.031$) was associated with DECT positivity.

Comparison of the MSU crystal deposit-positive and MSU crystal deposit-negative DECT groups in first attack

Next, we focused the patients with first episode of inflammatory arthritis or tendinitis. Among the 64 patients with a first gout attack, 21 showed DECT-positive results for MSU crystal deposits (Table 3). Similarly to the total group, the frequencies of renal insufficiency and serum urate level were higher in the patients with positive than in those with negative DECT results for MSU crystal deposits. Erosion on DECT was detected in 38.1% (8/21) of the patients with positive and in 2.3% (1/43) of the patients with negative DECT results for MSU crystal deposits ($P < 0.001$).

Factors associated with DECT positivity in the first gout attack

Table 4 shows the factors associated with DECT positivity in the first attack group. In the univariate analysis, serum urate level > 8 mg/dL was significantly associated with DECT positivity (OR 3.472, 95% CI 1.128–10.685,

Table 1 Baseline characteristics of the patients with clinical diagnosis of gout

Variable	DECT (+) (*n* = 64)	DECT (−) (*n* = 84)	p
Age (years)	71 (68.3–74)	71 (62.3–74)	0.122
Male sex	63 (98.4)	80 (95.2)	0.390
Comorbidity			
Hypertension	43 (67.2)	47 (56.0)	0.165
Diabetes mellitus	12 (18.8)	19 (22.6)	0.567
Renal insufficiency	29 (45.3)	20 (23.8)	0.006
Cardiovascular disease	15 (23.4)	18 (21.4)	0.771
Alcohol intake	4 (6.2)	11 (13.1)	0.172
Disease duration (months)	38.5 (3.3–120)	5 (1.3–33.3)	< 0.001
Frequency of attack			
First attack	21 (32.8)	43 (51.2)	0.025
Three or more attacks/year	11 (17.2)	11 (13.1)	0.488
Symptomatic joints			
First MTP	44 (68.8)	54 (64.3)	0.569
Midfoot	11 (17.2)	18 (21.4)	0.520
Ankle	8 (9.8)	8 (10.8)	0.828
Knee	1 (1.6)	3 (3.6)	0.634
Hand	0 (0)	5 (6.0)	0.070
Uric acid (mg/dL)	8.7 (7.7–9.5)	8.1 (6.8–9.1)	0.013
GFR (ml/min/1.73m^2)	58 (49–68.8)	67 (55–85.8)	0.005

Values are presented as number (%), or median (interquartile range)
DECT dual-energy computed tomography, *MTP* metatarsophalangeal, *GFR* Glomerular Filtration Rate

p = 0.030). In addition, age and renal insufficiency showed a tendency of association with DECT positivity. In the multivariable analysis, serum urate level > 8 mg/dL (OR 3.180, 95% CI 1.004–10.076, p = 0.049) were associated with DECT positivity.

Discussion

In the present study, MSU crystals were detected in 43.2% of the patients with clinical diagnosis of gout by DECT. The characteristics of the patients with MSU crystal deposit-positive DECT results showed higher frequency of renal insufficiency, longer disease duration, and higher serum urate level than those with MSU crystal deposit-negative DECT results. First gout attack was associated with a less likely MSU crystal deposit-positive DECT result.

According to the European League Against Rheumatism guideline, an effort to confirm the diagnosis of gout on the basis of the presence of MSU crystals is required [18]. However, there is a limitation in performing joint fluid aspiration in small joints, including the first metatarsophalangeal joint. Clinical diagnosis of gout without joint aspiration could be uncertain, and the effort to search for MSU crystal deposition using imaging continues to be necessary. DECT scan is a noninvasive test to confirm the presence of MSU crystals. The known specificity of DECT is 93–95% [19, 20]; thus, positive DECT results can be used in gout diagnosis. Furthermore, three-dimensional DECT color imaging of the MSU crystal could improve adherence to treatment with urate-lowering agents [21, 22]. However, the sensitivity is relatively low [15, 23], and the possibility of false-negative results should be considered. In a previous study, DECT showed high sensitivity in gout patients with tophi but low sensitivity in those without

Table 2 Factors associated with dual-energy computed tomography positivity

	Univariate			Multivariable		
	OR	CI	*P*	OR	CI	*P*
Age	1.043	1.008–1.078	0.016	1.030	0.994–1.069	0.106
Male sex	3.150	0.343–28.888	0.310			
Hypertension	1.612	0.819–3.171	0.167			
Diabetes mellitus	0.789	0.4351–1.774	0.567			
Renal insufficiency	2.651	1.313–5.356	0.007	2.110	0.994–1.069	0.055
Cardiovascular disease	1.122	0.515–2.445	0.771			
Disease duration	1.004	1.000–1.008	0.049			
Alcohol intake	0.442	0.1134–1.460	0.181			
First MTP joint involvement	1.222	0.612–2.441	0.570			
First attack	0.446	0.237–0.914	0.026	0.462	0.229–0.931	0.031
Three or more attacks/year	1.377	0.556–3.413	0.489			
Uric acid > 8 mg/dL	1.776	0.892–3.537	0.028			

OR odds ratio, *CI* Confidence interval, *MTP* metatarsophalangeal

Table 3 Baseline characteristics of the patients with clinical diagnosis of gout (first attack)

Variable	DECT (−) (*n* = 43)	DECT (+) (*n* = 21)	p
Age (years)	71 (59–74)	72 (68.5–80.5)	0.149
Male sex	41 (95.3)	21 (100)	1.000
Comorbidity			
Hypertension	23 (53.5)	15 (71.4)	0.170
Diabetes mellitus	9 (20.9)	6 (28.6)	0.540
Renal insufficiency	10 (23.3)	10 (47.6)	0.048
Cardiovascular disease	10 (23.3)	4 (19.0)	1.000
Alcohol intake	6 (14.0)	2 (9.5)	1.000
Disease duration	2 (2–4)	2 (2–4.5)	0.457
First MTP	29 (67.4)	13 (61.9)	0.661
Uric acid	7.6 (6.4–8.5)	8.6 (7.4–9.5)	0.045
GFR	72 (33–86)	60 (49–74)	0.078
Erosion	1 (2.3)	8 (38.1)	< 0.001

Values are presented as number (%), or median (interquartile range)
DECT dual-energy computed tomography, *MTP* metatarsophalangeal, *GFR* Glomerular Filtration Rate

tophi [15]. In addition, another study reported various sensitivity rates (35.71–92.86%) according to the first attack and early- and late-stage gout [14]. This indicates that the crystal size affects the sensitivity of DECT. In the present study, the proportion of positive MSU crystal deposition on DECT was 43.2%, which is a relatively low value. As > 40% of the patients we included were having their first gout attack, the crystal size might not be large enough to be detected on DECT. On the other hand, although we included patients with clinical diagnosis of gout, some of them might not have true gout. Thus, interpreting whether negative DECT results indicate a false negative or no gout is difficult, and the diagnostic role of DECT is limited. Thus, performing DECT seems useful in patients with a high probability of positive DECT results.

In the present study, the frequencies of renal insufficiency and serum urate level were higher in the patients with MSU crystal-positive than in those with MSU crystal-negative DECT results. The association of renal insufficiency and gout is well known. Among the patients with gout, approximately 20% had a chronic kidney disease (CKD) [24], and gout is associated with a higher risk of CKD [25]. Furthermore, recently, urate-lowering therapy has been found to be beneficial to renal function [26]. As two-thirds of urate is excreted by the kidney [27], patients with renal insufficiency might have a higher possibility of having a MSU crystal deposit in the affected joint.

A previous study reported that DECT positivity is associated with gout attack frequency [13]. In addition, short-term gout, especially the first attack, showed 35.7% sensitivity [14]. In the present study, the patients having their first attack showed 32.8% positive rate, and first attack was associated with a less likely MSU crystal- positive DECT result. Previous studies have reported that patients with asymptomatic hyperuricemia also showed 15–24% positive rate of DECT [28, 29]. Although the positive rates in patients having their first attack were slightly higher than those in asymptomatic hyperuricemia, the diagnostic role of DECT is limited in patients having their first gout attack. Thus, DECT might not be recommended in patients with a first attack. However, in the 2020 American College of Rheumatology guideline, patients with a first attack with CKD stage ≥3 or uric acid level > 9 mg/dl are recommended to start urate-lowering therapy [30]. Indeed, in the subgroup analysis, the patients with a first attack and positive DECT results showed higher frequency of renal insufficiency and higher serum urate levels than those with negative results. Thus, in the first attack, performing a DECT scan in patients with hyperuricemia or CKD could increase the positive predictive value. In addition, the frequency of erosion was 38.1% in the patients with MSU crystal

Table 4 Factors associated with dual-energy computed tomography positivity (first attack)

	Univariate			Multivariable		
	OR	CI	p	OR	CI	p
Age	1.058	0.998–1.121	0.057	1.052	0.992–1.115	0.089
Hypertension	2.174	0.709–6.666	0.174			
Diabetes mellitus	1.511	0.456–5.009	0.500			
Renal insufficiency	3.000	0.988–9.111	0.053			
Cardiovascular disease	0.776	0.212–2.846	0.703			
Disease duration	0.997	0.950–1.047	0.905			
Alcohol intake	0.649	0.119–3.529	0.617			
First MTP joint involvement	1.222	0.612–2.441	0.570			
Uric acid > 8 mg/dL	3.472	1.128–10.685	0.030	3.180	1.004–10.076	0.049

OR odds ratio, *CI* Confidence interval, *MTP* metatarsophalangeal

deposits in the first gout attack. In a previous study, DECT demonstrated a high reproducibility for joint erosion. The erosion was positively correlated with MSU crystal volume and indicated a high disease severity that might require intensive urate-lowering therapy [31]. Thus, in selective patients with a suspicious first gout attack, including hyperuricemia or CKD, performing DECT could provide more information about erosion and MSU crystal deposition.

The present study has some limitations. The presence of MSU crystals could not be confirmed on polarizing microscopy; thus, we could not evaluate the sensitivity or specificity of DECT for the diagnosis of gout in our cohort. Furthermore, false-positive or false-negative DECT results are also possible. Second, because of the single-center retrospective design of the study, the generalizability of the study results is limited. For example, the ages of the included patients were older than the expected age for gout.

Conclusion

The positivity rate by DECT was 43.2% in the patients with clinical diagnosis of gout and decreased more in the patients having their first gout attack. Positive DECT results were more frequently observed in patients with chronic kidney disease and hyperuricemia. When DECT demonstrates negative MSU crystal finding, diagnostic role of DECT is limited. Thus, performing DECT in selected patients with characteristics that have high probability of DECT positivity could increase the diagnostic value of DECT.

Abbreviations

CKD: Chronic kidney disease; CI: Confidence interval; CT: Computed tomography; DECT: Dual-energy computed tomography; MSU: Monosodium urate; OR: Odds ratio

Acknowledgements

The authors would like to thank Enago (http://www.enago.co.kr) for the English language review.

Authors' contributions

JSL contributed to data acquisition, data analysis and interpretation, article writing. WJS contributed to study design and article review. All authors take full responsibility for the integrity of the study and approved the final version of the manuscript.

Authors' information

Not applicable.

References

1. Kuo CF, Grainge MJ, Zhang W, Doherty M. Global epidemiology of gout: prevalence, incidence and risk factors. Nat Rev Rheumatol. 2015;11(11):649–62. https://doi.org/10.1038/nrrheum.2015.91.
2. Neogi T, Jansen TL, Dalbeth N, Fransen J, Schumacher HR, Berendsen D, et al. 2015 gout classification criteria: an American College of Rheumatology/European league against rheumatism collaborative initiative. Arthritis Rheum. 2015;67(10):2557–68. https://doi.org/10.1002/art.39254.
3. Dieppe P, Swan A. Identification of crystals in synovial fluid. Ann Rheum Dis. 1999;58(5):261–3. https://doi.org/10.1136/ard.58.5.261.
4. Perez-Ruiz F, Dalbeth N, Urresola A, de Miguel E, Schlesinger N. Imaging of gout: findings and utility. Arthritis Res Ther. 2009;11(3):232.
5. Rettenbacher T, Ennemoser S, Weirich H, Ulmer H, Hartig F, Klotz W, et al. Diagnostic imaging of gout: comparison of high-resolution US versus conventional X-ray. Eur Radiol. 2008;18(3):621–30. https://doi.org/10.1007/s00330-007-0802-z.
6. Ogdie A, Taylor WJ, Neogi T, Fransen J, Jansen TL, Schumacher HR, et al. Performance of ultrasound in the diagnosis of gout in a multicenter study: comparison with monosodium urate monohydrate crystal analysis as the gold standard. Arthritis Rheum. 2017;69(2):429–38. https://doi.org/10.1002/art.39959.
7. Wu M, Liu FJ, Chen J, Chen L, Wei C, Hu ZM, et al. Prevalence and factors associated with bone Erosion in patients with gout. Arthritis Care Res. 2019;71(12):1653–9. https://doi.org/10.1002/acr.23816.
8. Chou H, Chin TY, Peh WCG. Dual-energy CT in gout - a review of current concepts and applications. J Med Radiat Sci. 2017;64(1):41–51. https://doi.org/10.1002/jmrs.223.
9. Spermon J, Van Dijke CF. Dual energy CT: added value in gouty arthritis. Jbr-btr. 2013;96(1):34–7. https://doi.org/10.5334/jbr-btr.179.
10. Girish G, Melville DM, Kaeley GS, Brandon CJ, Goyal JR, Jacobson JA, et al. Imaging appearances in gout. Arthritis. 2013;2013:673401.
11. Mallinson PI, Reagan AC, Coupal T, Munk PL, Ouellette H, Nicolaou S. The distribution of urate deposition within the extremities in gout: a review of 148 dual-energy CT cases. Skelet Radiol. 2014;43(3):277–81. https://doi.org/10.1007/s00256-013-1771-8.
12. Bongartz T, Glazebrook KN, Kavros SJ, Murthy NS, Merry SP, Franz WB 3rd, et al. Dual-energy CT for the diagnosis of gout: an accuracy and diagnostic yield study. Ann Rheum Dis. 2015;74(6):1072–7. https://doi.org/10.1136/annrheumdis-2013-205095.
13. Gamala M, Linn-Rasker SP, Nix M, Heggelman BGF, van Laar JM, Pasker-de Jong PCM, et al. Gouty arthritis: decision-making following dual-energy CT scan in clinical practice, a retrospective analysis. Clin Rheumatol. 2018;37(7):1879–84. https://doi.org/10.1007/s10067-018-3980-y.
14. Jia E, Zhu J, Huang W, Chen X, Li J. Dual-energy computed tomography has limited diagnostic sensitivity for short-term gout. Clin Rheumatol. 2018;37(3):773–7. https://doi.org/10.1007/s10067-017-3753-z.
15. Baer AN, Kurano T, Thakur UJ, Thawait GK, Fuld MK, Maynard JW, et al. Dual-energy computed tomography has limited sensitivity for non-tophaceous gout: a comparison study with tophaceous gout. BMC Musculoskelet Disord. 2016;17(1):91. https://doi.org/10.1186/s12891-016-0943-9.
16. Neogi T, Jansen TLTA, Dalbeth N, Fransen J, Schumacher HR, Berendsen D, et al. 2015 gout classification criteria: an American College of Rheumatology/European league against rheumatism collaborative initiative. Ann Rheum Dis. 2015;74(10):1789–98. https://doi.org/10.1136/annrheumdis-2015-208237.
17. Wallace SL, Robinson H, Masi AT, Decker JL, McCarty DJ, Yü TF. Preliminary criteria for the classification of the acute arthritis of primary gout. Arthritis Rheum. 1977;20(3):895–900. https://doi.org/10.1002/art.1780200320.
18. Richette P, Doherty M, Pascual E, Barskova V, Becce F, Castaneda J, et al. 2018 updated European league against rheumatism evidence-based recommendations for the diagnosis of gout. Ann Rheum Dis. 2020;79(1):31–8. https://doi.org/10.1136/annrheumdis-2019-215315.
19. Lee YH, Song GG. Diagnostic accuracy of dual-energy computed tomography in patients with gout: a meta-analysis. Semin Arthritis Rheum. 2017;47(1):95–101. https://doi.org/10.1016/j.semarthrit.2017.03.002.
20. Kiefer T, Diekhoff T, Hermann S, Stroux A, Mews J, Blobel J, et al. Single source dual-energy computed tomography in the diagnosis of gout: diagnostic reliability in comparison to digital radiography and conventional computed tomography of the feet. Eur J Radiol. 2016;85(10):1829–34. https://doi.org/10.1016/j.ejrad.2016.08.004.
21. Breuer GS, Bogot N, Nesher G. Dual-energy computed tomography as a diagnostic tool for gout during intercritical periods. Int J Rheum Dis. 2016;

19(12):1337–41. https://doi.org/10.1111/1756-185X.12938.

22. Desai MA, Peterson JJ, Garner HW, Kransdorf MJ. Clinical utility of dual-energy CT for evaluation of tophaceous gout. Radiographics. 2011;31(5): 1365–75; discussion 76-7. https://doi.org/10.1148/rg.315115510.
23. Huppertz A, Hermann K-GA, Diekhoff T, Wagner M, Hamm B, Schmidt WA. Systemic staging for urate crystal deposits with dual-energy CT and ultrasound in patients with suspected gout. Rheumatol Int. 2014;34(6):763–71. https://doi.org/10.1007/s00296-014-2979-1.
24. Zhu Y, Pandya BJ, Choi HK. Comorbidities of gout and hyperuricemia in the US general population: NHANES 2007–2008. Am J Med. 2012;125(7):679–87.e1.
25. Singh JA, Cleveland JD. Gout is associated with a higher risk of chronic renal disease in older adults: a retrospective cohort study of U.S. Medicare population. BMC Nephrol. 2019;20(1):93.
26. Levy G, Shi JM, Cheetham TC, Rashid N. Urate-lowering therapy in moderate to severe chronic kidney disease. Perm J. 2018;22:17–142. https://doi.org/10.7812/TPP/17-142.
27. Maiuolo J, Oppedisano F, Gratteri S, Muscoli C, Mollace V. Regulation of uric acid metabolism and excretion. Int J Cardiol. 2016;213:8–14. https://doi.org/10.1016/j.ijcard.2015.08.109.
28. Dalbeth N, House ME, Aati O, Tan P, Franklin C, Horne A, et al. Urate crystal deposition in asymptomatic hyperuricaemia and symptomatic gout: a dual energy CT study. Ann Rheum Dis. 2015;74(5):908–11. https://doi.org/10.1136/annrheumdis-2014-206397.
29. Wang P, Smith SE, Garg R, Lu F, Wohlfahrt A, Campos A, et al. Identification of monosodium urate crystal deposits in patients with asymptomatic hyperuricemia using dual-energy CT. RMD Open. 2018;4(1):e000593. https://doi.org/10.1136/rmdopen-2017-000593.
30. FitzGerald JD, Dalbeth N, Mikuls T, Brignardello-Petersen R, Guyatt G, Abeles AM, et al. 2020 American College of Rheumatology Guideline for the Management of Gout. Arthritis Care Res. 2020;72(6):744–60. https://doi.org/10.1002/acr.24180.
31. Dalbeth N, Nicolaou S, Baumgartner S, Hu J, Fung M, Choi HK. Presence of monosodium urate crystal deposition by dual-energy CT in patients with gout treated with allopurinol. Ann Rheum Dis. 2018;77(3):364–70. https://doi.org/10.1136/annrheumdis-2017-212046.

Permissions

All chapters in this book were first published by BioMed Central; hereby published with permission under the Creative Commons Attribution License or equivalent. Every chapter published in this book has been scrutinized by our experts. Their significance has been extensively debated. The topics covered herein carry significant findings which will fuel the growth of the discipline. They may even be implemented as practical applications or may be referred to as a beginning point for another development.

The contributors of this book come from diverse backgrounds, making this book a truly international effort. This book will bring forth new frontiers with its revolutionizing research information and detailed analysis of the nascent developments around the world.

We would like to thank all the contributing authors for lending their expertise to make the book truly unique. They have played a crucial role in the development of this book. Without their invaluable contributions this book wouldn't have been possible. They have made vital efforts to compile up to date information on the varied aspects of this subject to make this book a valuable addition to the collection of many professionals and students.

This book was conceptualized with the vision of imparting up-to-date information and advanced data in this field. To ensure the same, a matchless editorial board was set up. Every individual on the board went through rigorous rounds of assessment to prove their worth. After which they invested a large part of their time researching and compiling the most relevant data for our readers.

The editorial board has been involved in producing this book since its inception. They have spent rigorous hours researching and exploring the diverse topics which have resulted in the successful publishing of this book. They have passed on their knowledge of decades through this book. To expedite this challenging task, the publisher supported the team at every step. A small team of assistant editors was also appointed to further simplify the editing procedure and attain best results for the readers.

Apart from the editorial board, the designing team has also invested a significant amount of their time in understanding the subject and creating the most relevant covers. They scrutinized every image to scout for the most suitable representation of the subject and create an appropriate cover for the book.

The publishing team has been an ardent support to the editorial, designing and production team. Their endless efforts to recruit the best for this project, has resulted in the accomplishment of this book. They are a veteran in the field of academics and their pool of knowledge is as vast as their experience in printing. Their expertise and guidance has proved useful at every step. Their uncompromising quality standards have made this book an exceptional effort. Their encouragement from time to time has been an inspiration for everyone.

The publisher and the editorial board hope that this book will prove to be a valuable piece of knowledge for researchers, students, practitioners and scholars across the globe.

List of Contributors

Jeremy Y. Ng, Alexandra Vacca and Tanya Jain
Department of Health Research Methods, Evidence, and Impact, Faculty of Health Sciences, McMaster University, Michael G. DeGroote Centre for Learning and Discovery, Room 2112, 1280 Main Street West, Hamilton, ON L8S 4K1, Canada

Gabriela Bittencourt Gonzalez Mosegui
Department of Health and Society, Community Health Institute, Fluminense Federal University, Rua: Marquês do Paraná, 303, 3° floor, annex building, Niterói, RJ CEP: 24033-900, Brazil

Fernando Antõnanzas
Department of Economy and Company, Economy Faculty, University of La Rioja, Calle la Cigüeña, 60, 26006 Logroño, La Rioja, Spain

Cid Manso de Mello Vianna
Department of Health Policy, Planning and Management, Health Medicine Institute, Rio de Janeiro Estadual University, Rua São Francisco Xavier 524 - Maracanã, Bloco D, 7° floor, Rio de Janeiro, RJ 20550-013, Brazil

Paula Rojas
Department of Economy and Company, Economy Faculty, University of La Rioja, Calle la Cigüeña, 60, 26006 Logroño, La Rioja, Spain

Eduardo Deves and Rodrigo Novotny
Urology Service, University Hospital Prof. Polydoro Ernani de São Thiago HU/EBSERH, Federal University of Santa Catarina (UFSC), Florianópolis, Brazil
Graduate Program in Medical Sciences (PPGCM), Health Sciences Center (CCS), Federal University of Santa Catarina (UFSC), Florianópolis, Brazil

Fernando Hartmann Barazzetti, Mara Cristina Scheffer, Maria Luiza Bazzo and Letícia Kramer Pacheco
Laboratory of Molecular Biology, Microbiology and Serology, Health Sciences Center (CCS), Federal University of Santa Catarina (UFSC), Florianópolis, Brazil

Adriana Fontes Zimmermann
Rheumatology Unit, University Hospital Prof. Polydoro Ernani de São Thiago HU/EBSERH, Federal University of Santa Catarina (UFSC), Florianópolis, Brazil

Ivânio Alves Pereira
Rheumatology Unit, University Hospital Prof. Polydoro Ernani de São Thiago HU/EBSERH, Federal University of Santa Catarina (UFSC), Florianópolis, Brazil
Universidade do Sul de Santa Catarina- UNISUL, Florianópolis, SC, Brazil

Fabricio Souza Neves
Graduate Program in Medical Sciences (PPGCM), Health Sciences Center (CCS), Federal University of Santa Catarina (UFSC), Florianópolis, Brazil
Internal Medicine Department, Health Sciences Center (CCS), Federal University of Santa Catarina (UFSC), Florianópolis, Brazil
Departamento de Clínica Médica, Hospital Universitário, Universidade Federal de Santa Catarina, 3° andar, Rua Profa. Maria Flora Pausewang, Florianópolis, SC 88036-800, Brazil

Samanta Daiana De Rossi
Division of Rheumatology, Hospital de Clínicas de Porto Alegre, Universidade Federal do Rio Grande do Sul, Porto Alegre, Brazil
Divisiont of Dermatology, Hospital de Clínicas de Porto Alegre, Universidade Federal do Rio Grande do Sul, Porto Alegre, Brazil

Penelope Ester Palominos, Charles Lubianca Kohem and Rafael Mendonça da Silva Chakr
Division of Rheumatology, Hospital de Clínicas de Porto Alegre, Universidade Federal do Rio Grande do Sul, Porto Alegre, Brazil

Tania Ferreira Cestari
Divisiont of Dermatology, Hospital de Clínicas de Porto Alegre, Universidade Federal do Rio Grande do Sul, Porto Alegre, Brazil

José Alexandre Mendonça
Department of Rheumatology, Celso Pierro Hospital, Pontifícia Universidade Católica de Campinas, São Paulo, Brazil

Ricardo da Cruz Lage and Gustavo Gomes Resende
Universidade Federal de Minas Gerais (UFMG), Alameda Álvaro Celso 175, Ambulatório Bias Fortes, 2° andar, Belo Horizonte, MG 30150-260, Brazil

Claudia Diniz Lopes Marques and Rafaela Silva Guimarães Goncalves
Universidade Federal de Pernambuco (UFPE), Recife, PE, Brazil

Thauana Luiza Oliveira and Marcelo de Medeiros Pinheiro
Universidade Federal de São Paulo (UNIFESP/ EPM), São Paulo, SP, Brazil

Carla Gonçalves Saad, Célio Roberto Gonçalves, Eduardo de Souza Meirelles, Cláudia Goldenstein Schainberg, Wanderley Marques Bernardo and Percival Degrava Sampaio-Barros
Universidade de São Paulo (USP), São Paulo, SP, Brazil

Antônio Carlos Ximenes
Hospital Estadual Geral de Goiania (HGG), Goiânia, Brazil
Centro Internacional de Pesquisa, Goiânia, Brazil

Washington Alves Bianchi
Santa Casa de Misericórdia (SCM) do Rio de Janeiro, Rio de Janeiro, RJ, Brazil

Mauro Waldemar Keiserman
Pontifícia Universidade Católica (PUC) de Porto Alegre, Porto Alegre, RS, Brazil

Adriano Chiereghin
Pontifícia Universidade Católica (PUC) de Sorocaba, Sorocaba, SP, Brazil

Cristiano Barbosa Campanholo
Santa Casa de Misericórdia (SCM) de São Paulo, São Paulo, SP, Brazil

André Marun Lyrio and Rubens Bonfiglioli
Pontifícia Universidade Católica (PUC) de Campinas, Campinas, SP, Brazil

Lenise Brandao Pieruccetti
Hospital Heliópolis, São Paulo, SP, Brazil

Michel Alexandre Yazbek
Universidade Estadual de Campinas (UNICAMP), Campinas, SP, Brazil

Rodrigo Luppino Assad
Ribeirão Preto, Ribeirão Preto, Brazil

Sônia Maria Alvarenga Anti Loduca Lima
Hospital do Servidor Público do Estado de São Paulo, São Paulo, SP, Brazil

Sueli Carneiro
Universidade Federal do Rio De Janeiro (UFRJ), Rio de Janeiro, RJ, Brazil

Valderílio Feijó Azevedo
Universidade Federal do Paraná (UFPR), Curitiba, PR, Brazil

Cleandro Pires Albuquerque
Universidade de Brasília (UnB), Brasília, DF, Brazil

Andrea Barranjard Vannucci Lomonte and Cristiano Augusto de Freitas Zerbini
Centro Paulista de Investigação Clínica (CEPIC), Rua Moreira e Costa, 342 - Ipiranga, São Paulo, SP 04266-010, Brazil

Emerson Gimenez
Instituto de Pesquisa Clínica e Medicina Avançada (IMA Brasil), São Paulo, Brazil

Antônio Carlos da Silva
Clínica Clinilive, Maringá, Brazil

Sebastião Cezar Radominski
Centro de Estudos em Terapias Inovadoras (CETI), Curitiba, Brazil
Universidade Federal do Paraná, Curitiba, PR, Brazil

Morton Aaron Scheinberg
Associação de Assistência à Criança Deficiente (AACD), São Paulo, Brazil

Kaiyu Pan
Department of Paediatrics, Xiaoshan Affiliated Hospital of Wenzhou Medical University, Hangzhou 311200, Zhejiang, China

Rongliang Tu
Department of Paediatrics, Zhejiang Xiaoshan Hospital, Hangzhou 311200, Zhejiang, China

Xiaocong Yao
Department of Osteoporosis Care and Control, Xiaoshan Affiliated Hospital of Wenzhou Medical University, Hangzhou 311200, Zhejiang, China

Zhongxin Zhu
Department of Osteoporosis Care and Control, Xiaoshan Affiliated Hospital of Wenzhou Medical University, Hangzhou 311200, Zhejiang, China
Clinical ResearchCenter, Xiaoshan Affiliated Hospital of Wenzhou Medical University, Hangzhou 311200, Zhejiang, China

Seong-Kyu Kim, Ui Hong Jung and Jung-Yoon Choe
Division of Rheumatology, Department of Internal Medicine, Catholic University of Daegu School of Medicine, 33, Duryugongwon-ro 17-gil, Nam-gu, Daegu 42472, Republic of Korea

Gustavo Nogueira Schincariol Vicente, Gláucio Ricardo Werner de Castro, Ana Paula Carnieletto, Dhara Giovanna Santin de Souza and Fabiana Oenning da Gama
Universidade do Sul de Santa Catarina- UNISUL, Florianópolis, SC, Brazil

Licia Maria Henrique da Mota and Cleandro Pires de Albuquerque
Hospital Universitário de Brasília, Universidade de Brasília, Brasília, DF, Brazil

Ana Beatriz Vargas Santos and Geraldo da Rocha Castelar Pinheiro
Universidade do Estado do Rio de Janeiro, Rio de Janeiro, RJ, Brazil

Manoel Barros Bértolo
Faculdade de Ciências Médicas, Universidade Estadual de Campinas, Campinas, SP, Brazil

Paulo Louzada Júnior
Universidade de São Paulo, Ribeirão Preto, SP, Brazil

Rina Dalva Neubarth Giorgi
Instituto de Assistência Médica ao Servidor Público Estadual, Hospital do Servidor Público Estadual de São Paulo, São Paulo, SP, Brazil

Maria Fernanda Brandão Resende Guimarães
Hospital das Clínicas, Universidade Federal de Minas Gerais, Belo Horizonte, MG, Brazil

Karina Rossi Bonfiglioli
Faculdade de Medicina, Universidade de São Paulo, São Paulo, SP, Brazil

Maria de Fátima Lobato da Cunha Sauma
Faculdade de Medicina, Universidade Federal do Pará, Belém, PA, Brazil

Claiton Viegas Brenol
Universidade Federal do Rio Grande do Sul, Porto Alegre, RS, Brazil

Jin Shang, Xiao-Hu Li, Shu-Qin Lu, Lu-Lu Li and Bin Liu
Department of Radiology, The First Affiliated Hospital of Anhui Medical University, 210 Jixi Road, Hefei 230022, Anhui, China

Yi Shang
Outpatient Department of The Second Central Division, The General Hospital of PLA, Beijing 100853, China

Piero Ruscitti, Alessandro Conforti and Paola Cipriani
Rheumatology Unit, Department of Biotechnological and Applied Clinical Sciences, University of L'Aquila, L'Aquila, Italy

Roberto Giacomelli
Rheumatology and Immunology Unit, Department of Medicine, University of Rome 'Campus Biomedico', Rome, Italy

Marco Tasso, Luisa Costa and Francesco Caso
Rheumatology Unit, Department of Clinical Medicine and Surgery, School of Medicine, University of Naples Federico II, Naples, Italy

Renato Vicente Ferreira
Rheumatology Division, Universidade Federal de Sao Paulo (UNIFESP), Sao Paulo, Brazil

Suely Roizenblatt and Vera Lucia Szejnfeld
Department of Internal Medicine, Universidade Federal de Sao Paulo (UNIFESP), Rua Angelina Maffei Vita 670, Sao Paulo, SP CEP:01455070, Brazil

Gustavo Citera
Instituto de Rehabilitación Psicofísica, Echeverría 955, Buenos Aires, Argentina

Wilson Bautista-Molano
Universidad Militar Nueva Granada and University Hospital Fundación Santa Fe de Bogotá, Bogotá, Colombia

Ingris Peláez-Ballestas
Hospital General de México "Dr. Eduardo Liceaga", Mexico City, Mexico

Valderilio F. Azevedo
Universidade Federal do Paraná, Curitiba, Brazil

Risto A. Perich
Hospital Nacional Guillermo Almenara Irigoyen, Lima, Peru

José A. Méndez-Rodríguez
Hospital La Católica, Guadalupe, San José, Costa Rica

Mariel S. Cutri and Cecilia E. Borlenghi
Pfizer, Buenos Aires, Argentina

Rafaela Silva Guimaraes Gonçalves, Jonas Braynner Carvalho, Maria Eduarda Lima Vidal, Marina Coelho Mores de Brito and Angela Luzia Branco Pinto Duarte
Hospital das Clinicas da Universidade Federal de Pernambuco, Recife, Brazil

Alice Heaney
Galen Research Ltd, Manchester, UK

Stephen P. McKenna
Galen Research Ltd, Manchester, UK
School of Health Sciences, University of Manchester, Manchester, UK

Hui-hui Li
Department of Obstetrics and Gynecology, Qilu Hospital, Cheeloo College of Medicine, Shandong University, Jinan 250012, Shandong, China
Department of Obstetrics and Gynecology, University of Wisconsin-Madison, Madison, WI 53715, USA

Jing Zheng
Department of Obstetrics and Gynecology, University of Wisconsin-Madison, Madison, WI 53715, USA

Xue-quan Li
Department of Gastroenterology, Shouguang People's Hospital, Shouguang 262700, Shandong, China

Lin-tao Sai
Department of Infectious Diseases, Qilu Hospital, Cheeloo College of Medicine, Shandong University, Jinan 250012, Shandong, China

Yi Cui
Department of Intensive Care Unit, Qilu Hospital, Cheeloo College of Medicine, Shandong University, Jinan 250012, Shandong, China

Jia-hui Xu
Shandong First Medical University & Shandong Academic of Medical Sciences, Jinan 250000, Shandong, China

Chi Zhou
School of Animal and Comparative Biomedical Sciences, University of Arizona, Tucson, AZ, USA

Xing-fu Li and Hua-xiang Liu
Department of Rheumatology, Qilu Hospital, Cheeloo College of Medicine, Shandong University, Jinan 250012, Shandong, China

Ying-jie Zhao
Department of Obstetrics and Gynecology, University of Wisconsin-Madison, Madison, WI 53715, USA
Department of Rheumatology, Qilu Hospital, Cheeloo College of Medicine, Shandong University, Jinan 250012, Shandong, China

Fernando Henrique Azevedo Lopes, Veralice Meireles Sales de Bruin and Pedro Felipe Carvalhedo de Bruin
Laboratory of Sleep and Biological Rhythms, Department of Medicine, Federal University of Ceara, Rua Prof. Costa Mendes 1608 - 4° andar, CEP 60430-971 Fortaleza, Ceara, Brazil

Max Victor Carioca Freitas
Dr. Cesar Cals General Hospital, Fortaleza, Ceara, Brazil

Taciana Fernandes Araújo Ferreira
Clinical Hospital of Federal University Triângulo Mineiro, Functional Units Rom, Av. Getúlio Guaritá, 130, B. Nossa Senhora da Abadia, CEP 38.025-440, Uberaba, MG, Brazil

Ana Paula Teixeira dos Santos
Clinical Hospital of Federal University Triângulo Mineiro, Uberaba, MG, Brazil

Alexandra Silva Leal, Gilberto de Araújo Pereira, Sheila Soares Silva and Helio Moraes-Souza
Federal University of Triângulo Mineiro, Uberaba, MG, Brazil

Florencia S. Pierini, Martin Brom, Marina Scolnik, Valeria Scaglioni, Javier E. Rosa and Enrique R. Soriano
Rheumatology Unit, Internal Medicine Department, Hospital Italiano de Buenos Aires, Perón 4190, 1181 Buenos Aires, Argentina

Francisco Vileimar Andrade de Azevedo
Department of Internal Medicine - Faculdade de Medicina, Universidade Federal do Ceará, Fortaleza, CE, Brazil

Hermano Alexandre Lima Rocha
Department of Global Health and Population, Harvard T. H. Chan School of Public Health, Boston, MA, USA
Department of Community Health, Federal University of Ceará, Fortaleza, CE, Brazil

Anamaria Jones and Jamil Natour
Division of Rheumatology - Escola Paulista de Medicina, Universidade Federal de São Paulo, São Paulo, SP, Brazil

Francisco Airton Castro da Rocha
Department of Internal Medicine - Faculdade de Medicina, Universidade Federal do Ceará, Fortaleza, CE, Brazil
Instituto de Biomedicina - Laboratório de Investigação em Osteoartropatias, Rua Cel. Nunes de Melo, 1315 - 1°. Andar, Rodolfo Teófilo, Fortaleza, CE 60430-270, Brazil

Sevtap Acer Kasman
Department of Physical Medicine and Rehabilitation, University of Health Sciences Ankara Dışkapı Yıldırım Beyazıt Trainig and Research Hospital, Ankara, Turkey
Present affiliation: Department of Rheumatology, University of Health Sciences Kartal Dr. Lütfi Kırdar Training and Research Hospital, Istanbul, Turkey

Özgür Zeliha Karaahmet, Ajda Bal Hastürk, Halise Hande Gezer and Aytül Çakcı
Department of Physical Medicine and Rehabilitation, University of Health Sciences Ankara Dışkapı Yıldırım Beyazıt Trainig and Research Hospital, Ankara, Turkey

Özge Başaran and Banu Çelikel Acar
Department of Pediatric Rheumatology, University of Health Sciences Ankara Child Health and Diseases Hematology Oncology Training and Research Hospital, Ankara, Turkey

John M. Stacy and Jacob R. Greenmyer
University of North Dakota School of Medicine and Health Sciences, Grand Forks, ND, USA

James R. Beal
Department of Family and Community Medicine, University of North Dakota School of Medicine and Health Sciences, Grand Forks, ND, USA

Abe E. Sahmoun
Department of Internal Medicine, University of North Dakota School of Medicine and Health Sciences, Forks, ND, USA

Erdal Diri
Division of Rheumatology, Trinity Medical Group, Minot, ND, USA

Binfeng Wang and Xiangwei Liu
Orthopaedic Ward 2 (Trauma Surgery), Chifeng Municipal Hospital, No.1, Zhaowuda Road, Chifeng City 024000, Inner Mongolia, China

Jung Sun Lee and Wook Jang Seo
Division of Rheumatology, Department of Internal Medicine, Seoul Veterans Hospital, 53 Jinhwangdo-ro 61-gil Gangdong-gu, Seoul 05368, South Korea

Index